T0381061

Forward Written by Amrik Walia, MD, PhD –
President of the American Health Research Institute & The Center For Mind Body Medicine

THE BALANCE DIET & LIFESTYLE

THE SECRET CHEMISTRY OF WEIGHT LOSS

New Studies Prove That Being Overweight Is Not Just About Your Diet, Medical Research has Discovered Ancient Secrets that Help You Restore Your Health, Slenderize Your Body and Soothe Your Mind

---

An Invigorating and Empowering Introduction to The Mind Body Weight Loss Program that Offers a Life-Balancing, Whole-Person Approach to Weight Management and Anti-Aging.

BONUS: Includes Tips to Help You Identify and Eliminate Mysterious Symptoms and Hidden Causes that are the Major Culprits of the Weight Epidemic and helps You Prevent Imbalances that are known to Destroy Health, Cause Disease & Accelerate Aging.

Joyce Peters, ND, CNC, PFT, CHT
Co-Authored By: Summer Perry, NC, CP

Precautionary Disclaimer:

The intention of this book is to inform and educate only. As with any exercise and weight loss plan, it is recommended that you visit and obtain approval with your physician before beginning the program. This book is not designed to be a substitute for professional medical advice. It is important for individuals with Illness to seek doctors approval and medical clearance before starting any new diet, especially, while taking prescription medication or if one or more diseases are present such as Diabetes, Heart Disease, High Blood Pressure or High Cholesterol in combination. All reasonable efforts have been made to ensure effectiveness, accuracy and safety. However, it does not prescribe or replace medical care. The author, publisher or printer is not responsible for any liability or misuse of information contained in this book. A "*Mind Body Fitness Trainer*" is recommended to assist you with proper form and technique and to avoid injury from improper exercise positioning and techniques. A "*Mind Body Weight Loss Counselor*" may be able to assist you with your "*Mind Body Weight Loss*" program as you personalize your individual "*Mind Body Weight Loss*" regimen.

Copyright Disclaimer

No portion of this book may be copied without written permission from the author. Every effort has been made to acknowledge and credit the people who have contributed to the information that the author obtained during research. Every effort has been made to approve the usage of the pictures contained in this book. Please, accept apologies for unintentional errors or accidental omissions. To anyone who has made a contribution to the research of the listed agencies and who may have been accidentally over sighted or were unintentionally not included on the list, we extend an apology and belated thank you.

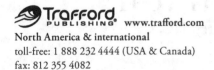 www.trafford.com
North America & international
toll-free: 1 888 232 4444 (USA & Canada)
fax: 812 355 4082

TABLE OF CONTENTS

RESEARCH REFERENCES

The American Health Research Institute

The American Naturopathic Medical Association & Board

Harvard University Medical Research "Research Matters" Program

The Mind Body Medical Institute of Harvard University

The American Accreditation & Certification Board of Naturopathic Physicians

The American Association of Nutritional Consultants

The Association For Research and Enlightenment (ARE)

The American Society for Metabolic & Bariatric Surgery

The World Health Organization

The International Holistic Health Summit

The California Naturopathic Medical Board

The Centers for Disease Control and Prevention

The National Centers for Disease Control

The National Institutes of Health

The US Department of Agriculture

The US Department of Health and Human Services

The Health Keepers Alliance

American Obesity Association

American Heart Association

American Naturopathic Medical Association

American Hypnosis Association

Hypnosis Motivation Institute-John Kappas, Phd & George Kappas, Director

American Psychotherapy and Medical Hypnosis Association

American College of Alternative Medicine

Associated Body Workers and Massage Professionals

Trinity College of Natural Health

National Association for Natural Health Care Practitioners

The National Association of Certified Natural Health Professionals

The National Foundation for Alternative Medicine

Biomechanics Clinic/Institute – Live and Dry Blood Cell Assessment REAMS

Certification in Advanced Biological Ionization

The Coalition for Natural Health Care Professionals

Aerobics and Fitness Association of America-AFAA

International Holistic Medical Association

American Holistic Medical Association

Holistic Medical Association of Alabama & Laura Heller

The U.S. Department of Agriculture/National Agricultural Library-USDA

The U.S. Department of Health and Human Services

The Surgeon General's Report

Weight-Control Information Network (WIN)

National Institute of Diabetes, Digestive, and Kidney Diseases

The Food and Drug Administration – Office of Food Labeling

Medical Esthetics Association – Certification Medical Esthetics Specialist

The Upledger Institute – Cranial-Sacral Therapy & Somato-Emotional Release

Parker, Life & Palmer Chiropractic Colleges

The Edgar Cayce Foundation, Virginia Beach

The Alabama State Chiropractic Association – Certified Assistant Program

The University of Texas-Addiction Science Research & Carlton Erickson, PhD

Parker Chiropractic College – Resource Foundation

Alabama State Chiropractic Association Auxiliary

Alabama Massage Therapy Institute-Certified in Advanced Techniques

AFAA American Aerobics and Fitness Association

Vanderbilt University – AFAA Personal Fitness Trainer Program

HCFA – Alternatives in Patient Care 2002 Compliance Law

Professional Lab Services/Clinical Laboratory International Association

National Institute for Natural Health Care Professionals

The Better Business Bureau – North West Alabama Advisory Board

BBB/Shoals Area Board of Directors

The Shoals Chamber of Commerce – Executive Board Members

SCC/Ambassador Committee Chairman and the Board of Directors

SCC Leadership Shoals Program

Alabama State Chiropractic Association Auxiliary and State Board

ACKNOWLEDGEMENTS

THE FOLLOWING ACKNOWLEDGEMENTS AND SPECIAL THANKS ARE TO CERTAIN IN-DIVIDUALS that without their support, I could not have devised this program and made it a success. There are those who assisted me in research, those who worked with me in clinical practice, those who inspired me directly or indirectly with their intellectual philosophies and there are others that I simply wish to express my appreciation for their friendship, love and kindness and to let them know that my life has been a brighter and happier place just by knowing them. Thank-You!

Summer Perry – Co-Researcher, Nutritional Consultant & Certified Hypnotherapist

Lillian Cole-Peters, Mother/Author/Poet

Dr. Amrik Walia, Medical Doctor, Researcher & Immunologist-UAB/AHRI

Scott Miller, Advisor/Confidant

Regan Lanier, CPT-The Center For Mind Body Medicine (Yoga Poses)

Pat Kirt & Norm Titcom – "Living Additions" Television Show

Leonardo Berezovsky-Chairman-AssistMed

Michael Denniston-Copyright & Trademark Attorney

Margaret & Ray Aderholt, Stephen, John & Pam Peters, Marie, Fredrick, Jillian & Amanda Tetro, Leiah, Nina, Doug & Lindsey Jackson, Stephanie, Randy, Hillary,

DR. JOYCE PETERS

Alex & Andrew Wood, Margaret, Jason & Ray Aderholt-my wonderful family.

Mike Kerr, Hospital CEO/Director

Gerald Edwards, Chiropractic Neurologist/Lifesaver

Tiffany & Jim Richer – "The Exposure Studio" Los Angeles

Tiffany Woodham-Richer – "Happily Ever After" (Healthy Children's Parties)

Beverly Hills Physicians Group

Roland Jeoffe – Producer/Director Light Motive Productions

Dr. Wendell Whitman, ND – Trinity College

James Solomon, N.M.D. & Glen Mahoney, M.D.

Harold Klassen, N.M.D. & Dr. Jed Adamson – Research Scientist

Dr. Marcus Mobley – Doctor, Acupuncturist & Kinesiologist

Dr. Asa Wrange "Optimal Health"/ Dr Alicia Burke "Absolute Health"

Dr. Lou Parbery – Psychologist & Greg Parbery – Confidant/Economics

Dr. Bruce Lipton, PhD-Cell Biologist/The Biology of Human Consciousness

Tobas & Elisha Crystal Company – "Art & Elenor" "Steve & Michael"

Bobby Levin, Attorney & Business Advisor Virginia Beach/Los Angeles

Ron Maestri-Infomercial Producer & Comedy Union Host in Los Angeles

Ian Rich – Music Composer/Producer of the Mind Body Weight Loss CD

Lee Waller-Advisor & Consultant/Melbourne Australia

Frankie Potts – Attorney Potts & Young Attorneys at Law

Karen Borick, Andy Clay & Monique Barrera-Mind Body Weight Loss Winners
Dr. Jeanne Northington, Mind Body Psychological Counselor in Psych-K

Nicole Pope & Mary Feltchner-Mind Body Yoga Exercise Instructors

Caylie Cavaco – Arthor/Editorials & Paul Cavaco-Allure Magazine

My adopted girls-Tina, Becky, Jennifer, Erica, Stacy, Lindsey, Victoria, Casey, Sarah, Lauren, Rachael, Andrea & Woo you always have a place with me.

Bridget Trapp-Crossroads of the World

FORWARD

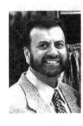

Amrik Walia, M.D. Ph.D.
President of the American Health Research Institute

MIND BODY MEDICINE IS NO MORE AN ALTERNATIVE OR COMPLIMENTARY medicine. It is a mainstream form of medicine, thanks to medical research. The research that is being conducted on Mind Body Medicine is being done in some of the most prestigious medical centers around the world. Dr. Joyce Peters holistic approach to weight loss addresses the root causes of weight gain and accesses the mind and body connection to remove the excess weight. The Mind Body Weight Loss Program is a powerful and inspirational program that can help you transform your life. For those of you who have gone through diet after diet with very little results, there is new hope. You are not alone in your struggle, in fact most dieters gain the weight back within three years of dieting. Some return to the same weight as before dieting and oftentimes, many will gain back even more weight than before they first started dieting. This program offers a permanent approach.

A large number of research studies have shown that emotional and environmental factors contribute to the epidemic of obesity and overweight phenomenon. Joyce's approach addresses these issues. I believe that her approach is a valid and perhaps one of the most effective approaches to healthy weight management that is currently available. In my opinion, her program may be the type of program that will finally be able to make a major difference in managing the weight control issues that we are facing. In her book, Joyce shares with us the synergistic activation of our metabolic processes through diet, exercise, yoga, meditation, breathing, stress management, healthy lifestyle and behavior modification. These mind body type techniques not only help in weight loss but are the essential elements in achieving overall good health, happiness, physical fitness, beauty and peaceful living. The goal of this book is to first bring your awareness to problem areas and then transform yourself and your lifestyle to create a new image of your hopes, dreams and desired health, image and life. Over the past several years, I have watched Joyce develop this system of weight loss. She has comprised this book utilizing a vast array of knowledge in various disciplines of medicine, working in most every aspect of health care gathering information to form an effective and systematic approach. This mind body approach has the potential of being the real answer to weight loss. That is why I encourage you to start using these principals and stay on the program. Joyce also, has a very motivational CD that can be very beneficial to your success, as well.

It is with great honor and pleasure that I introduce you to Joyce's book.

Amrik Walia, M.D.(C.A.M.),Ph.D. President
American Health Research Institute
The Center for Mind-Body Medicine

Spa Moksha[1]

Visit the Mind Body Health Programs Websites at:
http://www.mindbodyhealthprograms.com
http://www.shop.mindbodyhealthprograms.com
http://www.thebalancedietplan.com
http://www.drjoycepeters.com
http://mind-body-weight-loss.com
http://myspace.com/mindbodyweightlossprogram

---

1   Indian word meaning 'total bliss'

CHAPTER 1

Concepts Of The Balance Diet & Lifestyle

WELCOME, TO THE "BALANCE DIET & LIFESTYLE". IF YOU REALLY think about it, we are living in a revolutionary time of unprecedented technology and medical advancements. Many remarkable discoveries are taking place in the world. We have entered into an age of DNA, Genetic, Stem Cell and Anti-Aging medicine. The good news is Anti-Aging helps in the prevention of adult onset disease. Therefore, these advancements in medicine promise us less disease and longer life-spans. With the technology revolution speeding up the transmittal of this knowledge, "change" will begin to rain down upon us at a rapid flow instead of trickling down slowly as it has in the past, but, with an inevitably shorter adaptation time. In the midst of all the other change and restructuring that is taking place in the world. We should focus on staying balanced during change, because with change may begin to feel that we are struggling to keep up with the fastly-changing world. Change is good, change is necessary, but change can sometimes cause stress and stress can cause imbalance, and imbalance can cause the worst case scenario in every situation. Therefore, "Balance" is the reason that we must learn to adapt to change more quickly. The thing we will value most, with a longer Lifespan, is good health and quality of life. If you're going to live past a hundred don't you want to be healthy so you can get out and enjoy your long life? Adopting a healthier more balanced lifestyle, now, will help ensure a long healthy lifespan in later life. We are all becoming more aware of the consequences of the choices we make for disease prevention. We understand the effects that certain choices in the diet can have on our lives. Still over 80% of the population is over-weight, so, it seems that our biggest health problem is the continually rising epidemic of obesity. It is the number one preventable cause of death and it is the condition that is most affected by the choices we make in our diet and lifestyle. With all of the healthcare advances, obesity is still growing beyond an epidemic and cost the U.S. over $117 billion in obesity related healthcare cost, annually. Clearly, the biggest epidemic of our lifetime is obesity. No one wants to be overweight and everyone seems to always be on a diet but can't seem to lose weight permanently or effectively. Why? There is "a chemistry" to weight loss and there are hidden culprits that affect the body chemistry and every other aspect of health, including, a person's ability to control their weight. To shed some light on the concepts of The Balance Diet and Lifestyle there are some important aspects of imbalances that are usually known as the hidden culprits and causes that are believed to be linked to the weight epidemic that the world is facing, today. No matter what your dieting experiences have been in the past, there is always hope and there is always room for improvement in everyone. No one wants to be overweight and now, you no longer have to be. Read along and discover the secrets of good health that stem from maintaining balance in the mind and body. I hope that you are blessed with the successful results that you seek with this valuable information and that you maintain a healthy balanced weight for a lifetime.

As the author of this balanced approach to weight loss by Mind Body Health Programs, I want to guide you in every step of the way during your lifestyle transformation process. Use this information to help guide you to take the steps of change that are necessary to create a new image that is closer to the body of your dreams. It is my pleasure to assist you with this balanced lifestyle program that is designed to help you achieve your best self-image. You are now on your way to creating the new self-image that you seek in your personal weight management goals with a Mind Body Health Program that has helped many others, such as your self. I would like to help you find the calm from the raging storm

THE BALANCE DIET & LIFESTYLE

within your struggle with weight control with The Balance Diet and Lifestyle. I want to assure you, that it is not as hard as you may think it is to achieve successful weight management. As hard as it may have seemed to accomplish weight loss and to maintain a healthy steady weight, in the past, it can be achieved more easily with a healthy lifestyle plan in addition to dieting. It is much easier to maintain weight by adopting a healthy lifestyle than it has ever been with the dieting. The Balance Diet and Lifestyle is the basics of this Mind Body approach and can help show you how to create a lifestyle of peace and harmony by utilizing the information that it provides to educate yourself in how to live a healthier lifestyle to achieve and maintain your ideal weight.

Uncontrollable hunger is one of the main reasons that it is hard for people to lose weight. Hunger can feel like a storm raging out of control on the inside, but developing the power to tame your appetite is easy, all it takes is learning to recognize your real hunger. Satisfying true hunger is much easier than solving the mystery of false hunger signals. There are hidden culprits that can sabotage your diet and cause false hunger signals, but the power is within if you to learn how to tame these false hungers. You can learn to recognize your real hunger and access the power that you need to tame both types of hunger and often the power comes from within yourself. Some of the methods that do this require power from your mind and some of the techniques require power from within the body. The Mind Body powers must be balanced and this guide will help teach you balance in many areas of life as well as in your diet. You have the power within yourself to manage your weight and once you find an inner-balance, you can learn to exude the proper balance of energy toward achieving your ideal weight with more successful weight loss efforts. The great news is that once you find your inner power that is hidden within your own inner being it will help you bring balance to your overall health and well being. Once your body's true hunger signals are satisfied, you no longer have an uncontrollable urge to over eat and it helps to bring balance to your weight while enabling your whole being to feel a state of peace, tranquility and harmony within. Your body is the temple in which you reside, your mind is the thermostat of the sanctuary which can regulate its function and provide a state of balance on all levels. When we become imbalanced, our energy is thwarted and day to day living becomes exhausting and draining.

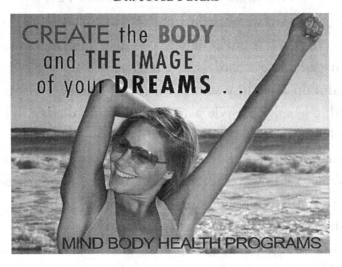

You can become a power house manufacturer of energy, burning away stored fat to invigorate your life and metabolism, which will reveal the slender beautiful you hidden underneath, when you follow the principles of The Balance Diet and Lifestyle. You can energize your life and gain the ability to accomplish and create your health goals. If you want to achieve your better health goal with all of your heart, mind, body and soul, you can do it! As you will soon recognize you are about to embark on a new approach in your personal weight control regimen. The same power that motivated you to pick up this book can be used to motivate yourself to start living a healthier lifestyle. You have already taken the first step to make yourself and the world around you a healthier place to live. The Balance Diet & Lifestyle is a safe, non-medical and natural approach to weight management. However, being overweight is not safe. People die from being overweight. Your personal weight-war can be won and it all starts with you and the choices you make. Being over weight is a multi-faceted issue, the original Mind Body Weight Loss Program is a multi-disciplinary system designed to be utilized in Medical offices and hospitals. As many dieters have found in the past, diet and exercise alone is not a permanent solution. However, understanding the delicate balance of your Mind and Body can help you control your hunger drive and help to achieve permanent results. Being over weight is a conglomeration of combined patterns which have to be identified and dealt with effectively on each individual level to achieve permanent success. For every physical aspect there is a mental aspect to correct imbalances in your health. Undetected imbalances in various aspects of life including diet, habits, lifestyle and other hidden imbalances of many sorts are culprits in being overweight. These imbalances may involve metabolic, hormonal, behavioral, physical, psychological, emotional, mental, spiritual, meta-physical, bio-chemical, and bio-rhythmic imbalances which may be hidden culprits in the formation of imbalances that lead to a condition of excess weight.

While preparing to begin your new approach to weight loss, feel assured that you are not alone. Weight problems are in epidemic proportion in this country and other countries, which mimic the American diet and lifestyle. There is an explosion of over weight people. Overweight and obesity are both an epidemic problem. It is believed that the biggest aspect to the epidemic is living an inactive lifestyle and overeating. There are over 300 fad diets on the market, at any given time. There are many self-medicating fad diets, which hold over a ninety percent failure rate. Fad diets are clearly, not the solution to the epidemic we are facing. Healthy living programs are of course, a key aspect in achieving permanent weight loss success. This program addresses the complexities in the "Mass Epidemic of Weight Related Problems" in the world, today. This program offers solutions and options for overcoming these health related issues that are linked to obesity and excess weight conditions. This program was designed to give the individual a powerful and effective weight-loss plan with successful lifestyle transformation with lasting and permanent results. There is an undisputable need for safer treatment plans with recent diet-pill travesties linked to chemically induced heart damage and ill side effects of the typical diet pill approach.

Diet pills and popular fad diets prove not to be the lasting answer to weight management as 80% of dieter's taking these types of approaches, gain back some or all of the weight they had lost while on their diets. In most cases, fad-dieters gain back the weight back in even greater quantities than was lost. Even the best physician can write a prescription, recommend a diet & exercise program and send the patient out the door to venture off to lose their weight on their own and the patient will lose weight, but without behavior modification the weight will gradually be regained. People can self medicate with over the counter medications, and usually when the person stops taking the medication the weight is regained usually with additional weight than before the person began dieting. Sadly, the statistics show that most fad-dieters gain back their weight in even greater quantities than they had originally lost. Each time people loose weight in this manner, it becomes harder to loose weight again without medication. The subconscious mind is 80% of the controlling factor of your success; your will power is 12-15% at

6 •

DR. JOYCE PETERSDR. JOYCE PETERS

over 80% the subconscious mind will easily over ride the will power or conscious mind. The self-sabotaging behavior needs to be addressed at the subconscious level. Sabotaging behavior has to be corrected at the subconscious level. The focus of this book is how to best keep the weight from coming back, without life long addiction to appetite suppressants or diet pills. A diet which closely resembles a Mediterranean diet has proven to be the best to guard against obesity, however, if it were that easy no one would be over weight.

DETERMINING YOUR GOAL WEIGHT AND IDEAL HEIGHT WEIGHT RATIO

According to the USDA Center for Nutrition, the following tables show the proper height weight ratio for women and according to the Merck Manual of medical information; the following height-weight reference chart indicates acceptable weight ratios for men.

Height Weight Ratio Chart			
Women		**Men**	
Height	Weight	Height	Weight
4'10	91-119		
4'11	94-124		
5'0	97-128		
5'1	101-132	5'1	105-134
5'2	104-137	5'2	108-137
5'3	107-141	5'3	111-141
5'4	111-146	5'4	114-145
5'5	114-150	5'5	117-149
5'6	118-155	5'6	121-154
5'7	121-160	5'7	125-159
5'8	125-164	5'8	129-163
5'9	129-169	5'9	133-167
5'10	132-174	5'10	137-172
5'11	136-179	5'11	141-177
6'0	140-184	6'0	145-182
		6'1	149-187
		6'2	153-192

THE BALANCE DIET & LIFESTYLE

Height Weight Ratio Chart			
Women		Men	
Height	Weight	Height	Weight
		6'3	157-197

My Height _____ My Goal Weight _____
Choose your goal weight from your height range to determine your goal weight.

Use the chart to set your weight loss and weight management goals.

The real challenge is to change eating habits. Even the Mediterranean diet should be individualized to your needs and geographical location. This is where the hidden culprits and causes come to recognition. Those culprits are related to imbalances in the lifestyle. Anytime that a person is overweight or obese, there is an imbalance. By adopting a healthier lifestyle, this can help in creating a more successful balance by achieving a more ideal weight. By adopting a healthier lifestyle similar to the European, a healthier diet similar to a Mediterranean style diet, and practicing portion control as recommended by the American Dietetics association, learning moderation of food consumption, decreasing your intake of processed foods, saturated fats and sugars and while improving the nutritional quality of the foods that you eat and utilizing habit control techniques it will help greatly in eliminating excess weight. Obviously, what this comes down to is, avoiding improper food consumption with a healthy active lifestyle being one of the key components and a major part of the real solution to effective weight control. The answer to developing a healthy lifestyle is by utilizing effective principles and methodology in the attainment of synchronicity of mind and body.

If you want your body to look a certain way, is important to develop a positive sense of self and thought consciousness. In behavior modification therapy, gaining "awareness" is important as it is to realize the consequences of bad habits. Many things can cause detriment and unfavorable manifestations in the Mind Body connection such as, negative self talk, bad eating habits, lifestyle imbalance, lack of exercise, lack of emotional support or neglecting the importance of a properly balanced diet. The most important imbalances to be corrected are negative self image and lack of lifestyle "awareness" of the significance of having a balanced lifestyle in achieving a good state of health, in Mind Body & Spirit. It is imperative in the treatment of weight related conditions that we develop a better self-image, more positive thinking, healthier lifestyles, and learn to meditate away stress and to achieve internal balance in order to maintain permanent successful weight control results that increase health, energy and endurance from our own inner Mind Body power to achieve successful weight management care plans.

This book is intended to help shed new awareness on the techniques that have been shown to reduce health risk and imbalances, which, correlate to many health issues including weight problems. There are many environmental distractions and culprits that may prevent us from achieving balance in our Mind Body. The balance diet and lifestyle can help to create a better or optimum state of health. The Mind Body Weight Loss Program was designed with the intent to empower those with weight related problems to effectively help them take control of their physical appearance and weight issues. With the Mind-Body Weight Loss program, you can loose weight and keep it off using the power of your own Mind and Body. The Mind Body Weight Loss Program reminds us that we are individually the powerful creator of all that we manifest in our lives. This book is a powerful reference tool to help the over weight individual take their life back into their own hands with full control over their weight and ultimately all aspects of life. In this book, my intention is to shed new & more positive "awareness" on how we think and treat, over indulgence, excess weight problems, obesity and the associated related health risk and with acknowledgement that weight involves issues with our whole being.

CONCEPTS OF THE BALANCE DIET & MIND – BODY WEIGHT LOSS PROGRAM

As a retired Doctor of Traditional Naturopathic Medicine, with specialty training in weight loss and weight management I began to recognize that there were many hidden causes, I noticed that many of the patients and clients who were visiting me for other health problems displayed a few common similarities, such as, being over weight, compounded by a habitually inactive lifestyle and a "can't lose" or self-defeating state of mind and that often was linked to an imbalanced body chemistry which I now believe is the main culprit in weight gain, disease and obesity . A huge prevailing cause of bio-chemical imbalances is stress in relation to almost every state of disease I realized that it was time to take a new approach to weight management and to focus on balance of body and mind. I founded the "Mind-Body Weight Loss Program". I designed The Mind Body Weight Loss Program

THE BALANCE DIET & LIFESTYLE

as an integrative well-rounded program. The "Balance Diet & Lifestyle" as a derivative of the Mind Body Weight Loss Program and is about bringing "Balance" back to your Mind and Body while recognizing that we are multi-dimensional beings with individual thoughts, emotions, behaviors, feelings and body types. Your "Mind Body Type" reveals the Causes of Your Weight Gain Issues. There are three easy profiles or identifiable groups that comprise a body type approach to your weight loss plan to ensure your weight loss success. Within these three categories there are general traits that will help you to identify your problem areas and resolve your weight gain issues, easily and permanently.

Mind Body Types

<u>Group One</u> – pertains to identifying the type(s) of imbalance(s) in the "Mind" and recognizing and eliminating sabotaging behavioral issues.

<u>Group Two</u> – pertains to identifying the type of imbalance(s) in the "Body" or Organ Systems resulting from Bio-chemical or Bio-hormonal imbalances that affect metabolism and weight gain patterns that result in the body's shape.

<u>Group Three</u> – pertains to how to determine your "Dieters Dosha Type" and how to identify and correct the imbalance(s) in your "Dosha" and how to correct "Lifestyle" imbalance(s).

In each group, you will find the correlating types to individualize your weight loss program and identify the causes of your weight gain which will ensure your weight loss success. The first step is to be prepared to overcome interfering obstacles, while on a weight loss program there will usually be obstacles to overcome, but, by utilizing these techniques you can overcome most interference. You can do it. I went through the process, too. I lost over 35 pounds and have kept it off for several years. The challenge of change is the challenge of a lifetime. I know that you are facing the challenge of change. I encourage you to make the necessary changes and you will defeat the obstacles and achieve your goal. Assess your activity factor, besides the diet; active living is a key aspect.

Dr. Joyce Peters

Determining Your Activity Factor

A.   Sedentary (Minimum Physical Activity)   9.1

B.   Moderate (Moderate Physical Activity)   11.4

C.   Very Active (Daily Rigorous Physical Activity)   13.6

My activity Factor is _____.

Anyone trying to lose weight can benefit from the active lifestyle tips in this book for the other two groups and for self improvement in regards to diet, exercise and motivational aspects. The first and most important step is to start correcting lifestyle imbalances by adopting healthier habits and that is something that we each have great personal control over. Recognizing the combination of your Mind-Body Types and your Ayurvedic DoshaType are the first steps in establishing your individual holistic weight control plan. By recognizing these factors you are bringing up to the conscious level things about yourself you may have never recognized before and this allows for self-empowerment, successful weight loss, healthy behavior modification and positive growth.

Determining Your Daily Caloric Intake

Caloric intake depends on age, sex, height, and rate of physical activity. Obviously, inactive people require less caloric intake than active people do. And athletic highly active people require more calories as they are burning off the energy at a higher rate. Therefore, daily caloric intake may vary in individuals from as low as 1,000 to as high as 4,000 calories per day according to the individual. Generally, young active men need approximately 2,400 calories a day where active women need approximately 2,000 amount of necessary calories increase with the increasing level of activity. When the physical energy output exceeds the caloric intake, weight loss occurs.

Multiply your activity factor times your goal weight:

AF_____ x GW_____=_____ your daily caloric intake.

(Goal Weight) _____ x (Activity Factor)_____= _____ Daily Caloric Intake.

THE BALANCE DIET & LIFESTYLE

To effectively personalize your weight loss plan, it is important to identify or determine which "Mind-Body Weight Loss" categories you are in out of each of the three groups. Once you identify your individual, unique and personal group types, you can focus your awareness on your individual problem areas, this will help you to maximize the effectiveness of your weight loss plan and ensure permanent weight loss success. Many experts predict that the twenty-first century medicine will focus on more of an integrative health care approach. As we combine alternative, complimentary, natural, traditional, eastern and western medicine to "Integrate", the best of these medical treatments that will provide successful and lasting results.

Determining Your Rate of Weight Loss

A pound of fat contains 3500 calories, therefore, to lose a pound of weight per week, you must eliminate 500 calories per day x 7 days in a week. You may eliminate calories by reducing caloric intake, by exercise or by a combination of reduction of calories and exercise. To lose 2 pounds per week, you must double your reduction of calories and exercise to eliminating 1,000 calories per day.

A Mind Body Weight Loss (MBWL) Formula For 1 or 2 Pounds of Weekly Weight Loss::

Daily Caloric Intake_____– 250 Calories by a "Reduced Calorie Diet" =_____
MBWL Daily Caloric Intake (from food consumption)=_____MBWL-DCI
MBWL Daily Caloric Intake_____– 250 Calories From Exercise=_____
Total Calories Per Day_____ x 7 days=_____– 500 calories daily (by calorie reduction & exercise)= _____
= 1 pound of weight loss per week.

Daily Caloric Intake_____– 500 Calories by a "Reduced Calorie Diet" = ____

MBWL Daily Caloric Intake (from food consumption)= _____MBWL-DCI
MBWL Daily Caloric Intake _____– 500 Calories From Exercise= _____

Total Calories Per Day _____ x 7 days= _____
-1,000 calories daily (by calorie reduction & exercise)=_____
= 2 pounds of weight loss per week.

Today's Date _____ My Current Weight _____

Goal Date _____ MBWL Goal Weight _____

Indicators of Imbalance in Weight Gain

For tips on how to restore balance to your body type, read the sections on bio-chemical imbalances, the importance of homeostasis and healthy diet for the individual body types. To understand and balance your Dieter's Dosha, see the chapter on Ayurveda. Ayurveda is an ancient healing art that began in India long ago. Many of the secret Ayurvedic principles and practices have been resurrected and prove to be beneficial in preserving and restoring health, today. Having balance in all aspects of life is an important part of the Ayurvedic lifestyle.

CHAPTER 2

The Hidden Causes & Dangers Of Being Over Weight

IF YOU ARE OVERWEIGHT YOU HAVE AN IMBALANCE. BEING OVERWEIGHT is an indication of imbalance within the body. Being "over fat" poses the greatest risk because it affects the heart and other organ systems. Imbalances in your weight may be due to more than one cause or hidden culprit. New studies reveal that losing weight is not just about diet and exercise and that there are hidden causes. It is dangerous to your health to be overweight as there are many negative health consequences from being overweight. People have all kinds of excuses and reasons to explain why they can't lose weight.

The Seven Main Excuses People Make To Put Off Losing Weight	
Fatigue –	Too Tired/Not Enough Energy.
Genetics –	I have hereditary factors but "it won't happen to me" do not want to face the fact that behavior is affecting your health or Beauty is only skin deep.

The Seven Main Excuses People Make To Put Off Losing Weight

Fear of Change –	What extra work do I have to do? I am comfortable with my current lifestyle. I like eating the foods I eat and do not want to stop eating them.
Hypochondria–	I have aches and pains. Therefore, I cannot exercise.
Procrastination–	I am going to lose weight but I have to take care of some other things, first.
Stress –	I am too busy to have a healthy lifestyle &diet. I do not have time to take care of myself I am taking care of business and other things.
Habits –	Enjoying and being accustomed to over indulgences and lifestyle that is out of balance and too difficult to change.

Most of these are excuses for a need of better self care and a lack of motivation to live a healthy lifestyle. The good news is, you can develop the motivation required to reach your health goals. Motivation comes from knowing what goal to set and believing the goal can be achieved. If you set a goal to do one simple thing to improve your health, increase your lifespan and decrease your risk of developing adult onset diseases, that one thing would be "prevent yourself from becoming obese". For starters, make simple goals and simple choices. For example, eating protein for breakfast which gives you more energy and boost metabolism to burn up to 60% more calories in a day rather than sugary refined carbs which sabotage weight loss. Becoming more dedicated to live healthier is more simple than you might think. just eating right and exercising on a daily basis is a simple first approach to a healthy lifestyle goal. As you start to look and feel better, you will see the results of the lifestyle changes you have made and seeing results offers the feeling of well-being, accomplishment and success. This is the reward that fuels continued motivation. As the results of your dedication shows, you will develop more motivation and a habit of healthy living. Once you are back in the habit of living a healthy, balanced, wellness lifestyle, stay motivated and stick to it. You can read more about developing motivation in chapter 15.

The number one killers of Americans are diseases related to obesity. Maintaining a healthy weight is the best anti-aging tip you can do to increase

THE BALANCE DIET & LIFESTYLE

longevity. Successful permanent weight management is a lifelong process that involves living a healthy lifestyle to keep your weight balanced. Awareness allows one to change, in this chapter we will take a look at the hidden health dangers of being over weight.

> Every extra pound of fat requires an additional mile of blood vessels! The Heart has to pump through an extra mile of blood vessels for every pound of extra fat on the body! This means, if you are 50 pounds over-weight your heart is pumping through 50 miles of blood vessels. Heart stress increases the risk of heart attack and weight related diseases!
> Fat around the abdomen means fat around the organs. Leptin is the hormone that regulates how much fat is stored around the organs.

ALL EXCESS CONSUMED CALORIES THAT ARE UNUSED ARE STORED AS FATTY BULDGES ON THE BODY

When we lose weight we trigger a fall in leptin, the brain receives the decline in leptin as a starvation signal that then begins to slow down metabolism and weight loss. This is why we hit a weight loss wall. When we hit this wall this is when most people go off their diet and that is why there is a high rate of yo-yo dieting. The metabolic systems then signals to the body to burn fewer calories so that it can gain the weight back. This is a hidden culprit that you must over-ride to deactivate these mechanisms and restart the weight loss process, this may take a couple of weeks to see results, your weight may seem stuck until the body feels that it isn't starving and begin the weigh loss process going again. During this phase you must stick to your diet and weight loss program. Once you get through the wall you will start to see the weight coming off again. Increasing exercise adding a little protein and decreasing the intake of refined carbs can help jump start your weight loss again, but you must stay on track with your diet as it is imperative to your success during this critical stage of weight loss.

> **Are You Shaped Like An Apple Around The Waist Line?**
> **FAT AROUND THE ABDOMEN = FAT AROUND ORGANS**
> **FAT AROUND ORGANS = DISEASE & OBESITY**

Fat Facts

A pound of fat=3,500 calories

To loose a pound of fat, you must eliminate 500 calories a day, every day for seven days, to loose one pound of fat in a week.

The best way to eliminate 500 calories a day is to exercise or reduce caloric intake or a combination of both.

Fat & Muscle Replicas

Another secret to weight loss is utilizing your body to work for you. Your Muscles can be a powerful aid to weight loss. Did you know that muscle can help burn off stored fat? As little as 2 pounds of muscle can burn off 10 pounds of fat in a year. A pound of muscle will also burn over 50 additional calories per day as fuel. Include light weight lifting in your exercise routine because by building muscle you can burn more stored fat if you keep your calorie intake in a range for the muscles to pull from energy reserves. This can help accelerate your weight loss progress. A proper diet and exercise will build more muscle.

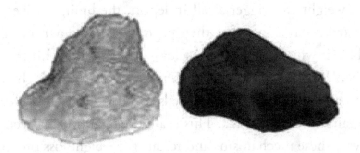

EATING FAT = FAT AROUND ABDOMEN
An Illustration of Replicas of ½ Pound of Fat and 1 Pound of Muscle…

Fat takes up twice as much space as muscle, therefore fat takes up more room than muscle in your clothes. Fat weight makes you look bigger than lean muscle at the same weight. Yet, muscle helps burns stored calories, such as fat, when you exercise. We tend to accumulate fat as we age, so it is important to control fatty weight gain to also control obesity related diseases. Fear cannot serve as the only motivating factor for weight loss and lifelong weight management. To ensure success, a goal and commitment has to be continually present in the mind. In other words, a personal lifelong commitment has to be made in order to maintain a healthy weight, for life. Goals must be set and a change has to be made. By setting realistic goals and being committed to a permanent lifestyle change, successful weight loss and weight management is yours with The Balance Diet & Lifestyle Program.

THE BALANCE DIET & LIFESTYLE

Changing Ineffective Weight Loss Methods Of The Past

Forms of healing practices brought to early America such as; Ayurveda, Homeopathy, Herbology, Naturopathy and all other Aboriginal Medicinal Practices were categorized as Alternative or Mind-Body Medicine. Alternative, Mind-Body and Traditional Medicine utilized as Preventative Integrative medicine, in combination, these healthcare forms are very effective in early detection and prevention of disease. Use the forms in this book to maintain health and balance to form your own integrative regimen. Integrative medicine is based on results and efficacy. Integrated medicine is comprised of combining the most effective methods of all forms of known health care practices in the world. By utilizing the power of mother-nature in combination with the technology of modern medicine we form a holistic integration of healthcare systems known as integrative medicine. As children we learn to go to the doctor, and are taught from birth to believe in medicine because we are born in hospitals. It makes since to use the best methods available and most patients who utilize Integrative Medicine are happier, healthier and more satisfied with their health care regimens than those who utilize only one form of health care.

Weight Loss Methods of the Past

Anorexia/Bulimia – mental disorders where one has no control over their behavior, and obsessively practice self – deprivation or forced purging causing illness and death.

Starvation Diet – going without food starving

Stomach Stapling/Gastric Bypass Surgery – Old procedures sewing off two thirds of the stomach (there are safer types of surgery now, such as lap banding)

Jaw Wiring – suck blended food through a straw risk choking to death

Aversion Shock Therapy – painful electrical shock is pulsed through the dieter.

HCG Hormone Injections – suppose to turn fat into waste.

Corsets – painful and uncomfortable binding of the body.

FAD Diets – Imbalanced food group gorging.

Liquid Protein – over 60 deaths have been reported.

Self Help Groups – Non-Medical approaches such as: Weight Watchers, Overeaters Anonymous and other similar groups appear to work. However, people tend to have problems maintaining their weight loss success after going off the program if a healthier lifestyle isn't ad-opted and reinforced.

The procedures that I have just listed are now considered potentially dangerous and sometimes even fatal methods by most medical standards and even diet and exercise programs haven't seemed to work as a permanent solution, either. Today, there are safer medical and surgical procedures, now that lifestyle pro-grams are being included. The weight epidemic is dynamic and that is why that many of the old or outdated methods are now considered to be drastic weight loss methods because they make no long-term consideration of the affects on future health, maintaining healthy weight for a lifetime, or with regard to the persons well being or as a whole being. The Mind Body Weight Loss Program offers these considerations and more and will help each person to shed light on hidden culprits to reveal the mysteries of the overweight epidemic in relation to not only a person's lifestyle but how it affects human body chemistry and explain how the amazing compensating ability of the body will enter into states of "imbalance" before disease as a compensatory effort to maintain its proper function in a state of "imbalance". When we realize that the body is a wholistic and synergistically functioning system, we can clearly see why, that when we correct one problem such as excess weight imbalance, another problem such as high cholesterol, high blood sugar or chronic pain condition will improve as well. There are thousands of examples of this with weight loss and healthy weight management.

Why Fad Diets Fail
Fad diets create unhealthy metabolic imbalances that oppose the normal func-tioning of the organ systems in the body. The body compensates by pulling out its reserves to handle the harsh chemical changes and therefore creates a meta-bolic imbalance sort of like "robbing peter to pay paul" effect. When the reserves

are depleted, the diet no longer works. And the health of the organ systems involved deteriorates. The heart, stomach and kidneys contain more alkalizing calcium and magnesium buffers than any other organs. Usually these organs are first affected by fad diets. Therefore, biochemical imbalances created by fad diets lead to the bio-hormonal imbalances that lead to disease, obesity or may even cause death. The result of the "yo-yo" diet and the health effects of loosing and gaining weight back in even greater quantities repeatedly may create detrimental effects on the organ systems and damage the overall health of the body leading to adult onset diseases.

Fad Diet Syndrome 98% Failure Rate

ALL LISTED MAY HELP YOU LOSE WEIGHT BUT MAY CREATE YO-YO DIETING

Infomercial diets, gadgets and gimmicks Latest Miracle Diet
Starvation Diets
Restricted or Reduced Calorie Diets
Lifestyle Plans Without An Exercise Regimine
High Protein Diets
Low Carb Diets
Grapefruit Diets
Non-Medical Weight Loss Centers
Laxatives & Purgatives
Prescription Diet Pills

CHRONIC "YO-YO" DIETING

Most fad or self-medicating methods of weight loss, fail because there is no behavior modification made to correct problem behavior. As soon at the diet is stopped, the weight is gained back and usually gained back in greater quantities than was lost on the diet. Breaking away from chronic yo-yo dieting is impor-tant. Behavior modification is necessary to break this pattern as it teaches one how to reprogram self-sabotaging behaviors into healthier thought patterns and habits.

All of the "Mind Body Health Programs" are based on integrative and whole person approach to help you bring balance back to your life and lifestyle. All of the "Mind Body Health Programs" are designed to help, you develop a healthier and more active lifestyle and to teach and empower you of ways to achieve a healthy balance within your Mind, Body and Spirit. The Balance Diet and Lifestyle focuses on helping you to detect and correct imbalances in these groups. In the original Mind Body Weight Loss Program, Group one and two are part of a medically supervised regimen, because testing is required to detect imbalances. Mind Body Weight Loss can help you do that.

Diet Reality Check List

At any given time upwards of 70% of the population is on a so-called "Diet".
Fad diets will seldom have permanent effects.
Radical changes in eating habits are difficult to continue long term.
Crash diets usually perpetuates a cycle of rapid loss, rapid regaining.
Sudden weight loss creates a rebound effect in the body, gaining back more than the original weight before the rapid weight loss.
Extremely low-calorie diets can deprive you of essential nutrients required by the body to maintain good health and proper organ function.
Crash diets have serious risk that should be utilized only under medical supervision.

In general, fad diets and quick weight loss diets do not work permanently. Once you stop the fad diet, the weight is usually gained back in even greater quantities.

The Mind Body Weight Loss Program was designed to integrate the most successful aspects of traditional and non-traditional healthcare with treatment protocols from eastern and western medical systems from around the world to form a method of achieving permanent weight loss and weight management. The Mind Body Weight Loss Program is an integration of the most effective healthcare and healthy living practices in the world. The Balance Diet will give you the basics of success with a brief description of the processes that are used in the medical programs. The great news is that you have options and there are many health professionals that are joining in this battle to help get the weight epidemic under control. Awareness and detection of the hidden culprits are the first step, knowing how far off baseline that we are before we start, allows us to see how far we have to go to get to our goal.

THE BALANCE DIET & LIFESTYLE

The coined term "Mind-Body-Spirit" is an eclectic method of healthcare designed to balance the body-physical, mind-mental, spirit-connected to all knowing. The Mind-Body Weight loss program is about empowering the individual with balance to maximize the innate healing potential of their whole being. Mind Body Weight Loss is a way of teaching one to utilize the full healing power of their Mind, Body and Spirit to achieve life long success in achieving their weight loss and weight management goals. Therefore, The Mind Body Weight Loss Program integrates a whole person approach to successful permanent weight management.

Weight loss occurs when there is insufficient energy consumption rate (ECR) Weight loss occurs when there is not enough incoming energy or calories to support the level of physical activity or the energy expenditure rate (EER). A simple formula may be monitored, and adjusted on a daily basis according to your activity levels for that day to determine your rate of weight loss.

WHY ARE 23 MILLION AMERICANS 100 POUNDS OVER THEIR IDEAL WEIGHT?

The type of weight gain that we see when people are a hundred or more pounds over their ideal weight, is not just about their diet, it's not just about overeating. In fact, this type of weight gain is not just about food. It is a medical condition that requires medical supervision. Bio-chemical and genetic factors are involved. In addition, when people appear bloated it is usually from toxic overloads in the body. The chemistry and metabolism is imbalanced due to a combination of many hidden culprits. When the body is bombarded with complex metabolic issues, the reason for extreme weight gain may include multiple food allergies, stress, metabolic syndrome, elevated cortisol levels and other complex inflammatory responses. This is a serious type of weight gain caused from imbalances in the chemistry that may cause misregulation of metabolic hormones that perpetually slow down the metabolism and trigger ever increasing weight gain. Obviously, abdominal weight gain is a cardiac risk factor that can be hazardous to your health but it also affects a person's sense of well being. There is hope for the morbidly obese. Obese people can get their weight under control with the right lifestyle changes and bariatric approach. It is always recommended that you see a doctor because obesity is considered a disease that may cause other diseases called co-morbidities, such as type II diabetes, heart disease or high cholesterol which are the number one killers of Americans. Obesity occurs around the world, like the 23 million Americans that are 100 pounds over their ideal weight, there is hope with the right treatment, and new methods are less invasive and more advanced. I feel confident that with today's medical advances and with the principles in the "Balanced Diet and Lifestyle" program, all obese people can lose this weight. Being obese can make one feel imprisoned by their weight, it affects your freedom of doing things like a pair of shackles Think of what a lighter world it will be to lose a hundred pounds. It would give your life many more freedoms.

THE WORST TYPE OF WEIGHT GAIN FOR ANYONE

Weight gain around the abdomen is the worst type of weight gain. Whether you are young or old, male or female, belly fat is the type of fat that poses the greatest health risk and it is the type of fat that should concern you most. There are two types of adipose tissue, brown and white; science has now discovered a hidden link to obesity and white adipose tissue. The reason why white adipose tissue or fat cell behavior has changed is still a mystery; therefore, hidden factors are involved. White adipose tissue is now considered to be as highly metabolically active as endocrine and paracrine organs. It interacts with other organs and tissues, and enables us to adapt to a wide range of metabolic challenges. White adipose tissue produces two known types of adipokines. The first type is hormonal so a feedback effect occurs between the fat cell and can cause major changes in metabolism, including leptin resistance which causes increased appetite and decreased in energy requirements resulting in body fat and weight gain. The second type is Pro-inflamatory cytokines which contribute to the inflammatory changes that occur in obesity; increased appetite, decrease in metabolic energy and medical conditions such as diabetes, pancreatitis, heart disease and osteoarthritis. Anytime the body is displaying a little too much belly fat, this type of weight gain is the type that is most harmful to your health and leads to heart disease. Heart disease strikes both sexes, but, it is the number one killer of women in the U.S. Visceral adipose tissue (VAT) is the name of the fat surrounds organs in the internal midsection. It is the kind of fat that kills as it leads to poor heart. No matter what age or gender this type of weight gain is the enemy and must be prevented or treated it at all cost. In addition, belly fat is associated with stress. Living a very demanding or stressful lifestyle causes the body to produce cortisol, which increases VAT fat storage. In other-words, the body cannot distinguish between psychological and physiological stress, it reacts to stress the same way. The body doesn't know if you are running from a Saber Toothed Tiger or over exerting yourself to the point of exhaustion due to an unhealthy lifestyle or if some chemical substance is causing a false signal to store more fat. When the body is exerted to physical exhaustion the metabolism slows down and redirects blood flow away from the digestive organs to the extremities, such as the legs and arms, the two main body parts, just like when someone is running to escape danger, the body stops thinking about eating and sends all the energy to the legs so you can run away, and the arms so you can fight and protect yourself. The bad part is digestion and metabolism slows down in this state of stress and when your not digesting you can be gaining weight. If two seasons of your life have been rigorous or tough you must break the stress cycle to prevent belly fat gain. Some of the things you can do are Mind Body exercises and practice better stress management. I believe this type of weight gain is the body's way of saying I am exhausted, slow down a bit. In addition, I am sure the competitive nature of today's economy and stress from the economic crisis is psychologically challenging which is an added stress. No matter how much dieting you do with severe stress, you will have more belly fat. I think in order to stop belly weight from escalating everyone could benefit from taking a "Mind-Body" approach to stress management and develop a adapting to life's pressures and stressful types of change to ensure a healthier lifestyle. Developing a more balanced and healthier lifestyle will be important to keep stress attributed weight gain under control. It appears that stress tricks the body to feel fatigue or exhaustion as though it has been working out, and probably cause us to stress eat. Emotional eating combined with a little more carb-calorie intake than is necessary will begin the appearance of belly fat. Watch the carbs, reduce the stress and add 10,000 steps of brisk walking to help your body deal with added stress and to look leaner, do some Pilates or yoga in addition to better managing your stress levels by doing relaxation breathing exercises to reduce the acid effects of stress and improve metabolic balance in the body. Inflammation can cause weight gain and can be increased through a process called glycation. Glycation occurs from consuming sugar or when excess sugar is in the blood. Sugars can attach to proteins when there is excess sugar in the blood. The protein molecules experience a "sugar burn" and are damaged. These damaged molecules are called advanced glycation end products, and they activate even more inflammatory response which can also lead to weight gain and other health issues.

POPULAR FAD WEIGHT LOSS APPROACHES:

The mind body connection must always be considered for any weight loss program to effectively work. Think very carefully about the name of any weight loss program and if it leaves you thinking of any negative thought, it is not a weight loss program that will work. Most rapid weight loss approaches are harsh, weaken or age the body. Personal training and coaching can be beneficial as an intricate part of a well rounded weight loss approach as long as guilt and shame are not used as key motivators of the weight loss program. Guilt is a negative emotion. Using guilt as a weight loss strategy is a recipe for disaster. Furthermore, failing at a popular approach, is typical because it is just another form of FAD dieting, which can be permanently damaging to metabolic set-points in the body and be detrimental to the dieter's view of themselves and their image, when they do fail. Some weight experts believe that going on a talk show to lose weight, is an unacceptable form of public humiliation, which is never an effective permanent weight loss solution. This approach will never work, especially for emotional eaters. Some shows on television encourage high pressured weight loss and weekly weigh-in's in an exposé' manner, others use the same-ole-same-ole diet and exercise approach. Exploiting a person's weight loss failures, public exposure or public humiliation is not a healthy solution for anyone's overweight problem. These types of techniques create embarrassment, shame and mental complexes about food, complexes about their body and may adversely affect a person's self-esteem. Most crash weight loss approaches do not offer real solutions; if they are broadcast, many are dramatized up to boost ratings and often are not a permanent solution to the participants or the overall weight epidemic. Fat Farms are not logical because, firstly the name is negative; again, always think carefully about the name of a weight loss label. After many participants have gone into a Weight Loss Camp that controls all food intake without the participant given the right or the choice of food selection, they come out feeling starved and deprived, people must go home and back to their old lifestyle after the camp, specific attention is required for those over-eaters who are binger's as many people relapse and go on a binge shortly after the camp is over. Little long-term success is achieved with no aftercare support system in place and this is where, unresolved bad habits may cause a relapse of weight gain, and lead to a feeling of lack of control and hopelessness. This is only one example of negative and harmful weight loss techniques. Lifestyle systems need to be put in place, as a healthier lifestyle is the only permanent solution. Adopting a healthier lifestyle will offer more than just weight loss, it offers, better health and anti-aging benefits, as well.

ONE SIZE FITS ALL DIET

There is no one size fits all diet. This is one of the main culprits that has caused the weight epidemic. When you visit a fast food restaurant, you get a one size fits all meal; everyone gets the same size, and usually people try to eat everything in the meal. If you think about it, one fast food combo meal usually contains far too many calories for the average person. An example, a 30 year old, 120 pound female and her twin brother who is a 30 year old male who weighs 175 pounds, they are twins but the female does not need all of the calories that is in a double burger with cheese and fries, and in most other cases at any age a man can usually eat more calories without gaining weight due to muscle mass and female hormones which cause the body to retain more fat than males. Learning to manage portion size and selecting smaller sized menu items will help reduce the risk of overestimated portion sizes in restaurants. In addition, talk to your doctor, nutritional consultant, nutritionist or dietitian about your individualized dietary needs, caloric requirements, specific diet restrictions, food allergies, allergies and an individualized diet that may be best suited for your individual state of health in regards to specific health conditions and nutritional needs. If medication is prescribed, be sure to ask about possible side effects and food interactions with current health issues or with the medications which you are taking. Always consult a healthcare provider before taking any dietary substance and contact your doctor immediately if you experience negative side effects after taking anything, even if it was recommended by a health professional. There is no one size fits all diet and it may be hard to lose weight eating out at establishments where all of the meals are the same size.

HIDDEN FACTORS THAT CAN AFFECT WATER WEIGHT GAIN

When we go on a new diet, the first thing that we lose is water weight gain. What causes and symptoms of water weight gain and what makes the body appear to be retaining water, Dietary imbalances can cause approximately 10 pounds of water weight gain in everyone with a poor diet. High sodium in foods such as canned soup, prepackaged prepared foods, sodas and snack chips, all can contribute to water weight gain. Watch the sodium content of processed foods. For example, one cup of soup may contain up to 1100 mg. of sodium the maximum daily intake of sodium is 2400 mg. In addition, these types of foods usually contain food additives, preservatives and transfats, all things that can cause imbalance within the body.

CLUES FOR VARIOUS TYPES OF IMBALANCE

Wondering What Is Making You Feel Sick, Tired & Overweight? You are not only what you eat, you are what you think! Everything you think, eat, drink or consume; physically or mentally, has an effect on your health, weight, chemistry, DNA, cells, pH, moods, internal balance and lifespan. Restore Balance to Your Diet and Lifestyle and Get Well!

The areas affected by a bloated appearance on the body can indicate the type of imbalance the weight gain is due to and is a clue to why the weight gain has occurred. For Example, weight gain in the thighs or in the "pear-shape" body type of weight gain may indicate a hormone imbalance. Most Females with this type of "thigh- area" weight gain usually happens due hormonal imbalances. In addition, weight gain that causes a spare tire around the middle or "apple-shape" can indicate nutrient deficiencies, genetic factors and dehydration. Conditions such as PMS can be a factor in women, as well. In Males, Poor diet, excessive sweating from sports and repeated loss of vital nutrients or electrolytes and not replenishing the bodies nutrient reserves after depletion, leads to water weight gain and causes slow metabolism that results in weight gain. I have seen this type of weight gain in athletic males and females who are stressed to exhaustion. Therefore, lifestyle imbalances can be a major culprit for these types of weight gain. Often when the body appears to have some fluid retention it causes an appearance of a lack of muscle tone, this type of water-weight gain is usually hormone related and may be due to a loss of electrolytes or from excreting too many trace minerals so it can raise serious health concerns. If you

THE BALANCE DIET & LIFESTYLE

have edema you should see a doctor. In addition, to hidden health concerns, eating salty carbs can create bloating due to an imbalance in the sodium levels which causes puffy looking fingers and ankles. Stress can also, be linked to this type of weight gain. Proper diet and adequate nutrient intake is important.

EFFECTS OF NUTRIENT DEFICIENT FOODS

Nutrient deficiencies can cause food cravings because if your filling your body with foods that are lacking essential nutrients the body cannot function if it is missing a nutrient that the body requires in order to maintain good health and proper organ function. Potassium, sodium and magnesium imbalances can affect kidney function and fluid retention can sometimes result. Eating more mineral rich foods and drinking kidney tea can sometimes help get rid of bloating and water weight gain. Fast food and junk foods do not supply enough nutrition for athletes or say a dancer. Such physical activity will require extra nutrition; otherwise an athlete may end up having uncontrollable food cravings and eating the wrong foods. When we sweat from exercise or dancing we lose sodium, potassium and electrolytes, and to be low on these nutrients may make you crave crunchy salty foods, because after all minerals are rocks that plants absorb and convert into krebs cycle inorganic minerals for human absorption. Plants provide the right types of minerals for humans. Eating the wrong foods such as snack chips, add extra fat and sodium leaving you looking bloated. If you clean the junk food out of your diet, you can usually lose 10 pounds in a couple of weeks. Plus, drinking water and electrolyte replenishing fluids during exercise sessions help muscle definition and you will look less puffy. Swelling and edema can be a sign of something more serious, always see your doctor about edema.

Vitamin Deficiency Example
A vitamin deficiency can be serious and cause multiple symptoms. Just one example of how a vitamin deficiency can affect you, is the signs or symptoms caused as a result of Vitamin B12 deficiency which are as follows:
- Apathy or Malaise
- Mood Changes or Depression
- Fatigue or Low energy
- Lack of appetite
- Eye or Vision Disturbances

- ❧ Imbalanced Gait, stumbling or staggering
- ❧ Muscle weakness
- ❧ Feeling Disoriented and Dementia
- ❧ Phobias or Psychoses
- ❧ Bladder or Bowel Incontinence
- ❧ Low Blood or Anemia
- ❧ Sore tongue or mouth
- ❧ Shortness of breath
- ❧ Slow Thinking or Inability to concentrate
- ❧ Behavioral Changes and Mood swings

This multitude of symptoms are the signs of a B-12 deficiency. You can imagine how you would feel if you had multiple vitamin deficiencies. B-12 regulates many functions and is needed for the healthy production of cells and DNA. Similar symptoms may also be caused by other medical conditions, too. That is why; if you experience symptoms like these you should consult your health care professional before self-medicating. Foods rich in vitamin B-12 are Curry dishes which contain lamb, chicken or other meats such as fish, liver, and dairy such as yogurt, cheese, milk and eggs contain B-12, too.

THE MYSTERY QUESTION OF THE CENTURY-

Jay Leno once did a skit where he asked former President Bill Clinton a question that has been perplexing the nation for a long time, "Why chubby girls"? But, the question of the century is no joking matter, why are there so many chubby and obese people? No one knows for certain because so many factors can be linked to this epidemic. What we do know is obesity is a killer; it causes the diseases that are the number one killers of Americans. Yet, it is an enigma, a puzzle and even scientist and doctors haven't figured it out, completely? If you ask all the obesity experts in the world this question you will not get a simple answer or get the same answer. It's a complex puzzle. If you wonder why the nation is overweight, and why obesity is an epidemic, there are hidden causes, there are hidden culprits, but it's not just one, it is from a complexity of many hidden factors. The "Hidden- causes" are the number one culprit of obesity. New studies indicate diseases may have vast hidden factors linked to everything from genetics, our habits, our lifestyle, our dietary choices, our food supply, and not only because of food additives, but because of food growing practices, food packaging and food advertising, too.

THE BALANCE DIET & LIFESTYLE

Is Obesity Hidden In Food, Food Packaging, Personal Care Products & the Environment?

There are many substances that can cause health risk that are found in foods and condiments. It is not easy to identify where all the risk are, more food labels should contain warnings such as on saccharine based artificial sweeteners have clearly marked on each package this substance has been known to cause cancer in laboratory animals. Burning meat also creates carcinogens, so how we prepare our food is important in reducing health risk. Cooking starches can cause cancer, too. French fries are high in Acrylamide, which is a carcinogen that is found in starchy foods from being fried, baked and cooked at high temperatures. The amount of acrylamide in a large order of fries is at least 300 times higher than the amount allowed by the Environmental Protection Agency for a glass of drinking water. The cancer scare is only the tip of the iceberg. There are many known and unknown risk factors. Another hidden risk in the development of metabolic disorders is Bisphenol A (BPA), a chemical used to manufacture plastics that is commonly used in plastics that are used for packaging foods and beverages. A study on BPA's link to metabolic disorders was conducted at Peninsula Medical School, in Exeter, U.K which indicated that BPA exposure is evident by the number of people with documented presence of detectable levels in at least 90 percent of the entire population in the United States. BPA has been associated with the development of type II diabetes and liver-enzyme imbalances and abnormalities. BPA exposure is widespread and continuous because plastics are used in packaging many foods, beverages, drinking water, implant devices and body and personal care products and even things such as shoes, clothing, furniture and cars pose dermal exposure.. The research is new and further research is ongoing to identify the real risk factors. Until then, it makes since to use "green" or natural "sustainable" products whenever possible. Do not microwave foods or water in plastic containers or leave them in a hot car as out-gassing becomes more of a risk when plastics are heated. In fact, balance your diet with raw uncooked well washed foods and lightly cooked foods. Heating chemicals change the molecular structure. Foods that are heavily laden with chemicals should be cooked with extreme caution and never over cooked. Why is it added to foods? Usually as a preservative or flavor enhancer. MSG (monso-sodium-glutamate) is in many of the foods we eat and it is added to foods to make us like the flavor and to make us eat more, no one can eat just one potato chip. If there is one food additive that you should choose to eliminate for appetite control, you would choose to eliminate MSG because it is considered by many health professionals and scientist to be a chemical with a suspected link to the obesity epidemic that is hidden in many foods. For the general public, Pub Med is a great resource for research references from the National Library of Medicine. You can read hundreds of medical studies at http://www.pubmed.com then click on search for "Obesity" or "MSG". Mice usually are not naturally obese, so research scientists give the test-mice chemical substances to fatten them up for use in hundreds of obesity studies scientists have literally created obesity in their test subjects. They can make mice morbidly obese by injecting them chemicals such as MSG which triples the amount of insulin the pancreas creates, causing the experimental mice to become obese. Therefore, you might easily wonder that perhaps, these substances may cause obesity in humans, too? The Glutamate Association lobby group argues that eating more benefits the elderly. One can only speculate what it does to the rest of us? Snack food advertisers come up with slogans such as 'No One Can Eat Just One' and if flavor enhancers are added to the chips you probably will eat more than just one. That is why, it is considered to be one of the hidden causes of obesity and it is masked behind alternate names. Flavor enhancers can enhance cravings for certain foods. Cigarette manufactures added other substances to cigarettes to make them more flavorful and addictive. Flavor enhancers are a similar ploy for FOOD sellers! Flavor enhancers were added to the American food supply many years ago and are being added in greater quantities as time goes on. Most prepackaged meals, soups, snacks and fast foods that we are tempted by daily, contain flavor enhancers that are considered, by many scientists, to be neuro-excitatory substances. Other Neuro-excitatory toxins are common substances that have been approved for human use, but that carry label warnings such as artificial sweeteners. I highly recommend that everyone research into the effects of "neuroexcitatory substances" and their effects on human health. What you will find is frightening because there are too many to list here. Other substance such as amalgam dental fillings contain a combination of chemicals and metals that are neruo-toxins, may cause metabolic disturbances. One of the more toxic substances is liquid mercury, combined with tin, copper, silver and zinc to make amalgam dental fillers. Ask your dentist for safer fillings such as gold, porcelain or resin composites. There are many books on the market referencing these substances and other neuro-endocrine disruptors, neuro-toxins and neuro-excitatory substances. The FDA is now investigating into many of these risks and may set new labeling guidelines or limits on use and how much can be added to food and other products at safer levels for humans. Change takes time, and in this field of science, only time can tell. Special interest groups have often falsely led decision makers to believe that these toxic things are safe for use at any amount. This is not about conspiracy, education is the solution, if we see that a substance is not as safe as once believed then regulations can be mandated. Hundreds of scientific studies cannot be denied and will serve as proof to prevent these problems and change usage guidelines. In the meanwhile, make healthier choices, and detox your body the best way available. As the medical research communities document the side effects of these things "manufacturers" have to change. Instead of banning its use, most proponents of these substances claim it's a personal choice. The most simplistic solution is to protect yourself from these multiple hidden factors by making educated and healthier choices as part of a healthy lifestyle; make it a habit to go green, organic and sustainable with all food and personal products whenever possible!

Cracking Label Codes?

It is standard knowledge that you should always read product labels be it medications or nutritional supplements. Now it is important to read the lables for cautionary warning statements and additives disguised under alternate names. Just as reading all food labels makes good sense, is a good habit to read personal care product and clothing labels, too. In fact, it should be considered to be part of a healthy lifestyle and it is recommended as a precautionary measure. Likewise, to ensure that your weight loss journey is a success, do research on your personal diet for food additives and other substances, before you consume them. Anything with known risk, because there are so many things out there that we don't know the risk, it becomes a compound and complex issue that cause complex metabolic imbalances. It is easy to eliminate something once you know the negative health effects when the research shows that there is a known side effect, health risk of that a food additive may increase your appetite. Therefore, research the ingredients if you don't know what they are because your diet may be sabotaged. Certain common flavor enhancers may make your hunger soar out of control, what more reason do you need to eliminate it from your diet when you are on a weight loss plan. Check all of your food sources for MSG as it may be hidden in foods under many other different names or disguised as Hydrolyzed Vegetable Protein; Start you additive research in your own kitchen by checking all foods in your cupboards and fridge. MSG is also considered a flavor enhancer so it can be found in almost everything! Soups, Snack Foods, Chips, Cookies, dehydrated noodle products, boxed and canned macaroni dishes, canned sauces or gravy, frozen meals, pre-prepared meals, salad condiments and salad dressings, especially the 'healthy low fat' ones. Children are at a higher risk for exposure as kid's foods are purposefully made more colorful or sweeter and more flavorful to entice finicky little eaters. It may be alarming to see how many typical children's foods are filled with flavor enhancers such as these, in combination with artificial food colors, high fructose corn syrup and sugar. In addition, a food item that may not be labeled as containing MSG usually contains hydrogenated fat as a flavor enhancer that robs the liver of enzymes and takes over 50 days to digest. The hidden culprit phenomenon doesn't stop in your kitchen. When your family goes out to eat, order your foods without MSG. Read labels and eliminating these hidden culprits from your household as well as your diet. As it is true, we all must assume greater "Personal Responsibility in Food Consumption" Our health is in our own hands and we are the most important teacher to our children in helping them not to be cursed with obesity. Since personal choices are so important to your health, decide for yourself? You can view the website sponsored by the food manufacturers which explains the reason they add additives. In addition, a study of elderly people revealed that elderly people eat more of the foods that contain MSG and some say that it is a good thing for elderly people to prevent weight loss. If this is the case, then maybe the food containing these substances should be labeled "scientifically proven to increase weight gain and food consumption in elderly populations". Or a better option for the rest of us would be a warning label, something like this "WARNING: Contains MSG which has been proven to increase eating WARNING: Eating this food contains additives that may result in weight gain or obesity. WARNING: This food carries an "O" risk factor rating because it offers an increased risk of your health of developing obesity from eating it. CAUTION: No one can eat just one, or control portion size, this may wreck your diet and cause weight gain and obesity and inadvertently obesity related diseases with regular consumption. We are the one who ultimately controls what we put in our mouth, but we need cautions and warnings to let us know the true risk. WARNING: May contain addictive substances that increases food cravings. There is a wealth of research that is available regarding Obesity related diseases and conditions. Obesity related conditions are the top killers of Americans, such as heart disease. Based on the research, some authors say that MSG is not only linked to Obesity, but is a hidden culprit to many other metabolic imbalances and conditions. Therefore, the best way to stop the food manufactures from hiding flavor enhancers, simply stop buying these items. The additives are found mostly in junk foods, and inadvertently fatten us up like test mice. The most important thing is that we need greater awareness about substances such as MSG and other flavor enhancers are put into our food supply because they may be one of the hidden causes the obesity epidemic? The studies are ongoing. Food additives should not be taken lightly. In addition, some additives are labeled as natural food additives, but just because something is natural don't always mean it's good for you. MSG is a drug-like substance that increases feeding and the urge to eat and it is only one hidden culprit in the obesity epidemic. Some view MSG as a poison, perhaps the food industry could learn a lot from the mistakes of the tobacco industry. In the meanwhile, there are several online resources that expose alternate names for MSG that may be hidden in foods. This is why "Food-label reading" is a crucial part of the Balance Diet and Lifestyle and your weight loss success.

WHAT'S IN THE AIR?

We breathe continuously and there are hidden risks in the air we breathe, too. According to experts at leading universities, the effect of low levels of particulate pollution found in many urban areas is not unlike secondhand smoke. In Canadian studies on Addictive Behaviors, a joint study from nine Canadian institutions found that second-hand smoke may trigger symptoms of nicotine dependence in children by causing symptoms that reflect nicotine withdrawal such as: depressed mood, trouble sleeping, irritability, anxiety, restlessness, trouble concentrating and increased appetite. It makes sense because many people gain weight when they stop smoking. This raises concern that non-smokers who are exposed to second hand smoke may have an increase in appetite which may contribute to weight gain. In addition, there may be other things that we breathe in from the environment that may increase appetite. We know that the aroma of food stimulates appetite. Many other factors in the air may be hidden culprits, too. Air pollution isn't just outside – the air inside buildings can also be polluted and affect your health. Allergies cause inflammation in the body and inflammation is a factor in weight gain. Clean air is must for good health. Avoid exposures whenever possible and use air purifiers and filters.

Viruses Linked To Obesity- Obesity is now classified as an epidemic. How can there be an Obesity epidemic around the world even in countries that are not influenced by the high-fat American diet, such as Somoa? Some scientist believes obesity may be linked to a virus and others fervently rebuke these claims. No scientist wishes to be responsible for panic or pandemonium, viruses are contagious, some are highly contagious. The link to obesity and viruses is still a mystery because more epidemiologic studies must be conducted on humans to determine if viruses are one of the main causes of obesity. Linking viruses to human obesity started in the U.S. but the research was fueled by something strange that happened in India, a strange viral epidemic in Bombay, India that left thousands of chickens dead which triggered the scientific curiosity of Sharad Ajinkya, a pathologist who noticed that there was something strange about the dead chickens, they were extremely fat when they should have lost weight from being sick with an adenovirus. Adenoviruses are a class of viruses with double-strand DNA genomes that cause intestinal infections in humans. This sparked an experiment, the pathologist then collaborated with Nikhil Dhurandhar, PhD, a viral and obesity researcher who conducted a reenactment study by injecting half of a test group of chickens with the virus and sure enough after six weeks, the injected test subjects had 50% more fat than the non-infected test group. The researcher from India could not afford to continue research due to lack of funding in India so he began writing U.S. Obesity researchers and luckily made contact with an interested Obesity Researcher who was already on a similar path of thinking, from the University of Wisconsin named Dr. Richard Atkinson, who was already conducting research and aware that viruses have been shown to cause obesity in animals due to the damage to the appetite control centers in the brain. Dr. Dhurandhar then moved to Madison to work with Dr. Atkinson and together they began a research study on available adenoviruses and discovered adenovirus-36 (Ad-36) which is a virus that is capable of producing obesity in animals turned out to be a common human virus, too. Since human research wasn't possible, animal research studies were conducted and revealed that mice, monkeys and chickens all gained weight after being infected with the virus. In addition, the research revealed that the virus changes the metabolism of fat tissue and increases the size of fat cells in addition to increasing the number of fat cells, too. After this discovery the scientists tested fat tissue from these animals in comparison to obese humans and found 30% of the humans to be infected with the virus. The scientist found the viruses' genetic material or DNA present in the fat tissue of the infected animals and found Ad-36 DNA in the human fat tissue, as well. While this concept is gaining credibility in medical communities more research needs to be done and effective treatments developed. However, testing is now available for people who want to be tested for the virus. While living a healthy lifestyle is always important those who test positive may wish to pay careful attention to their diet and lifestyle to help in preventing obesity and all of its associated risk.

NEW DIET AND LIFESTYLE ADJUSTMENT EASING TIP

Taking an Idebenone supplement helps repairs the damage from excitatory amino acids and other substances such as or "hydrolyzed vegetable protein" or street drugs such as Ecstasy it is also good for helping people who have eaten a lot of junk food with flavor enhancers such as MSG in helping to repair any damage of the myelin sheaths of the brain or nerves. It is an anti-aging compound that can help lessen feeling mentally fatigued while on a diet or detox program. It helps information transfer across the corpus-callosum, into the learning centers of the brain improving balance between the left and right brain hemispheres making behavior modification easier. Therefore, It may help ease the transition between lifestyle changes and enhance the mind body connection. Taking an Idebenone supplement may ease the transition of adopting a healthier new diet and lifestyle because it protects against the effects of cellular hypoxia that may occur after exercise. Especially, in people who are out of shape that are beginning a new exercise program and who are changing their physical activity while trying to get back in shape. Therefore, it is great for helping sedentary people or so called "couch-potatoes" in getting back into an exercise routine.

DNA & GENES, GENETICS, GENETIC CODES, GENOTYPES AND PHENOTYPES

DNA is Deoxyribosenucleic Acid. DNA tells cells how to make cells and proteins based on your genetic makeup, environmental factors and lifestyle. DNA contains genes and structures that regulate genetic instructions and healthy cell replication. Genes carry information for making all the proteins required to improve how well the body metabolizes food, how it heals itself, how it fights infection, and even affects how we behave. A gene is a region of DNA that controls hereditary characteristics. Scientist have discovered the human genome and about 25,000 genes that control everything in the body along with 600 enzymes or other chemicals in the chemistry that control many body functions. In addition, to nutritional deficiencies, genetic factors can cause disease and can cause enzymes to work poorly in the body, scientist are researching how to take out defective genes and some scientist believe that by adding vitamins they may be able to decrease or reverse genetic defects. The only problem is figuring out how to alter the genes without causing adverse mutations. Gene mutation may occur from nutritional deficiencies and can lead to cancer or other conditions such as Alzheimer's, cardiovascular disease, diabetes, obesity and may even affect how you look and feel. Genetic flaws can improve with a healthy lifestyle. Genetic flaws may improve with specific vitamins but if you take too many vitamins, they can build up to toxic levels. Taking vitamins is not the solution. If you take the wrong vitamins or if you take too many vitamins, it can do more harm than good; high doses should be monitored. Some studies indicate that someday, physicians may use specific vitamin based compounds in genetic-medicine to altering genes. In the future, access to individualized genomic based medical treatment will be very readily available for the general public and to those who can afford it. A person may be genetically pre-dispose to becoming obese but lifestyle is a factor in the development. Scientist at Oxford University have discovered another link to obesity, FTO is the gene linked to obesity (you don't even want to know the story about how it got its name or what it stands for, it sounds quite ridiculous, but here goes, a group of German researchers, reported in their research findings that after removing the gene from the DNA in the region, the mutations in the mice test subjects occurred and their toes fused together resulting in the name FT because of the effects on Chromosome 8 in mice, later when other researchers discovered the link to Obesity the O was added and now it is commonly referred to as FTO or FATSO) FTO is a gene linked to obesity on Chromosome 16 in humans, which is one of the 23 pairs of chromosomes which contain the building material of DNA in humans. Dr. Gerd Birkenmeier, a research scientist from Germany, conducted a research study on Leptin, a hormonal product of the obese gene that is secreted from adipose tissue. In mice, Leptin acts on the central nervous system to regulate body weight through the control of appetite and energy. In mice and humans, the level of leptin is highly correlated with the size of the body fat mass. Recent data suggest a Leptin imbalance as a possible cause for obesity, as the research indicates that it is not the absence of leptin but the presence of leptin resistance that appears to be one of the causes of obesity. The cause of a leptin imbalance may be linked to a suppression of an enzyme affecting hypothalamic regulation. Other genetic factors are being researched in Genetic variants of an enzyme that adjust the rate of balance of metabolism between gluconeogenesis and glucose assimilation which suggest another possible link to obesity. The discovery of FTO will reveal clues about how the brain and body regulate weight and will help scientist to begin to develop effective treatments for obesity.

Obesity is a disease with many hidden aspects bundled together. Scientist discovered ways that genes can be altered and are seeking ways to recode genes and are seeking to find ways to alter genes or program genes to improve health and to prevent obesity and other diseases. In addition, this only makes us recognize that hidden culprits may cause imbalances and DNA damage in humans which may alter genes and trigger disease, too. Improper diet, lifestyle, environmental factors, bio-chemical factors and toxic exposures are often hidden risk factors. However, obesity is a complex condition that is far beyond simply being overweight. Obesity causes co-morbidities, these are diseases linked to obesity, such as diabetes and obesity increases the risk factor for some cancers. Becoming obese is one of the worst things to decrease lifespan; therefore, obesity is not a friend to an anti-aging lifestyle. Genotyping identifies what region of the world that the majority of your genetic makeup originated from. Your Genotype is your full hereditary information as stored within your DNA, even if not expressed. Your Phenotype is your actual observed properties, such as development and behavior. Therefore, if you know your genotype it's easy to eat a diet consisting of the region of the world.

DIET AND GENETIC FACTORS AND PHENOTYPE HAVE AN EFFECT ON WEIGHT AND AGING

There have long been hidden factors regarding human health, until now, we are fortunate to be living in the age of DNA science with Genetics as the priority in the future of medicine. Our Genetic make-up often dictates our body size and shape. If both of our parents are overweight due to genetic build, then we are more likely to have weight issues. Our genetics and DNA affects our metabolism, our behavior and how we age, as well. However, now it is possible to improve our DNA and our overall health with certain natural substances, which can be provided by a healthy nutrient rich diet. The Diet is an important factor for healthy DNA transcription, production and repair, but, diet alone isn't the only factor, a healthy lifestyle is important as well. Scientific research proves, proper nutrition and a balanced diet, is important to good future health, healthy aging and for DNA replication and repair, even during weight loss. The Human Genome Project has concluded that genes can be altered through gene therapy but due to a few research catastrophes using retroviral vectors which resulted in death or near death reactions in the test subjects, the genetic movement has been slowed down by the governing powers that be. Therefore, the Food and Drug Administration has not yet approved very many, if any human gene therapy products for consumer sale. The good news is, progress is being made and the ban on gene therapy trials using retroviral vectors in blood stem cells, making way for more advances to be made. Until this branch of healthcare matures, the rest of us can focus on natural and safe means of improving our DNA weaknesses and also, increase our natural Stem Cell production by including specific substances in the diet and decrease our known risk with healthy lifestyle practices. If heart disease runs in your family, it would make good sense to protect your heart and eat a diet that promotes good cardiovascular health

Lifestyle is very important because it determines your Phenotype. Understanding how your Phenotype is affecting your DNA and how it has affected your genes, is a little more complex, as most of us are living in other places than where our ancestors originally descended from. It would make sense to eat a diet which consists of foods that support your genetic makeup and adopt a lifestyle that helps us develop a healthier phenotype. Caution is to be used and not to be mistaken with stereotyping. Personality traits will vary by an individual. However, Danish people, for example; historically, people from Denmark are from a rich cultural and intellectual heritage, it is acceptable in their culture to speak their mind, and do so without the intention to insult, rather to be honest. Denmark was once a seat of the Viking raiders. Denmark is now a major north European power. The climate of Denmark is temperate and humid with mild, windy winters and cool summers. The landscape of Demark is low and flat with gentle slopes bordering the sea, and surrounded by other countries and cultures. Fish and fowl would be part of the diet and animals such as rabbit, deer, sheep and game animals would live in that terrain and certain plants and cabbages would grow in that climate. These would serve as food for that geo-graphical location and would have been eaten for thousands of years, they have a diet consisting of certain foods native to that geographic location, in addition as people from that region of the world evolved, their body developed strong build and physical features to hike or climb, strong legs would typically be one of their physical features and therefore people of this genotype would benefit by doing exercises that mimic dwelling in a sloping terrain would help balance your genomic or phonemic type. The environment has an effect on the emotions, the Danish do not consider themselves to be a particularly warm people, but, family relations are important. Hygge is a word that describes the fundamen-tals of the Danish culture. Hygge is a description of the manner in which they conduct their social interaction and home relations. It is a cordial demeanor meaning a complete absence of anything annoying, irritating, or emotionally overwhelming, and they enjoy pleasure from comforting, gentle, and soothing things which they surround themselves and their home environment. Hygge is a typical aspect of their lifestyle. Therefore, a fifth generation Danish-American person with a genotype from this part of the world, living in a hectic U.S. City, would need to adjust their lifestyle to accommodate innate genotypic needs to support their phenotype and create an environment, that will help bring balance to their current life situation. Tracing your ancestral family tree is a good way to get in touch with your, heritage, discover hereditary factors and adapt your life-style to your genotype, and learn traditions and customs of your ancestors that can help improve your environment and balance your life. All of these things have an effect on health and future health.

3 STEPS TO HEALTHIER DNA

1. Educate Yourself- Research your family tree and family health history. Your "Jeans" size may be due to your "Genes". Ask questions, lots of questions. Find out what types of health conditions are most prevalent in your family. Read up on preventative measures that may help pre-vent or delay the onset of any health conditions which you may find to be common or reoccurring in your family. Visit your health care provider for regular visits. An ounce of prevention is worth a pound of cure.

2. <u>Change Your Lifestyle!</u> Adopting a healthy lifestyle by following the principles and health practices found within this book along with other Mind Body practices and regular medical care can help to improve your DNA and overall health. Be active, get out and enjoy life. Practice Prevention. Do satisfying activities to boost, nourish and supplement your mental state.

3. <u>Change Your Diet!</u> Eat a well balanced diet and avoid high fat in your diet. Avoid eating foods that could lead to adult onset disease which you have a known genetic risk of developing. Eating certain foods containing specific nutrients can improve metabolism and the efficiency and repair damaged DNA. In addition, diet restrictions by not eating certain unhealthy foods can decrease future damage. Starvation type diets are never healthy; being nutrient deficient is the worst diet habit as it can cause out of control hunger and because your body needs the building blocks to be healthy and energized. If, necessary, supplement your diet with dietary supplements to prevent nutritional deficiencies. Live an anti-aging lifestyle and look for new advances in nutrition, as they develop. Take a different approach to food and eat to improve health.

CHAPTER 3

Balance Is The Key To Weight Loss

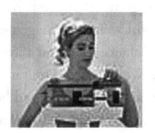

SOMETIMES IT MAY FEEL THAT THE DOOR TO WEIGHT LOSS is locked shut, when weight control has been a major struggle in our lives. It is not hard to find the key to unlock the door to weight loss. We simply need to find the motivation to stick to the weight loss program until we reach our goal. The Balance Diet and Lifestyle can help you find the courage and strength within yourself, to improve your health and lifestyle creating a powerful balance in body and mind so that you can have the satisfaction of knowing that you have the personal power which is the key to conquer your weight loss battle. This motivation is waiting for you to tap into it; you already have everything you need to achieve your goal. This balanced lifestyle plan can show you how to stick to a fitness plan, adopt healthier eating habits, set personal health goals, practice "weight gain" prevention and to adhere to a healthier lifestyle for a lifetime. Along with regular medical care, you can achieve successful results in the lifelong management of your weight with your desired outcome. Balance is the goal to strive for in order to achieve successful weight loss and healthy weight maintenance. Staying interested in maintaining good health is a good motivator in developing a healthy lifestyle that helps you feel balanced as a whole person.

Lack of Balance is the Problem

Excess consumption of the wrong foods and not getting enough of the right foods is a problem. Fast food is a culprit for encouraging a diet of low nutritional value and high fat and calorie content. Eating fewer calories than your body is using allows the body to dip into the stored fat reserves and burn stored fat for energy.

You can create more balance in your life by adopting a lifestyle that is preventative to gradual or perpetual weight gain. This lifestyle would naturally include healthier habits and behaviors balanced with a healthy diet, proper nutrition, adequate exercise, stress management and rest. Many of these key ingredients in achieving lifelong successful weight management and creating a balanced lifestyle are revealed in The Balance Diet and Lifestyle which are foundational aspects of "The Mind Body Weight Loss Program". These Programs can help you to realize the need to set attainable goals and help you reach those goals to achieve weight loss and permanent weight management.

BALANCE IS THE SOLUTION TO THE OVER WEIGHT EPIDEMIC

Scientific studies have shown that few people are overweight due to genetic or disorders. The detrimental effects of refined and processed food diet trigger the majority of people that are overweight due to metabolic and glandular disorders that were not present from birth. The solution to the overweight epidemic will come with knowledge. We have to adopt the mind-set of Hypocrates "Let your food be your medicine and your medicine be your food". The proper combination of the proper foods can be the solution of the overweight epidemic.

THE BALANCE DIET & LIFESTYLE

The Basis of the "Balance Diet & Lifestyle"

How is overweight and obesity related to disease? They are signs of excess, sometimes associated with deficiency due to an imbalance within the body. The body requires certain "essential nutrients" to maintain good health and proper organ function. Essential nutrients are required to maintain optimum organ function. If our body is not receiving the essential nutrients it needs, the body will incessantly hunger for those nutrients. Homeostasis is a state of harmonious balance within the body. The longer the body is not in homeostasis the ferocious the appetite will become, the pounds pile on over time, and being overweight becomes more of a perpetual problem as the deficiency becomes chronic. Without the required essential nutrient, and with depleted nutrient reserves, the organ becomes dysfunctional and eventually leads to loss of organ function and disease.

Throughout history the evolution of weight management has been through many unnatural and unsuccessful treatment plans. There are over 300 diet books on the market at any given time. Evolvement of modern medicine, is now occurring, it has become clear that the solution to many health problems including being overweight can be as simple and natural as creating a healthy lifestyle that identifies and addresses the major causes of becoming overweight. Fad diets are not the solution to this epidemic. The fact is clear that broad scale behavior modification is needed to regain control of our weight and health. We must utilize every means possible in the prevention of over weight conditions before they develop into serious weight related diseases. In weight control lifestyle education is a major step in winning the battle of the bulge.

"The doctor of the future will interest his patient in the care of the human frame, in diet and nutrition and the cause and prevention of disease." Thomas Edison

As so eloquently stated, by the world-renowned as the infamous and brilliant inventor of the light bulb and the originator of this statement. Many of us in the healthcare field see this as a prediction that is just now coming true. Edison has shed light on our existence in more helpful ways than the one way that he is most infamously credited. As Edison describes if we recognize the cause we can develop the cure or prevent the disease before it occurs by practicing prevention. Being overweight or obese is one of the major culprits of disease in today's society. The next step is to find the cause so that we can prevent ourselves from becoming over weight. It is not as simple as a balanced diet, avoiding obesity is one of the surest ways to avoid the major causes of disease. Hundreds of diseases and the top three health related causes of death either stem from being over weight. In order to maintain good health and the cause of disease is to maintain a healthy weight permanently. To do this, a person must be interested in avoiding one of the major causes of disease; an Imbalanced diet. Healthy natural foods contain the basic primary and essential nutrients that are required by the body to maintain good health and proper organ function. The essential nutritional needs of the body must be met, or excessive hunger will persist causing cravings and uncontrollable withdrawal type symptoms for food. Processed foods contain so many food additives and chemicals and lack the digestive enzymes that are needed to properly break down nutrients in your stomach. Lack of enzymes stresses your liver robbing it of metabolic enzymes which will hinder, interrupt and slow down the metabolism. There is really no way to achieve balanced nutrition and good elimination of waste by eating a heavily processed food diet on a daily basis. In addition, highly processed foods are usually laden with hidden diet-wrecking ingredients such as, sugar, flour and fat that sabotage your weight loss.

There is a link to health related disease and being overweight that can clearly be seen before the resulting disease states are set into motion within the human body. Most of us were not born with disease unless we have hereditary factors in play. We tend to develop "Adult Onset" conditions as we age and hormones begin to decline. What changes in our body to "trigger" the onset? How can we prevent these changes or at least slow down the aging process.

FORGET MYTHS AND REMEMBER TRUTH!

Weight Loss Myths

"If you try this fad-diet you will lose weight and keep it off for life".
"All foods that are labeled "low fat" will help you loose weight"
"High protein, animal meat diets are not dangerous to your health or cardiovascular system"
"Highly processed foods containing refined carbohydrates do not cause, obesity, heart, liver, and pancreatic damage.
"Diet foods help you stay healthy and permanently loose weight if they are labeled healthy, low-fat, sugar free "

THE BALANCE DIET & LIFESTYLE

As metabolism slows due to imbalances we tend to gain weight. Being over weight can be related to stress, fatigue, low energy, anxiety, depression, chronic pain syndromes, chronic infections, immune dysfunction, auto immune diseases, bio-chemical and bio-hormonal imbalances as well as most adult onset diseases. We are not usually born with adult onset disease something changes in the chemistry to trigger these conditions and at some point we are diagnosed with one or more of these conditions. If we do not take preventative measures to keep ourselves healthy as we age we will tend to develop more adult onset diseases. Being overweight increases the risks of developing these types of diseases and other diseases which are associated with obesity.

Weight Loss Truths

Food products that are labeled "low-fat" usually contain simple carbohydrates that are loaded with amylase that convert to sugars at a rapid rate releasing too much glucose causing the pancreas to overproduce insulin which is stored as fat and leads weight gain, pancreatic damage and eventually adult onset diabetes.

There is an obvious food-labeling problem that urgently needs to addressed and corrected. Some processed diet foods may make you fat. Read labels.

There is no scientific evidence that supports the claim that high-protein diets enable people to maintain their initial weight loss. However, there are reports that it can be damaging to your health and that on record there are over 60 people who have died from high protein diets and many more from other fad diets. Some of the most famous advocates of high protein diets have gained their weight back after coming off the diet and others actually died grossly overweight or from heart disease and heart attack.

FAD diets may work at first but they rarely have a permanent effect. High protein items of animal source usually are high saturated fat as well. High fat diets raise the cholesterol and acid levels in the body, causing damage in the vascular walls and can raise blood cholesterol resulting in an increased risk for heart disease and cancer.

A reduced calorie, balanced, healthy diet has more effective long-term results, than any fad diet. Moderation in lifestyle and behavior modification is the key.

THE SIMPLE NUMBER ONE WEIGHT LOSS FACT

The number one weight loss fact to remember is to keep your weight loss plan simple. Einstein was once quoted saying "keep it as simple as possible but not more simple than that…" You cannot permanently, lose weight by eating a daily diet that is high in "dead" or processed foods without the proper balance of "live" healthy foods. It doesn't take a scientist to figure out that the body simply needs food for one reason, to sustain life. Sometimes less is more, the more natural energy in the food the better it satisfies and helps maintain a balanced metabolism. A balance of good food and water are foods that are rich in vitamins, enzymes, minerals, proteins carbohydrates and that are low in saturated fats. Following the Balance Diet and Lifestyle will help assist you in making successful and healthier weight loss and weight management choices. Listening to motivational speakers are another way to increase your motivation as you begin your new health adventure. You may find it helpful to utilize the "Mind Body Health Programs" weight loss CD in addition to the book. The CD has subliminal messages that may help as reinforcement to accelerate your success in achieving your weight loss goal. Make a commitment to yourself to adopt a Mind Body lifestyle. Commit to achieve better health and a better more relaxed state of mind, commit to achieve your weight loss goals and for making an individual conscious decision to improve your personal health and the health of your family and future generations to come.

The Mind Body Weight Loss "Better Commitment" is all about you!

Lose weight because you want to be better.
Lose weight so that you look better
Lose weight so that you feel better
Lose weight so that your health is better
Lose weight so that your energy is better
Lose weight so that your strength and stamina is better
Lose weight for yourself not for anyone else or because of what anyone else thinks.
Be committed to yourself. You deserve to have the life and the looks you desire.
By being committed, to be your best and using the Mind Body Weight loss program you can achieve your weight loss goals.

THE BALANCE DIET & LIFESTYLE

Your individual effort and commitment is important in improving your health statistics for achieving a steady weight in the future. You make a major difference and impact on others, by losing weight, you are improving, not only your current health status but your future health status and longevity. Weight control is the single most effective health practice to improve your long term health. The key to gaining control of weight is achieving balance in life. Many people do not have a balanced lifestyle and this is very important aspect of being healthy.

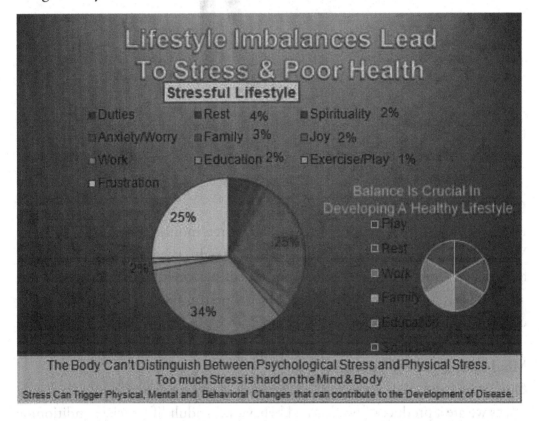

The Balance Diet & Lifestyle is a spin off of my Mind Body Weight Loss Program that is available through thousands of medical sites. This basic foundational consumer version, is a informational guide for understanding the basics of the integrated "Mind Body Weight Loss Program" approach. I hope that this information will help you transform your life into one of health and fitness.

DR. JOYCE PETERS

Before and After Pictures

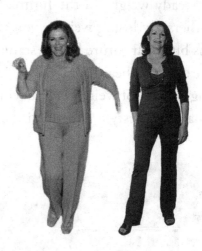

"I feel so much better. I love the way I look and feel after losing
weight on Dr. Joyce's Program" *Karen Borick*

Reclaim your figure an image of youth!

Karen Borick lost 25 pounds in less than three months on the Mind Body
Weight Loss Program! Not only did she loose weight, she is happier with herself
because she looks younger, she is more toned, healthier and fit. The best part
about it all is that she is actually is a healthier person than she was before going
on the Mind-Body Weight Loss Program.

Mind Body Food For Thought

Our eating habits start at birth. We learn how to eat in infancy from our caregivers, as we are a product of our learned behavior. In adult life, social conditioning
and brainwashing or hypnosis influences our eating habits by bombardment of
food advertisements, tradition and other influences. We must forget learned behaviors from childhood that have a negative effect on our diet that are creating
self-sabotaging adult behavior. The solution is the eating habits and behaviors
which lead to weight gain and obesity. There are many ill health consequences
linked to obesity. Obesity causes other health conditions, which are the leading causes of death in the USA, today. The Federal government acknowledges
the tremendous tax burden associated with excess weight and correlating health

related conditions in the USA. We have the best medical care on the planet however; we are the sickest population in the world. We have diseases of royal dynasties at every level of our population. These diseases are diseases of gluttony, excess and overeating.

As a society, we must get our weight problems under control, the health consequences, tax burden and federal cost for governmental health programs are becoming phenomenal. Insurance rates are becoming astronomical due to the rate of occurrence of weight related diseases. This is why, to help and encourage our society, the federal government in corroboration with the IRS passed legislation that gives tax exemptions to patient's who are obese and who are under "physician assisted" weight loss and maintenance care programs to reduce the growing healthcare cost associated with the treatment of obesity and weight related diseases.

Diet Awareness

Weight loss is usually temporary for dieter's. Adopting healthy eating habits can be permanent. It is true, we are what we eat. That is why it is so important to eat nourishing nutrient rich foods that are healthy and in moderation quantity wise. Our liquid intake is as important as the foods we eat. Fresh, pure cleansing water is necessary to maintain balance in the chemistry and to flush out toxic waste. You would not water a plant with cola; you can imagine what would happen. Nor should you rely on sugary drinks to hydrate your body's cells and tissues.

However, it is important not to drink icy cold drinks when eating meals, in particular protein rich meals as it slows down metabolism and neutralizes the gastric juices required for proper digestion. When making food selection and while designing your weight loss regimen, remember this; FAD diets do not permanently work. After coming off most FAD diets, the weight is usually gained back in even greater quantities. Some people become intimate with food when they are in lack of intimacy with a loving & caring partner. With the divorce rate at over 50% of the married population is challenged, it is ever more difficult to break away from past learned behavior from the post depression influence in our culture. The last world war triggered a spurt of growth, which resulted in the baby boomer generation. The culture has been greatly influenced by this generation because it allowed us to focus on the material world and the gain of wealth instead of spirituality to recover from the depression. We went from keeping up with the Jones, to everyone is king an a culture with the mindset of "the more the merrier". The mindset of constantly wanting more may show up as weight on the body, from a metaphysical perspective.

In brain scans, that monitor brain waves during an activity or during thinking about the same activity, there is very little difference between thinking about doing the activity or actually doing the activity, they look the same or similar, However, there are actually visible changes within brain activity of the individual who is in compulsive mode. If some one is in a compulsive eating binge the brain scan shows a distinctive pattern similar to that of an addict. Similar patterns are noted in the brain of sex addicts viewing pornography in the foreplay state of arousal and during sexual activity or drug addicts in the process of preparing their fix and taking their fix. This means that addictive behaviors, in pre-action phase, display similar brain scans as displayed during the addictive activity. Watch your thoughts carefully, your thoughts lead to action and become reality.

Awareness Meditative Phrase

Repeat this phrase daily as you meditate to increase your success potential:

> "I have removed the filters that usually separate my conscious mind from my subconscious and super conscious mind to heighten the awareness of how I can achieve my fullest potential in successful weight management."

Instead of having dinner table discussions over a home-cooked meal, we evolved to microwave TV dinners. As our culture has evolved, we have desensitized ourselves to our families and matters of the heart. We have sacrificed our time spent in cultivating family relationships, for the sake of gain of the almighty dollar and material wealth. We have all become work-a-holics to make more and more wealth after the great depression. We wanted to please our parents because we as children never want to disappoint their parents and children want to please and make their parents proud. Having a fast paced, stressed out, work-a-holic lifestyle may lead to eating the wrong types of food for the wrong reasons or for emotional comfort. The dining experience is to be savored and enjoyed, a hectic lifestyle can wreck the experience and our health if we do not take the time to sit down and listen to our body's true needs, chew our food, and be conscious of our inner needs and out true selves. We must get in touch with our higher self to get in touch with what our body, mind and spirit need to survive in a health and balanced state of existence. We need balance in everything, otherwise, life becomes unhealthy, unproductive, obsessive compulsive or habitual. These are behaviors that are difficult to recognize and break away from and if food is our chosen comfort to compensate for some unmet emotional need, we then become overweight and obese.

The Benefits of A Mind Body Weight Loss Program

The Mind Body Weight Plan educates the individual of how to develop a healthier lifestyle in order to successfully gain personal control over weight problems and maintain the positive results for a lifetime. Primarily, It helps the individual understand why they became over weight by launching a self-discovery and self-realization program.

The "Mind Body Weight Loss "program is an Eclectic and Integrative, Mind-Body Medicine approach to achieving and maintaining the individual's Ideal weight through self discovery for the development of a healthier lifestyle.

The Mind Body Weight Loss Program consist of achieving balance in Mind, Body & Spirit by bringing a "Whole Person Conscious Awareness" to the "real cause" or hidden cause of most excess weight conditions.

The Mind Body Weight Loss Program takes an in depth look at the typical modern diet and addresses how learned behaviors, habits and negative emotions create imbalance which contribute to "Weight Gain", Obesity and other "Related Health Problems".

The Mind Body Weight Loss Program gives useful recommendations in overcoming the "battle of the bulge." by correcting imbalances in the Mind and Body.

The Mind Body Weight Loss Program teaches the individual how to achieve successful and permanent weight control, by utilizing a dynamic action plan of proper nutrition, exercise, behavior modification & lifestyle adjustments.

The Mind Body Weight Loss Program creates a more positive conscious awareness about food and our food choices. And gives us a new awareness about how we approach health and fitness to achieve weight loss and maintain balance in Mind & Body for a lifetime of good health and fitness.

DR. JOYCE PETERS

Heavily processed junk foods and drinks are both major contributors of the epidemic of overweight and obese conditions

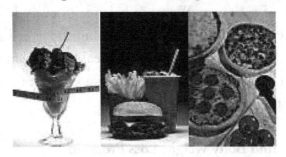

Do these pictures look familiar? It is important to acknowledge and to understand the real health risk factors of the typical American diet. Consuming junk and processed foods and drinks can be linked to the development of overweight conditions and obese conditions.

Conscious Awareness of the American Diet

It is important to acknowledge and to understand the real health risk factors related to being overweight and the ill health consequences linked to obesity. Obesity causes other health conditions, which are the leading causes of death in the USA, today. The national centers of disease control issued a report that 207 million Americans are believed to have excess weight problems and about 300,000 Americans die each year of obesity related problems. Not to mention, the upcoming generation in which research studies show that more than one-in-eight teens and children are over weight and three in five adults ages 20-74 are currently overweight. Which averages out to a one in four Americans are considered not just over weight, but clinically OBESE. What this means is that the number of overweight related deaths are increasing with time when compared to current studies.

The dietary guidelines for America have drastically changed in comparative studies of the U.S. Department Of Agriculture Reports and The U.S. Department of Health and Human Services Reports just since 1995 and current studies. The Surgeon Generals report is available for public review it is titled "Call to Action" to Prevent and Decrease Overweight and Obesity. There is no discrepancy of the urgency of governmental agencies in dealing with this perpetuating health issue.

THE BALANCE DIET & LIFESTYLE

Research shows that Americans spend over 39 billion annually on self-medicating weight loss products. Most of these products are gimmicks and have a 90% failure rate. Health Professionals realize that Yo-yo dieting is not the answer. Federal and State Government paid 43% of the 1.3 trillion dollars spent on health programs related to obesity. This means that our tax dollars are being spent on diseases of overindulgence.

We have the long over due need to develop programs that will help us change our habits, compulsive behavior and excessive lifestyles to regain our health in America. The Mind Body Weight Loss Program is a program that can help. A public report of the seriousness of weight related disease is available online at http://www.cdc.gov?nchs. This report shows that the primary cause of death is obesity related diseases. Obesity related conditions and diseases are astronomical in comparison to all other risk factors such as smoking, homicide, infant mortality rates, infectious disease, accidents and injuries. In light of this information, loosing weight does require an Integrative approach. The truth is there are no short cuts or magic pills to keep excess weight off for a lifetime. We have to face reality of our overweight crisis to achieve a permanent solution to this epidemic. Using an Integrative approach, setting reasonable goals, changing eating behaviors and habits, exercising and adopting a healthier lifestyle is key.

Change Is In The Air
Along with making your personal commitment to a life long weight management program, it is important to recognize the transition that is occurring in medicine, today. Many forms of medicine have evolved. When we combine the most effective treatments that are available from each form of the healing arts and merge them together we form Integrative Medicine. Integrative Medicine is a Holistic approach to healthcare. The Mind Body Weight Loss Program takes an Integrative approach in helping you to achieve your weight loss goals. The birth of Integrative medicine stems from holistic healthcare practices. This program is considered to be a "whole person" approach; this is derived from the word "Health" in old English as being linked to the word "Whole" which translates to being whole or at one with self in "Body, Mind and Spirit" or "Holistic Health". As western medicine developed and became widespread world-wide, it was labeled traditional medicine. Traditional medicine has been accepted and considered mainstream medicine until it was recognized that it did not

consider preventative medicine, effectively. It is also, important for everyone to protect their own health over the past generation, people in Alternative and Complimentary health fields have fought legal battles and patients have struggled to maintain their rights to approach their healthcare issues with various unorthodox methods that were not considered mainstream medicine, this resulted in "freedom of choice in healthcare" acts, bills and laws. The continual support of congressmen and local politicians of the "any willing provider and freedom of choice laws" are what and who protects your freedom of choice in healthcare rights.

Many health professionals are now recognizing the benefits of implementing integrated medicinal practices into the medical treatment plans of their patients and are making more healthy daily lifestyle tips because as their patients began to show improvement and crediting it to Alternative Medicine they began to recognize the true value of health management and prevention practices. In addition, medical research at major universities began t support the claims of improved health with integrative methodology. The Mind Body Weight Loss Program is designed to be implemented in a medical setting under the supervision of an MD. Along with the doctors traditional medical care, specific healthy lifestyle methods are integrated to empower each individual in utilizing his or her own personal power of the mind & body practices help give the patient knowledge and conscious awareness of the effect that their lifestyle has on their health and patient outcomes tend to improve better than with traditional care only. The Mind Body Weight Loss Program enables one to overcome self-limitations and combine their creative will-power with the most effective methods of Integrative medicine, to help them win their individual battle with weight control.

CHAPTER 4

Balanced Nutrition for Weight Loss and Weight Management

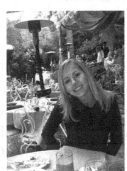

"The down fall of man's health began with the consumption of the first processed food... BREAD."
Quote from co-researcher Summer Perry, NC

PROPER NUTRITION IS IMPERATIVE FOR SUCCESSFUL LIFELONG WEIGHT MAINTE-NANCE. MANY diets stress the body leaving the dieter looking weak and un-healthy. With the Balance Diet and Mind Body Weight Loss Program, you can loose weight and look youthful and healthy all at the same time. We have to have a proper balance of vitamins, minerals, enzymes, electrolytes, amino-acids, proteins, fats, carbohydrates and water, to maintain good health. Information obtained from the U.S. Food and Drug Administration, revealed that research studies of the National Weight Control Registry involving the weight-control behaviors of more than 3,000 people showed that people who have successfully lost an average of 60 pounds of weight and kept the weight off for more than six years, reported that they successfully lost their weight and kept it off by eating a low calorie, low saturated fat, high-complex-carbohydrate diet in combination with being highly physically active.

A Happy Medium is a Balanced Diet

The body has to have a balance of carbohydrates, proteins, fats, vitamins, minerals, enzymes, amino-acids, electrolytes and water. It only makes since that a balanced diet is the answer for health and healthy weight. It is important to understand that carbohydrates are an important part of human nutrition. Carbohydrates provide the feel good hormone, serotonin. All carbohydrates are not equal. The mind body weight loss program allows you to eat good carbohydrates and teaches you how to avoid bad carbohydrates. Complex carbohydrates are natural carbohydrates that are loaded with anti-oxidants. Anti-oxidants stop free radical damage. Free radical damage is what causes the aging appearance. The anti-oxidants that are found in good carbs are a major part of anti-aging nutrition, rich in fiber and are digested easily for better health.

You Are What You Eat

There are some basic dieting tips that will help you to loose weight. We are what we eat, when we eat fattening foods we become fat. It starts when you make the food choices at the grocery store or market. Do not allow poor food choices in your shopping cart, much less your home. Remember, our eating habits are learned behaviors, save your children a struggle in their adult life's and allow the whole family a healthier diet menu. Choose foods that are going to be healthy and good for the whole family.

WE ARE WHAT WE EAT!

EATING FATTY FOODS=BEING FAT

THE BALANCE DIET & LIFESTYLE

Good and Bad Food Facts:

"The healthiest way to lose weight is to remember this quite simple fact. If the body is over-weight then there is an imbalance and the body is being over-loaded by an excess of hidden calories, usually from processed foods. Learn the difference between what are healthy <u>good</u> foods and drinks from what is un-healthy and <u>bad</u> foods and drinks. Recognize that there are in fact, good and bad eating habits. Eating in moderation is a <u>good</u> healthy habit and eating in an overindulgent manner unhealthy <u>bad</u> habit. Create a lifestyle that includes the <u>good's</u> and eliminates the <u>bad's</u>.

Drink lots of water and <u>good</u>, healthy liquids that flush, detox and purify your system. Avoid drinking liquids that are unhealthy or bad for you. Decrease your intake of <u>bad</u> carbohydrates, increase your intake of <u>good</u>, carbohydrates, reduce the intake of <u>bad</u> proteins while increasing your intake of <u>good</u>, healthy proteins and decrease your intake of <u>bad</u> fats while increasing the intake of <u>good</u> healthy fats. And ultimately, make sure your body is getting enough vitamins, minerals and other essential nutrients. Exercise daily. Get adequate rest and sleep as well as take steps to make the necessary behavior modifications to adopt a healthy lifestyle."

10 WAYS TO IDENTIFY THE REASON WHY YOU ARE EATING

1) Identify the reason you are eating – before eating anything, ask your self this question. "Is the consumption of this food healthy for me and will it be beneficial to my weight goals." Listen for your answer from within and adhere to healthy food selection.

2) Avoid dehydration – 80% of hunger pangs are really from dehydra-tion, not hunger. If you get dry, cottonmouth, your body is reabsorb-ing toxic fluid from the bowel, which can cause torpid body chemistry. Drinking water, Colon cleansing and keeping the body flushed and clear aids digestion.

3) De-Stress your life – if you are a Stress eater, you must identify and eliminate as much stress as possible.

4) Behavior modification – identifies your self-sabotaging eating behav-iors and eliminates them.

5) Sleep well – Hunger cannot be satisfied without adequate rest. If you are tired, you are more tempted to eat for energy when sleep is what is needed

6) Correct relationships. – When we need love and are not getting enough, we may be hungering for love instead of food.

7) Lifestyle Adjustments – Enjoy your natural surroundings, observe the beauty of nature, the sky, earth & water. When bored or driving find ways to feel peace and contentment in your life so that food and food advertisement signs are not the only scenery we notice along the way.

8) Avoid Substance Abuse of Food. Use caution in using for other reasons than nourishment to sustain life & health.

9) Nurture Your Emotional, Spiritual, Mental and Physical Health – Feel and Identify your emotions. Refrain from using food for emotional comfort. Do not feed your body with food, when it is your mind, body or spirit that is hungry for things other than food.

10) Do not feed your body to satisfy any other needs. Identify what your necessities are in life. Provide yourself with your individual needs. Meet your needs in a positive way and eliminate negativity. Recognize your need for Love, Food, Water, Air, Shelter, Sex, Spirituality, Peace, Hope, Joy, Faith, Supportive Relationships, Family, Friends and, whatever you need to bring happiness and peace into your life so that you can focus on being your best self and reach your higher self potential. Seek satisfaction from the simple joys in life, on a daily basis to avoid false hunger pains when it may be something other than food that you are truly hungering for. Seek out what you are truly hungry for.

THE MOST IMPORTANT FOOD & LIFESTYLE TIPS FOR WEIGHT LOSS

The most important foods to avoid while losing weight are, products containing white sugar, processed flour products, products containing high fructose corn syrup, hydrogenated, saturated or molecularly altered fats.

It is important to practice good food combining and it is important to eat a diet that supports balance of your chemistry and your Mind-Body type.

It is important to drink lots of water, exercise and manage stress in a healthy manner. It is important to keep your physical and mental energy at their peak with the proper herbs or nutritional supplements.

It is important to cleanse and detoxify the eliminative organ systems to speed up metabolism and waste removal as you lose weight.

THE BALANCE DIET & LIFESTYLE

Fiber is a Fat Zapper

The average person is not consuming enough fiber. Fiber is a fat magnet. Fiber is a fat sponge. Fiber can pull fat from the body and it keeps you feeling full. A man should consume 40 grams of fiber daily on any weight loss plan and a woman should consume at least 30 grams of fiber on her weight loss plan.

The fiber content of the food has to be considered as well. Fiber adds very few calories yet lots of bulk. The bulk that fiber creates in the stomach and intestines, leave you feeling full. It keeps you feeling full while it absorbs fats and flushes it from the body. The more fiber a food contains the better a diet food it is. Processing a food, usually destroys the fiber content in the food.

Food Item	Fiber Content
Wheat pasta	4 grams of fiber
Regular pasta	1 gram of fiber

The more processed a food is the more concentrated the carbohydrate becomes. Extracting the fiber increases the concentrations of calories and carbohydrates. The higher the gram of carbohydrate increases the glycemic rate and quickens the release of sugars into the blood stream, increasing the conversion and storage of fat on the body.

When a food is labeled "instant", it has been heavily processed and it is not recommended for consumption on this program. The less processed the food and the higher the fiber content, the better it is for you. The two preferred grains are natural rolled Oats, Soy, Fruits, Vegetables and Nuts. Unlike most other grains they are loaded with good dietary fiber that can help lower cholesterol and fat. White flour is not recommended under any circumstance whatsoever and is discouraged as it creates inflammation, water retention, fat and weight gain on the body. Corn and Rice are better tolerated by most people and therefore are listed as a close second, consumed in moderation while always observing and limiting caloric, starch and sugar content.

Low fiber, simple carbohydrates fried in hydrogenated trans-fatty oil

Pancakes   33 grams of carbohydrate=27 Teaspoons of Sugar.
French Fries   27 grams of carbohydrate=7 Teaspoons of Sugar.
Pizza   84 grams of carbohydrate=21 Teaspoons of Sugar.

These foods will tend to give you a spike in sugar levels that will cause the body to convert the excess sugars into fat. Continual consumption in these foods will result in a steady rise in body fat and weight gain over time. Overly processed potatoes, grains, flour, bread noodles and pasta are high in toxins and anti-nutrients compounds which rob metabolic enzymes away from healthy metabolism and digestion. They are poor sources of vitamins and minerals and bombard the diet with sugars causing fat storage and weight gain. There are enzyme blockers in these processed foods that commonly block the stomach enzyme pepsin that helps digest protein. They also effect the small intestine enzymes trypsin and chymotrypsin, which are made by the pancreas and help to produce insulin. Therefore, you should only eat these substances in extreme moderation and you should take digestive enzymes throughout the day on a daily basis to help your body to properly digest them. For maximum digestion of protein, you should not eat protein with these types of carbohydrates.

Simple carbohydrates pose a great health threat and are largely responsible for the fat epidemic that we are facing today as they release sugars too fast for the human body to properly digest them. Natural or complex carbohydrates release the sugars more slowly Fat accumulation occurs on the body after consumption of too many unused calories. When simple carbohydrates are over consumed, a pattern of syndrome-X type metabolic dysfunctions begin to occur as a result. These types of metabolic dysfunction can trigger an imbalance that may lead to adult onset stomach, intestinal, heart, liver, pancreatic and hormonal disorders.

Foods That Stabilize Blood-Sugar Levels and Offset Fatigue While Dieting

Common examples of foods that keep blood sugar levels more stable are whole grains, plant oils and fresh vegetables.

Food Item	Portion Size	Calories	Carbohydrate
Fish			
Tuna	3 ounce	85	0.5g
Salmon	3 ounce	150	0g
Sushi/Sashimi	3 ounce	190	10g
Vegetable			
Cucumber	1-cup	15	3g

THE BALANCE DIET & LIFESTYLE

Food Item	Portion Size	Calories	Carbohydrate
Salad Tomatoes	12	43	9.50g
Lettuce (leaf)	3-cups	23	3.45g
Soy/Beans			
Soy Milk	1 cup	100	8g
Tofu	3 ounce	60	3g
Hummus	2 T.	50	6g
Kidney Bean	¼ cup	50	10g
Dairy			
Yogurt	4 ounce	55	9g
Cottage Cheese	1 cup	160	6.5g
Ricotta Cheese	1 cup	255	10g
Poultry			
Chicken	1 breast (4 ounces skinless)	180	0g
Eggs	1 large(poached/boiled)	75	0.50g
Nuts			
Peanut Butter	2 T.	190	6g
Almonds	20 nuts	150	5g
Walnuts	¼ cup	180	4g
Oils			
Olive oil cooking spray	spray	10	0g
Walnut oil	1 T.	120	0g
Fish Oils	1 t.	90	0g

The foods listed above slowly release sugars into the blood stream delivering steady stream of energy. The following release the sugar more quickly the more natural foods are perfectly designed by nature for human consumption and digestion. Carbohydrates, in their naturally occurring state, are always better for you than processed carbohydrates regardless of their glycemic index rate.

Fruit			
Watermelon	1 cup	50	11g
Strawberry	1 cup	45	10g
Peach	1 (medium)	40	9g
Bread/Grains			
Crackers	3 whole wheat	55	8.5g

Food Item	Portion Size	Calories	Carbohydrate
Bread	1 piece(low carb)	60	10 g
Cereal	1 cup (wheat)	40	8g
Deserts			
Gelatin	1 cup sugar-free	20	0g
Popsicle	1 sugar-free	20	3g
Pudding	1 cup sugar-free	50	7g

FRUIT SORBET RECIPES

Put 8 ounces of fruit in a food processor, blend with four ounces of yogurt and freeze limit to a 3 ounce or less portion. Use stevia instead of sugar alternative to sweeten. These concoctions equal 1 ½ fruit serving.

Mellon Sorbet-Honey Dew, Caneloupe or Watermelon
Berry Sorbet – Raspberry, Strawberry, Blueberry
Peach Mango Sorbet – Peach, Mango
Orange, Lemon and Lime Sorbet – Juice without rind and freeze

HOT COBBLERS

Apple Cobbler – Mix three ounces of apple with 1 teaspoon of stevia or honey sprinkle cinnamon and bake until hot and bubbly cool and enjoy.

Berry Cobbler – Mix three ounces of blueberries, strawberries or blackberries with one teaspoon of honey bake until hot and bubbly, cool and enjoy.

Peach/Plum Cobbler – Mix three ounces of peaches or plums with a teaspoon of stevia or honey or sprinkle on nutmeg & cinnamon, bake until bubbly, cool and enjoy.

THE BALANCE DIET & LIFESTYLE

THE MIND-BODY FOOD COMBINING METHOD

One of the best Naturopathic approaches to weight loss is Food-Combining. There are a few basic rules while choosing the proper food combinations to maximize metabolism and digestion.

The basic food combining rules are:

Eat small portions per meal.
Eat several small low calorie meals a day to keep digestion going.
Allow time for meat proteins to completely digest before consuming them again.
Do not eat proteins and starchy carbohydrates in the same meal.
Eat only one meat protein per day.
Do not mix extra fats with meat protein.
Do not mix multiple proteins together.
Only mix non-starchy/mildly-starchy vegetables with meat protein.
Bread should not be mixed with meat protein.
Bread should not be mixed with starchy carbohydrates.
Eat only whole grain breads in moderation.
Whole grain bread is a meal with cheese or nut butter.
Fish protein is preferred over meat protein requires less than 10 hours for digestion.
Ocean Fish proteins naturally contain omega 3 fatty acids that send a "full signal" to the brain.
Eggs and fish eggs contain brain food, lecithin and fatty acids.
Fish and Eggs are brain foods and block mental fatigue while dieting.
Research studies have not shown that people eating eggs cause more heart attacks than people who avoid eggs in their diet.
Eating a boiled egg or an egg fried in olive oil, is a better breakfast choice than eating a fat free white bagel because of the glycemic index.
Eggs are exempt from food combining rules and can be mixed with most things.
Meat proteins require 12-14 hours for digestion.
If you eat red meat, you must eat an organ meat to get the enzymes to digest it.
Water and juice fast a day between heavy meat protein meals.
When juicing, recognize it as a meal.
Pineapple contains bromelain an enzyme which aids protein metabolism.

DR. JOYCE PETERS

Examples of proper natural food combinations:

Source of Protein	Good Protein Combinations	Poor Protein Combinations
	(not in any particular food combining order)	
Cheese	Corn	Potato
Coconut	Spinach	Bread
Eggs	Tomatoes	Beans
Fish	Lettuce	Cereal
Poultry	Garlic/onion	Grain
Nuts/Nut Butters	Celery	Pumpkin
Soybean	Broccoli	Split Peas
Yogurt	Cucumber	Avocado

2 Hours between other meals:

Whole grain/slice of bread-90 calories	1-T. of Peanut Butter 90 calories or
	1-T. of Farmer Cheese 20 calories or
	1-T of Cream Cheese 30 calories or
	1-T. of Natural Fruit Spread-30 calories.
Fresh Juice Recipe	3 ounces as a meal by itself
Natural Fruits-Mixed	4-5 ounces as a meal by itself
Half an apple sliced – 50 calories	" or
Celery Stick – 20 calories	"

The idea to trigger weight loss on the Mind Body Weight Loss program, is to not mix proteins with carbohydrates in order to trigger lipolysis. This is when the body starts burning calories from stored fat reserves. The body normally burns carbohydrates for energy. The body will revert to the stored fat when processed carbohydrates and sugars are eliminated if proper food combining is utilized. This can take up to 15 days into the diet to see a change. Good carbohydrates do not increase insulin levels in the manner that processed carbohydrates do, this is why heavily refined processed carbohydrates must be eliminated. The heavily refined carbohydrates peak insulin levels too fast for the body to sufficiently process and digest the rapid release of sugars into the blood stream and this is when the body converts the sugars into fat or alcohols damaging the organs and pancreas. Good carbohydrates release insulin more slowly and do not result in fat conversion and can actually help you loose weight. Good carbohydrates are usually high in fiber, which also aids in the digestion of fat.

Einstein once said, "keep it as simple as possible but not more simple than that…" Simplifying your diet with natural non-refined carbohydrates are acceptable diet foods and processed and refined carbohydrate foods should be avoided as much as possible during your diet. It is the refined carbohydrates and lack of exercise that sabotage weight loss. The proper amount of non-refined complex carbohydrates is approximately 45% and no more than 8% refined carbohydrates. Carbohydrates that are processed, such as white sugar and flour convert to sugars that are too hard to digest and covert to stored fat in the body. These simple carbohydrates leave you feeling bloated and will cause weight gain, disrupt the immune system, adrenals and insulin levels.

The types of complex carbohydrates that are acceptable are non-processed, such as: leafy green vegetables, corn, peas, beans, potatoes and whole grains fresh raw fruits and vegetables. These digest more slowly allowing the body time to utilize the sugars. The simple carbohydrates release the sugars too quickly causing problems with digestion. Examples of simple carbohydrates are foods or drinks containing white sugar, white flour, white rice, white pasta, syrup and processed fruit juices from concentrate. Simple carbohydrates are not acceptable foods and should be avoided during your weight loss program. Listen to your body, if you have symptoms of fatigue, bloating, sugar cravings you are probably consuming simple carbohydrates because they zap energy with a hangover effect. Always decrease or eliminate the refined carbohydrates first and then fruit before the non-refined and complex carbohydrates until you find balanced energy.

Eating to Maintain a Healthy Weight

Only eat when you are truly hungry.
Avoid hidden sources of calories.
Sit down when eating. Dine.
Eat slowly. Food is not intended to be eaten fast.
Chew your food. Masticate foods for an extended time.
Do not talk when chewing and swallowing.
Stop and wait 5 minutes when you are 5-10 minutes into your meal.
Savor your dining experience.
Taste the flavor of your food. Experience all the flavors of your meal.
Feel the texture of your food.

Feel your food as you swallow it and feel it fill up your stomach.
Acknowledge that the food that you ingest is becoming part of you.
Confirm that your food selection will create radiant energy for you.
Do not use meal times for problem solving discussions.
Do not eat when you are emotionally upset.
Eat in a pleasant and peaceful atmosphere.
Leave part of your stomach empty; do not eat until you "feel full".
Confirm that your food selection will not create fatty accumulations
on your body.
Burps are a sign that you have filled the stomach up to the natural
layer of air space within the stomach. Listen and feel for the expelling
of the air from the stomach. Burping acts as a cue that signals the hypothalamus to send the signal of cessation or fullness to the stomach.
Stop eating when you burp or belch and wait ten minutes before
resuming your meal. Burping is pushing the natural layer of air out of
the stomach signaling that you are approaching a state of fullness, that
you are overloading the stomach.
Drinking carbonated drinks desensitizes the body's natural signals and
creates excessive belching. Avoid carbonated drinks with meals.
Rest 30 minutes after eating a healthy meal and feel the sensation of
satisfaction.
Exercise 30 minutes after your meal take a 30-minute walk.
Do not eat another meal until you body fully digests the previous
meal.

Balancing Recipes

Fat Burning Vegetable Dip

Cucumbers are fat burners because of the phyto-hormones they contain that are
similar to insulin. At approximately 15 calories per 5 ounce serving they are full
of bulk fiber. Can be eaten whole or blended with yogurt and dill and used as a
vegetable dip for other vegetables.

> 1 large cucumber (grinded in food processor)
> 2 tablespoons of fresh dill
> ½ fresh lemon juiced
> ½ cup plain yogurt
> 1 tablespoon of olive oil

Mix and chill for 2 hours – serve as a vegetable dip for raw vegetables.

THE BALANCE DIET & LIFESTYLE

Non-starchy alkalizing complex carbohydrates are lettuce, spinach, cucumber, onions, green beans, garlic, zucchini, broccoli, celery, cabbage, turnip greens, sprouts, eggplant and parsley. Mildly starchy alkalizing complex carbohydrates are artichokes, carrots, corn, peas, and cauliflower. Starchy complex carbohydrates are cereals, potatoes, split peas, beans, and grains.

Simple carbohydrates are processed, and not recommended or in extreme moderation such as white pasta, rice, bread, instant oats and cereals. Good examples of good snacks or mini – meals in food combining are:

Fresh/Raw	Steamed/Sautéed
Cubed Cucumber	Baby Zucchini
Cubed Roma Tomato	Sweet Kernel Corn
Purple Onion	Diced Sweet Onion
Lemon Juice	Black Olive & 1T. Olive Oil
Salad Vinegar	Salt, Pepper, Garlic

You can mix all of the above ingredients and eat them raw or steam them. Fruits should be eaten as a separate meal. With the exception of pineapple which aids in protein metabolism. Juicing is a great meal replacement. When juicing vegetables add just enough fruit to accent the flavor. Juicing is high in energy giving nutrients and is low in fat. Fruits are categorized in alkalizing, acid and sub-acid groups. Acid fruits are sour apple, strawberry, tangerines, kumquat, pineapple and blackberry. Sub acid fruits are, apple, kiwi, mango, nectarine, peach, pear, papaya, cherry, grape and fig. Alkalizing fruits are, melon, cantaloupe, watermelon, casaba, and honey dew. Some acid fruits have an alkalizing effect in the body such as lemon and orange. Lemon is closest to our own hydrochloric acid and is a good substitute for salads including tuna salad. It is the one exception when fruit can be mixed with meat or dairy protein as it aids in digestion. Fats are necessary and good fats are beneficial and aid in digestion and immunity. Good fats are avocados, cold pressed olive, sesame, natural organic butter, cheeses, fish oils omega 3 and 6, and nut butters. The processed oils and saturated fats must be avoided.

MIND BODY WEIGHT LOSS IS FOOD COMBINING

The impact of proper food combining and eliminating heavily processed foods may produce profound long-term or permanent results.

> When you eat Protein, you must allow eight hours for digestion
> When you eat Carbs, you must allow four hours for digestion
> When you eat processed foods, you may allow your body more than 50 days to digest hydrogenated fat, artificial preservatives, anti-biotics pesticides & herbicides, hormone and steroid traces in commercial livestock and produce.
> Avoid mixing commercially grown, genetically altered food sources that are genetically modified.

The Importance of Food Combining

It is important to practice food combining. It takes more energy for the digestion of food than most any other bodily function. When we are becoming fatigued after a meal, we have not experienced proper food combining. The digestion of some foods, for example a large portion of meat with saturated fat, takes more energy than cycling or running. Therefore, energy needed to eliminate toxic waste, acid is shifted to digesting the heavy food, and we become sleepy or tired after consumption.

Alkaline and Acid Foods Chart

All food creates either an alkaline ash residue or an acid ash residue. All animal protein forms an acid ash residue. All chemically altered food additives form an acid ash residue. Very few food items are neutral in ph. The following is a list of alkaline and acid foods.

Alkaline	Acid
Herb Tea	Coffee
Almonds	Sugar (processed)
Carrots	Chicken
Cucumber	Turkey
Cabbage	Red Meat
Corn	Poultry
Mellon	Beef

THE BALANCE DIET & LIFESTYLE

Alkaline	Acid
Honeydew	Pork
Water Mellon	Tuna
Green or String Beans	Ham
Sweet Potato	Bacon
Squash	Lamb
Radish	Fish
Turnip	Banana
Orange	Deer
Apple	Peanuts
Raspberry	Shrimp
Pear	Beans (most)
Green Beans	Alcohol
Mushrooms	White Flour
Onion	Tomato
Eggplant	Wheat
Grape	Rice
Ginger	Red Beans
Spinach	Chocolate
Potato	Baking Powder
Lettuce	Dairy
Honey	White Sauces

Weak alkaline forming in the body:	Weak acid forming in the body:
Yogurt (whole)	Cottage Cheese
Soy Milk (Fructose Free)	Egg White
Cheese (Cheddar)	Cheese (American)
Celery	Grains
Broccoli	Goat's Milk
Corn	Butter
Coconut	Dried Figs, Dates & Raisins

High Protein Diet Fads

Protein is great, but, high protein diets that omit the intake of carbohydrates and allow the consumption of rich meaty protein, are not balanced. Food group gorging is never a permanent answer. Meat is an acid forming food. The taste buds may like it but the kidneys sure don't. Without raw veggies there are usually not enough alkaline buffers and enzymes to properly digest protein. Therefore, the body dips into its own alkaline reserves and pulls buffers from the bones, organs and chemistry to digest the protein excess. Excess acid ash residues that build up in the chemistry from eating a diet high in acid forming animal proteins can cause the body to pull alkalizing buffers that are needed to regulate homeostasis, one of the first places the imbalance affects is the kidneys. The kidneys contain high amounts of alkalizes and calcium that is robbed as the body goes into ketosis and the body tries to compensate to maintain homeostasis due to the acid imbalance that the high protein creates as an overload to the system and this contributes to acid build-up in the kidneys which usually causes mysterious pain syndromes and even may cause kidney stones. High Protein diets allow you to only eat high quantities of acid forming protein such as burgers, cheese, bacon and other fatty meats with no consumption of alkalizing complex carbohydrates.

The alkaline and enzyme reserves of the body and organ systems become severely depleted when eating a high protein diet for a continuous amount of time. The body goes into ketosis. Ketosis is a reaction of the kidneys when the blood ketone levels are too high, the kidneys start excreting the ketone waste through excessive urination, while the kidneys are in this mode, and the excessive water loss creates a potassium and electrolyte loss. Next, the heart is affected because the body starts robbing alkalizers from the organs; the heart has to have potassium, magnesium and calcium to maintain normal function without these nutrients and acidic blood pumping through it due to the purely acid forming diet, and causes damage to the heart and cardiovascular system. As this occurs oxidative, stress and lipid imbalances may lead to heart disease and heart attack. Next, the pancreas, brain and cells lose response to insulin forcing the body to produce more insulin, which is what leads to fat accumulation, erratic blood sugar fluctuations and eventually diabetes. This occurs when the reserve systems are very depleted and there are not enough carbohydrates to regulate normal organ and metabolic function. The endocrine system is detrimentally affected, as these organs are all part of the hormonal system of the body. Only a small quantity of a heavy food is acceptable, to maintain optimum energy and digestion. Instead of a six-ounce steak, only three ounces should be consumed per meal and it should be a lean cut, and cut away excess fat before and after cooking. When eating heavy meat proteins, limit intake to two meals per day should contain healthy sources of good protein. Good protein sources are soy, fish, eggs, nuts, nut butters, seeds, seed butters, yogurt, natural cheeses or meats such as tuna, chicken or turkey, with emphasis on organically grown and free range. These protein/acid meals should not be mixed with starchy carbohydrates. Mix proteins with non-starchy alkalizing complex carbohydrates. The heaviest meal in the day should be when the conversion of calories is at its peak in the human body. From 6 until 11 each morning is the time to eat the heaviest meal of the day because very little will convert to fat on the body. Avoid laying down full at night this is the slowest conversion time. According to scientist, Dr. Carey Reams, the body cannot properly digest pork, and it may actually age the body due to the extreme effort required to digest it. Therefore, the consumption of pork may create slowed weight loss.

Healthy Protein Selection

The body needs protein it is important to maintain a healthy diet consisting of balanced nutrition. However, one of the most important nutritional weight management tips is to avoid excessive intake of one of the recommended food groups. To maintain a healthy weight, eat a balanced diet and avoid FAD diets. FAD diets usually consist of creating an imbalance of one or more food groups. High protein diets force the kidneys to try to get rid of the excess waste byproducts of protein and fat, called ketones. This buildup in the blood is called ketosis. Ketones can dangerously cause the body to produce high levels of uric acid and urea's, which can lead to kidney stones, heart attack and gouty arthritis or gout. Ketosis is risky for people with diabetes because it can speed up the progression of diabetic renal disease and may lead to kidney damage and failure in diabetics. Unhealthy high protein diets may actually create a bio-chemical imbalance within the body that adversely affect the kidneys. The kidneys filter out liquid acid waste to maintain homeostasis in the body chemistry. An imbalanced chemistry can lead to bio-hormonal imbalances within the endocrine system, which the kidneys are a part of. The compensating nature of the endocrine system may create imbalances in the other organs within the endocrine system.

No more than eight ounces of lean meat protein should be consumed in a day. Fish, lamb, seafood. Free range poultry and cattle that consumed field grasses increase the quality of the meat where grain fed beef is more toxic and harder to digest and is more fatty. Soy, whey and egg proteins are similar in value.My favorite soy foods are tempeh and edamame. Moderation is the key to all food intake and thus, the same with soy. Fermented soy products are tofu, miso, tamari are said to be better for you. The FDA, American Heart Association, and leading health experts recommend that Americans eat more soy protein to lower their cholesterol, protect their heart, and reduce menopausal symptoms. New research shows that eating soy is associated with weight loss, stronger bones, reduced menstrual disturbances like PMS, and improved breast, endometrial, colon and prostate health. However, use your head when selecting soy protein. Soy is processed in many ways. Always avoid soy products containing sugar, select plain, sugar free or natural soy, that is organically grown such as edamame. Regardless, soy is a good diet protein but should not be your only source of protein. Soy protein powder can be added to your own juice concoction. There are many sorts of soy products available on the market, cautiously make wise soy selections. Soy lacks the amino acid methionine and therefore should not be the main source of protein in the diet, if soy is your main source of protein methionine should be supplemented in the diet. Select soy products that are as natural as possible and that support your weight loss program. There are few individuals who do not tolerate soy very well the majority of the public tolerate soy very well. However, if you have a mental or nervous condition, suffer from panic attacks, adrenal burnout, chronic fatigue, or suffer from narcolepsy, caution should be used and soy consumption should be minimized. Not eliminated, minimized, soy should only be consumed in small specific quantities such as tofu, edamame or tempeh. In some cases, the elimination of wheat products can resolve soy intolerance and most symptoms of being gluten intolerant. Regardless, soy is a better substitute for wheat and a good alternative source of protein compared to fatty meats and dairy. Soy offers a good source of protein for vegetarians. Vegetable protein is always better and the fiber content is high which is good for fat elimination.

THE BALANCE DIET & LIFESTYLE

High Carb Diets

High carb diets generally allow you to eat all the carbohydrates that you want but they have to be fat free. These are usually processed food items that create sugars in the body leading to storage of fat, stress on the hormonal system. These diets affect the pancreas in a detrimental way, which may lead to adult onset diabetes. The main problem with these diets is that they encourage the consumption of the processed diet foods that are labeled low carbs, low fat or fat free. These pre-packaged foods are full of artificial flavor enhancers, food additives, preservatives, are refortified with nutrients and are missing the digestive enzymes and nutrient balance that only natural foods can deliver. These foods are mostly chemicals that disrupt the metabolic functioning of the body. Not only is the weight gained back after coming off a high carb diet usually more weight is gained than before going on the diet.

The body becomes less insulin resistant causing fat accumulation on the body. Consuming a high carb diet with processed simple carbohydrates creates hormonal imbalances that stress and ages the body to digest them. It also, leads to toxic conditions in the body, digestive track disturbances and a gradual decline in the overall health of the body as well as, fatigue, food allergies, sugar imbalances, and adult onset disease. All of these may occur from long term consumption of high carbohydrate, processed food diets. Carbohydrates use to be valued as complex or simple carbohydrates based on the sugar and starch content of the food item, as research continues and more awareness is surfacing on how we digest foods, there is a shift occurring and the glycemic index is more of the current focus on carbohydrate food items.

As you know by now, grain products are one of the culprits of obesity and obesity related diseases such as adult onset diabetes. "G" is for grain "G" is for glycemic. "G" is for gain and "G" is a major part of the diets of the world. We have an overgrowth of grains, our market is flooded with grain based products, we are over consuming grain, based products, we are over feeding our livestock with grains and are shipping grains to third world countries to stop world hunger.

The "G" Force-

The "G" force/factor must always be considered in making healthy food choices for weight loss and weight management. The glycemic index of a food is the rate in which the food or carbohydrate raises blood sugar levels. Eating low glycemic index foods release a slow rise in blood sugar levels while eating high glycemic index foods release a rapid "G"-force rise in blood sugar levels. High glycemic foods blast our blood sugar levels up so rapidly that it creates shock to the pancreas that can eventually can damage and destroy its natural functioning. Because some of the same foods can have a different glycemic rate based on how the food is processed. Instant white rice releases sugars at a higher glycemic index rate than whole grain brown rice. Processed grains leave you feeling wired up and then washed out. High glycemic rated foods spike blood sugar levels and then bottom out on you giving you what can feel very much like a "food hang-over" effect. Examples of bad high glycemic index foods are white bread crackers, instant oats, white flour, five minute white rice and junk snack foods. Good examples of high glycemic foods are, bananas and carrots. The reason that these are good are that they also contain the fiber and enzymes for proper digestion. Obviously, some high glycemic index foods should be avoided as they do not digest as efficiently as the more natural high glycemic foods. Some are in the top three foods you should not eat and others should be consumed under proper food combining techniques. Such as a fruit would be, two hours after or 2 hours before the next meal.

"The most major factor to remember when considering the G-factor is that some of the same foods can have a high or low glycemic index rating depending on how it is processed or prepared the more refined a food is the worse it is for you".

The glycemic index of pasta can be lowered simply by serving it aldente' in other words by undercooking it. This is the ONLY way white pasta should be consumed. It takes the body a little longer to digest it when it is still a little hard from being undercooked therefore, it lowers the glycemic index by way of the way that it is prepared. When you are eating flour products such as pasta, think of it as bread, because that is what it is in an altered form. When you eat pasta eat much smaller amounts. The problem with pasta is that we tend to over eat by social conditioning, because it is cheep, many times restaurants pile pasta on the whole plate. The main thing to remember is to keep the portion size very small, pasta and bread swells up to over ten times the size you see on your plate in your stomach. Conduct your own experiment, fill a large mixing bowl with water drop a slice of bread, a bread stick, or ½ of a bagel in the water and look at it in an hour, the bread will usually expand to the size of the bowl. Many times, this is one of the reasons why we feel bloated after meals. If you eat these foods at all you should eat only very small portions and with pasta or rice eat it only aldente'. During the intial phase of weight loss they should be avoided, or if you hit a wall during weight loss they should be avoided, completely.

Aldente' Pasta Calculator

¼ -½ cup for children and small adults with high activity levels.

½ cup for over weight adults who are on an active exercise routine.

½ – ¾ cup for average sized adults with high activity levels.

¾ – 1 cup for athletic adults. (White is Discouraged Quinoa or Whole Grain Is Preferred)

Low Glycemic Index Foods Hit the Spot – Slow Rising "G" Spot Foods -

Not all carbohydrates are the same. Some hit the spot, just right and release long lasting, satisfying energy, all day long for sustained nutritional benifits. Low glycemic carbs are the carbs that leave you feeling healthy, full and satisfied after consumption. Low glycemic index foods are; peas, lentils, red potatoes, cherries, granny smith apples, and most vegetables. Because some of the same food can have a different glycemic rate based on how the food is processed. The glycemic index of whole grains is lower than the glycemic index of refined or processed grains. Whole grains are slower to digest and therefore take more time to release sugars more slowly into the blood stream than the processed, refined and instant grain products. The body can more effectively digest and handle the slower release of these types of sugar and utilize it more efficiently. The slow-rise low-index carbohydrates are best. These are foods such as fresh raw celery and salads. The pancreas cannot regulate rapid-rise high-glycemic index foods such as pasta and bread as effectively as slow rise low-index foods. The rapid rise of blood sugar levels causes the body to make conversions from starch sugars into weight gain and fat storage. The body can more efficiently handle the rate of sugar release from the complex carbohydrates in comparison to the rate of sugar release from simple carbohydrates with less conversion and storage of fat.

Good Fats

Certain naturally occurring fats contained in healthy foods provide satisfying long lasting energy and stamina. Good fats slow down the rise in blood sugars allowing foods to stay in your stomach and small intestine for a longer period of time allowing the body to absorb more nutrients and leave you feeling fuller longer. This may decrease the desire to continue eating after you are full therefore can be a deterrent of overeating. Good fats usually pose no risk of cardiovascular disease. Healthy fats such as omega 3 fats can help you lose weight. Omega 3 fat contains brain nutrients keeping the brain full with nutrients that it uses to combat mental fatigue and increase mental alertness and focus will increase you chance of weight loss success by reducing the brains starvation signals. Healthy fats these usually come from fish such as salmon and plants such as avocado, in comparison to dairy which contain very little of these types of healthy fats. Grass fed beef has more good fats than grain-fed beef. When it comes to livestock the quality of meat for human consumption, is determined by the way the animal ate and lived. If the animal ate healthy and had a happy life having a lifestyle that was natural to its existence, the meat it is more healthy for humans to eat than those animals that were raised in imprisoned environments and injected with toxic substances and synthetic hormones. Good fats should be included in your diet.

Good Fats

EFA – essential fatty acids

CLA – conjugated fatty acids

Omega 3, Omega 6, – found in ocean fish and salmon

ALA – alpha Lipoic acids

GLA – Gamma-linolenic acid

OA – Oleic Acid found in Olives

LA – Lauric acid found in coconut, normalizes lipids in the body

Good fats can be found in:

    Flax Seed Oil

    Fish Oils

    Olive Oil

    Evening Primrose Oil

THE BALANCE DIET & LIFESTYLE

Ocean Fish and Salmon (PCB & mercury free)
Eggs (Organic & Free Range)
Grass Fed Beef and Livestock
Borage Seed Oil
Nuts & Lentils
Black Current Oil

Making healthy food choices

Conscious awareness that making healthy personal choices in the diet on a daily basis and elimination of the improper use of food can affect the long term outcome of successful weight management.

Choose to eat a variety of healthy foods
Choose foods that are low in saturated fats
Choose food without a lot of food additives, salt, sugar or preservatives
Choose drinks without sugar, sodium, caffeine or alcohol
Choose to eat foods that help you loose weight
Choose to eat only when truly hungry
Choose to drink distilled water instead of sugary processed drinks
Choose healthy natural snacks instead of refined carbohydrate junk foods

DAILY BALANCE DIET & MIND BODY WEIGHT LOSS LIFESTYLE REGIMEN

Wake Up –	½ cup of lemon water – Do the Mind Body Stretches & Exercises
Breakfast –	3 eggs/whites and one whole free range organic egg (scrambled with veggies in olive oil & sprinkled with Dosha Balancing Spices)
	1 slice of dark gluten free whole grain toast/or flourless bread
	1 cup lite brewed black coffee
Mid-Morning –	Cup of yogurt with nuts, fruit/berries.
Lunch –	Large salad with mixed field greens and veggies topped with 3-4 ounces of Salmon and fresh herbs & ayurevedic spices. Fresh squeezed lemon juice and a tablespoon of red wine vinegar
Afternoon Snack –	Mellon smoothie/Veggie Greens (see juice section for more variety)

**Late
Afternoon
Snack –**   ¼ cup of almonds & 1 small apple (slices)

Dinner –   6 ounce bowl of Mind Body Weight Loss vegetable stew and 1 ounce slice of cheddar cheese.

**Early
Evening
Snack –**   4 celery sticks with cucumber dip, cottage cheese or fruit cobbler

Bedtime   ½ cup of lemon water, brush teeth and go to bed.

(For other menu options see exchange list or nutrition for weight loss chapter for recipes)

Your Daily Balanced Diet & Lifestyle Regimen

Behavior-   Do your behavior modification: Do not eat after 6 pm. Hunger Control-Keep a granny smith apple in a zip lock bag and graze on it a little throughout the whole day (sprinkled with Dosha spices)

Hydrate-   Drink your distilled & mineral water between 6am-6pmpm to flush the digestive track on a daily basis. Optional – Cup of soothing diet or chai herb tea. Allow an hour for urination before bed each night.

Exercise –   Do your body exercise (an hour of stretching & physical exercise in the morning and do the relaxing yoga exercises every evening)

Lifestyle-   Reinforce the Balanced Lifestyle – Listen to The Mind Body Weight Loss CD or Say your Weight loss mantras/vows.

Meditatation- Do your mind exercise. Meditate daily on your weight loss goals just before sleep and upon awakening.

CHAPTER 5

The Balance Diet Food Pyramid
& Recipes

THE ORIGINAL FOOD PYRAMID IS HIGHLY INEFFECTIVE FOR WEIGHT LOSS purposes. It is more important to consume foods that are rich in essential nutrients. The recommended portions of the original food pyramid can actually lead to overweight conditions if followed according to the daily-recommended intake of the major food groups. Another reason that the original food pyramid is not balanced in acid/alkalinity ratios. Therefore, most of the essential vitamins minerals, enzymes are not prioritized by essential nutrient consumption values. In order for a nutrient to have been deemed "an essential nutrient" by the FDA, the nutrient was scientifically proven to be required by an organ or gland in order for the organ or gland to maintain proper function. Without the essential nutrient an organ cannot maintain its proper function or maintain disease free health. In the old food group pyramid, the recommended amount of consumption of the original major food groups is deficient in valuable essential nutrients and excessive in fat and calories for most individuals. One should calculate their proper caloric intake based on activity level, frame size, normal body weight and height per individual.

In the original food pyramid, recommendations were made to consume 6-11 servings of pasta, rice, bread or cereal daily. Anyone can assume that much refined carbohydrate will make you fat unless the rest of your day is spent exercising those carbohydrates off. In the Mind Body Food Pyramid, commercially grown processed meats and processed starchy foods such as white pasta, white sugar, white rice and white bread and processed white potato products should be avoided as much as possible as well as most other snack type processed food sources. The original food pyramid suggest using all fats and oils sparingly. The low-fat craze has been a major culprit in the development of obesity and diabetes, due to the flood of low fat products that usually were full of simple carbohydrates that converted to sugar and fat in the body after ingestion due to the high glycemic index. In the Mind Body Weight Loss Pyramid, natural fats are good, it is the saturated fats that should be avoided. Complex Carbohydrates raise levels of Seratonin. Seratonin lowers levels of acid producing cortisol. Therefore, the consumption of alkalizing complex carbohydrates, may aid in breaking the pattern of stress related weight gain and bio-chemical imbalances that block essential nutrient absorption. Saturated fats and starchy carbohydrates are usually hidden. Balance is the Key.

The Mind Body Weight Loss Pyramid is a safe and effective guide in aiding successful weight control, naturally, while maximizing nutrient saturation in the body. People with disease should always take precautions and everyone should seek medical clearance, consent and supervision prior to beginning any diet and exercise plan. Consult your physician if you suffer with any disease before following the Mind Body Food Pyramid guide and obtain medical clearance.

THE BALANCE DIET & LIFESTYLE
"THE BALANCE DIET FOOD PYRAMID"
The Balance Diet Equation is 80% – 20% Alkaline/Acid Foods

Eat
an
80/20
Balance of
Alkaline/Acid
Foods

Avoid or Minimize the Intake
of: Refined Sugars, Salt, Caffeine
Refined Starches, Processed
Meats, Saturated Fats & Heavily
Refined Pasta, Breads, Processed Foods &
Processed High Glycemic Carbohydrates.

Good Fats: Plant Oils, Ocean Fish, Wild Salmon,
Eggs & Naturally Processed Hormone & Fat Free Dairy,
Yogurt, Lean Organic Meats, Whole Grains, Rice, Pine Nuts,
Avocado, Coconut, Fiber Rich Whole Fresh Fruits, Mellon,
Berries, Pine Nuts, Nuts, Seeds, Soy, Quinoa, Oats, Beets, White
Potatoes, Amaranth, Corn, Yams, Squash,, Peas, Lentils & Beans
(natural, organic, flourless, unprocessed & free range if possible)

Fresh, Whole, Natural, Alkalizing & Enzymatic Foods
Vegetables/ Salads/Raw Fiber/Greens/Sprouts
Raw, steamed, cooked & seasonal veggies: Tomatoes, Celery, Cucumber, Spinach,
Alfalfa Sprouts, Bean Sprouts, Water Cress, Cabbage, Broccoli, Lettuces, Onion, Garlic,
Parsley, Cilantro, Peppers, Nutritional Supplements & Fresh Herbs & Ayurvedic Spices

LIQUIDS
Steam Distilled Water/Purified Water/Natural Mineral Water
Herb Teas/Broth/Soup/Fresh Vegetable Juices from Organic Produce
Kombusha Tea, Effervesent Mineral Water Tablets, Cleansing
Broths, & Balancing Mind Body Health Program Juice and Smoothie Recipes

Eat a well balanced diet
Adjust Alkaline and Acid Consumption to Maintain Homeostasis in the Individual.

The Mind Body Food Pyramid focuses on liquid consumption and a balanced diet. High water-content foods are usually fresh whole foods and the overall diet consist of a varying range of Complex Carbohydrates 50-55%, 25-30% Protein and 15-20% Good Fats. The range is adjusted according to your specific dietary needs, your lifestyle and your activity factors.

50/30/20 55/30/15 or 80/20-70/30

The Balance Diet Pyramid is not just about balancing your Fat, Carbohydrate and Protein intake. The Balance Diet is about a new way of balancing the chemistry of the foods you eat and a new way of categorizing carbohydrates. While on a weight loss program, the balanced diet should consist of 50-55% Carbohydrates, 25-30% Protein and 15-20%Good Fats. Fluctuating by activity factors. On days with high activity you would eat a little more protein, or you may have more carbs and a little more good fats. On days with little activity or if you miss exercise, the calories are reduced even more.

A Healthy Daily Diet

A weight loss diet can vary depending on a person's body type, metabolism, fitness goals, genetic make-up, and nutritional needs, but, should consist of no less than:

5-8 servings of Raw or steamed vegetables.
1-3 servings of Fish, Eggs, Chicken, Turkey or Soy Protein or Meat Alternatives.
1-2 servings of Whole Grains
1-2 servings of Healthy Fats (Avocado, Olive or Flax Seed Oil)
1-2 servings of Fruits.
1-2 servings of Dairy (skim milk, bio-k/yogurt/Kefir)

In Addition, the diet should be balanced in acids and alkaline consisting between 70% alkaline 30% acid foods or 80% alkaline 20% acid for those under stress. The Carbohydrates should be broken down in three divisions and consumed as follows: 25 % should be high water and fiber content Vegetables such as lettuces, fresh herbs, seaweed, algae, broccoli, cucumber, onions, artichoke, asparagus, peppers and cabbages. Fiber is important, 15 % percent of the daily carbohydrate intake should be complex Carbohydrates, such as whole grains, oats, brown rice, bread and potatoes. 8 % should be fiber rich whole-fruits such as grapefruit, apples, pears and high fiber alkaline fruits and less than 2% percent high sugar fruits like grapes, peaches and fruits such as mangoes should be eaten with the skin. Protein should consist of lean cuts of meat, turkey, poultry, fish, lamb, eggs, tofu, soy, whey, nuts, soy or beans which are a complex carb that is balanced with high protein and can be exchanged for protein. Avoid high fat meat, choose leaner cuts of beef, use extreme caution with pork and beef

THE BALANCE DIET & LIFESTYLE

selection and do as the French and choose wild game such as pheasant, rabbit and venison or try exotic foods such as ostrich, kangaroo, crocodile or bison instead of chicken, beef and pork; which have been the staple meat proteins of the American diet for years. Change selections for greater variety, choose USDA alternatives whenever possible, chicken, beef and pork are fine, but avoid as many growth hormones and other additives, as possible. Whole grains are fine, but avoid as many heavily refined carbohydrates as possible. Dairy is fine, but, all dairy should organic, hormone free, fat free or skim or at least no more than 1-2% milk fat while on a weight loss plan. In addition, try other types of dairy such as goat cheese which is closer to human polypeptides and easier to digest. Good fats are in nuts, seeds, fish, avocado, ect. Basically, Eat the foods that are in season, to know what is in season, simply visit your local organic farmers. Nature, offers us a variety of foods as the seasons change, observe and adhere to Mother Nature's food advice. This is not a food elimination diet, it's a toxin elimination diet, and it's a balanced healthier selection diet combined with a healthy lifestyle that requires a life-long commitment. It's not just a diet, it's a lifestyle.

Eating A Balanced Diet Means Eat This:

You should have a variety of foods from each of the food groups, on a daily basis, at least one multi-vitamin per day. Fresh fruits and vegetables that are high in fiber, low in saturated fats and healthy sources of nutrients and protein. Good fats and whole grains curb the appetite and help reduce belly fat. Always avoid heavy sauces, gravy and dressings, while on a diet. Calcium and Magnesium rich foods such as broccoli and low fat dairy, potassium rich foods, such as Cantaloupe and Bananas help balance the diet. Good fats such as olive oil, fish oil or avocado slow digestion increasing nutrient absorption decreasing hunger. Most importantly, avoid fried or fatty foods, and empty foods such as heavily processed white flour, sugar and high fructose corn syrup as found in soda, during weight loss and as a permanent healthy lifestyle practice. In addition, you should protect your Digestive tract with digestive enzymes, bio-K and yogurt, which aid digestion and helps make a healthy digestive tract. Probiotics add good bacteria to aid digestion and reduce food allergies.

Good Food Choice Examples

Appetizer Selections

Ceviche', sushi, sashimi or a shrimp cocktail.

Tossed or vegetable salad with vinegar, lemon, olive oil and herbs or non-fat dressing on the side

Raw vegetables such as carrot or celery sticks

Broth's which are vegetable or tomato based or non-creamy soups.

Main Course Selections

Entrees containing a small meat portion or tofu with steamed vegetables. Lean Meats, Tofu or Fish prepared in broths or tomato based sauces Bakes, broiled, roasted or steamed fish, poultry, lean meat or tofu (without sauces or gravies)

Breakfast- 2- Egg omelet with broccoli and onion

Rough Oats sweetened with Fruit instead of sugar.

Shish kabobs or meat skewers with grilled veggies

No- shell taco salad

Whole Grain Pasta Such as Quinoa 1 cup portion size with tomato sauce and with turkey, fish or meat substitutes

Veggie plate, Veggie Burger, Tofu or Vegetarian dishes

Condiments/Accompaniments

Salads (Fresh Greens & Veggies) use lemon instead of dressing and aged or fermented cheese for flavor

Boiled rice (not fried)

Baked, broiled or mashed potatoes (use herbs, lemon, pepper, yogurt, salsa or 1 pat of butter)

Steamed, stewed, boiled or broiled vegetables without butter or sauces

Bread of rolls (preferably fermented bread bases such as rye) with olive oil & herbs or without butter

Noodles without butter, oil or cream sauces

Desserts

Fresh fruit, such as melons, citrus or berries

Frozen Fruit Ice, Sherbet, sorbet or, fruit popsicles

Flourless, Sponge or angel-food cake

THE BALANCE DIET & LIFESTYLE

Beverages (when made at home use distilled water)

Sugar Free Teas, Iced or hot tea
 Club Soda with Lime or Lemon
Sparkling water with lime
Coffee (decafe)
Fat Free or Skim Milk
Dry red wine or Unfiltered Beer

Medicinal Foods:

Eat Indian spices, Italian herbs, greens such as kelp, seaweed or algae, garlic and onions, and Mediterranean foods on a daily basis as these foods help improve metabolism and decrease inflammation and food allergies.

Medicinal Drinks:

Fermented drinks such as Kefir Cultures and Yogurt, Kombusha tea, green tea, acai berry juice and lemon water.

Food Hygiene:

Hygiene is important with recent bad bacteria and e-coli bacterial threats found in natural foods such as spinach and tomatoes. Wash all foods, thoroughly. Try not to eat undercooked meats, because it may release toxins, microbes and other poisons into the body and be too much work for your system to digest and eliminate with all of the extra toxins and waste your body will release during dieting or when on detoxifying cleanses and when fasting.

Portion Control

When dieting the typical approach is cutting back on calories and portion sizes, because a today's sized triple decker hamburgers are typically three times the size than they originally were. Therefore, it is important to eat normal sized portions and it is equally important not to cut back on nutrition to ensure that you are getting a sufficient supply of essential nutrients. In some cases, the body may need even more nutrition than the minimal daily recommended allowance of nutrients. However, to lose weight, you shouldn't add extra quantities of food over standard portion sizes. Therefore, weight loss can be a balancing-act between balancing calorie intake and exerting yourself physically for calorie expenditure. Nutritional supplements may help fill in nutritional gaps during dieting but do not skip or replace essential foods by supplementing vitamins or minerals.

Supplementing an Unhealthy Diet and Lifestyle:

We work our body and mind very hard in today's world. If you have eaten junk food and do not regularly eat a variety of nutritious foods, you should take a daily dietary supplement and change your diet. Dietary supplements are appropriate for people who are:

> People who are chronic junk food eaters.
> People under extreme stress.
> People under extreme physical labor or athletes.
> Poor eaters, who don't eat well or who skip meals.
> People who are anemic or who are suffering from a condition that inhibits them from digesting or absorbing nutrients properly.
> Bariatric surgery patients, recovering from gastric bypass.
> A vegan-vegetarian who does not complement their diet with sufficient protein.
> Women Trying to get pregnant or who are pregnant or who are breast-feeding
> Women who experience heavy menstrual bleeding and PMS.
> Peri-menopausal and Post-menopausal women
> People with certain medical conditions that affects how your body absorbs, assimilates, uses or utilizes nutrients.
> Excreting too many nutrients, by excessive sweating, vomiting or chronic diarrhea.
> People who cannot eat all food groups, those with food allergies or food intolerance.
> People with a disease of the kidneys, liver, gallbladder, digestive tract, intestines or pancreas, such as diabetes or hepatitis.

Foods For Balanced Weight, Better Health, Anti-Aging & Healthier DNA

Your Diet is important and you couldn't possibly add nutritional supplements of all of the plant compounds that aid the body's anti-aging systems. Therefore, it is important to add Certain "Anti-Aging" Foods such as Spices, Herbs and Plants that help protect the Body's DNA against damage while you boost metabolism to a maximum level to accommodate healthy weight loss without depleting your body and wrecking your metabolism on starvation or other insane or imbalanced diets. Simply, by adding organically grown foods you can improve your metabolism, enhance your body's weight loss mechanisms and slow aging by nourishing the cells to replicate healthy tissues and DNA. These foods are foods such as:

Foods That Help In Weight Management, DNA Repair, Stem Cell Production and Slow Aging

Green Tea – powerful weight loss agent and protects human DNA from the formation of lesions.

Red Grapes and Red Wines – Contain Resversatrol and Saponins. Resversatrol increases physical endurance and one of the best anti-aging compounds known found in red wine. Test rats ran three times as far as rats without resversatrol. Saponins decrease the risk of cardiovascular disease by preventing the absorption of cholesterol in the body. Red wines contain high levels of saponins. Most red wines contain 3 to 10 times as much saponins as white wine.

Peas and Soybeans – If you do not wish to drink wine, high energy foods like and peas and soy contain saponins and protein.

Curcumin Spice – an Indian spice in curry and turmeric with incredible anti-aging health benefits. It is also, an anti-inflammatory and helps in reducing weight gain from inflammatory reactions to food allergies. It is very beneficial to the colon improving metabolism.

Cruciferous vegetables – cabbage, leafy greens contain (DIM) Diindolylmethane an anti-aging hormone balancer.

Algae- – Canadian Researchers have discovered that a whole food, Super Blue Green Algae increases Stem Cell Production by 30 percent. Stem cells help the body repair itself. Another beneficial algae that can be eaten as a food is the type of algae that Sushi is wrapped in, this Seaweed contains iodine and boost thyroid function.

Fatty Acids – Conjugated linoleic acid (CLA) and DHA (docosahexaenoic acid) as found in fish, meat and dairy reduce body fat in studies by thirty percent and helps to protect DNA.

Grasses & Lettuces – Alfalfa and Barley Grass-Some Leafy Lettuces protect DNA and helps cleanse and detoxify the body. Chlorophyll is a building block of life.

Mushrooms – mushrooms are used often in Chinese medicine these are the non-poisonous, edible mushrooms which actually boost the immune system, aids metabolism and offer compounds that help repair cells and DNA

Nuts – Pine Nuts contain pineolinic acid which greatly reduces appetite, enhances fat metabolism and curbs hunger.

Seeds – Flax Seeds, Sesame Seeds, Sunflower Seeds and Grape Seed extract contain high levels of anti-oxidants, and are good for curbing the appetite, good for DNA and Anti-Aging of Cells.

Seaweed Salad – Same benefits as marine algae and is an easy way to include fresh algae in the diet.In addition, take algae supplements, such as Super Blue Green Algae, which not only helps detox the body, it is almost a whole food that is proven to increase Stem Cell production. Stem cells seek to repair other damaged cells.

Spirulina – contains chlorophyll that cleanses toxins from the body. Algae's help repair damaged DNA in Cells because they contain Polysaccharides.

A Few Natural Supplements That Protect Your Chemistry, Speed Metabolism, Slow Aging and Improve DNA:

Herbs: Herbs contain plant compounds and enzymes in perfect balance which helps increase the absorption of nutrients.
> *Ginkgo Biloba-* the oldest of all tree species helps protect Mitochondrial DNA against age-related oxidation.
> *Lions Mane and Skullcap-* helps to repair damaged DNA.
> *Cat's Claw and Pau D'arco-* helps to prevent damage to DNA and helps boost immunity due to repair viral damages.

Food Substances That Enhance Healthy DNA Production and Cell Repair:

Amino Acids: – Are the building blocks of protein. All amino acids are important as there are 20 important amino acids that transfer codes through ribosome's to form DNA and to form hemoglobin the cells in our bone marrow which release trillions of molecules per second. Carnosine is one of the best anti-aging compounds known it is a dipeptide combination of the amino acids beta-alanine and histidineAcetyl-L-Carnitine inhibits and reverses damage to DNA. N-Acetyl-Cysteine protects DNA from damage needed for production of DNA as a methyl donor..

Enzymes – More than 2,700 different enzymes are necessary for the adequate functioning of our whole metabolism and they keep our vital functions in order.

1. Monosaccharide Carbohydrate: Ribose-   is a component of DNA that is in RNA, too (ribonucleic acid) both are carriers of information.
2. Minerals: Magnesium, Selenium and Zinc assist an enzyme that produces DNA.
3. Proteins: Colostrum, Lactoferrin facilitates endogenous DNA production.
4. Vitamins: Choline, Folic Acid, Vitamin A, Vitamin B3, B6, Vitamin B12, C, Vitamin E is essential for the synthesis of DNA. Vitamin A, Beta Carotene, Vitamin D; all taken as a good multi-vitamin.

DNA Repair

DNA repair is an important factor in healthy aging and may be considered a major factor in weight control and in gene regulation in treatment programs for obese individuals. Therefore, part of maintaining a healthy weight and part of an anti-aging and disease prevention lifestyle is adding DNA support to your diet. Food is not the enemy; food provides nutritional constituents for the body to repair itself. Preventing obesity inadvertently helps healthy aging and helps prevent the proliferation of some cancerous mutations in the cells. Anti-aging is mostly about helping the body to regenerate healthy cells and maintain healthy organ function throughout a lifetime though disease prevention, well living and healthy lifestyle. Getting proteins into cells sustains continued healthy cell production. Proteins are made out of amino acids that execute many functions in cells. DNA makes each protein do a specific job so the correct amino acids must be joined up in the correct particular order sequences for this to work. Many hidden things can adversely affect metabolism of amino acids and cause poor cell renewal and accelerate aging. Often things that we can't see, can damage our

DNA, and not only things such as radiation, but thoughts. In addition, trace amounts of chemicals, biological transmutation of hormones, preservatives or environmental substances such as herbicides, pesticides, toxic out-gassing and other substances. Heavy metals, toxins and pollutant compounds are considered damaging to DNA and affect the body's ability to manufacture healthy cell and tissue renewal and some affect hormone balance within the body and these endocrine disruptors can affect aging. Dr. Leonard Horowitz is a Harvard graduate and public health expert who has a unique perspective on DNA repair worth checking into as he researched sound tones for use in DNA repair. Another Doctor who has developed an interesting approach to DNA repair and approach to health and wellness is Dr. Bruce Lipton, who explains how DNA is influenced by thought, and he doesn't stop there, our cells are affected not only our own thoughts but the thoughts of others that are directed toward us. Dr. Lipton is a former college professor of cell biology who resigned his position refusing to continue to teach med students what he viewed as false information about how cells really work inside the body and the curriculum not being correctly taught to med students, if you wonder why some doctors do not understand, they may not have been taught the truth and was not properly educated in med school. There are many damaging agents that we are exposed to on a daily basis but the good news is, developing a healthy lifestyle helps and as medicine advances, and other frequency type treatments emerge, there will be many options in DNA and genetic medicine. For now, there are a few natural substances that can be beneficial to help cleanse the body of the adverse effects of toxic exposures and in ridding the cells of age accelerators. There are some natural substances that can help with the removal of toxins and endocrine or DNA disruptors and it is of equal importance to live a healthier lifestyle which can help, too.

Various Food Substances and Supplements For Weight Loss, Anti-Aging & Healthy DNA:

Adaptogens

Triphala – an Ayurvedic combination of three herbs and fruits originating in India adapts to correct imbalances. Russian Rhodiola or Golden Root- helps repair damaged DNA and helps prevent future damage.

THE BALANCE DIET & LIFESTYLE

Panax , Chinese or Korean Ginseng - inhibits the oxidative damage caused by Free Radicals.

Allicin and Diallyl suphide — are contained in the vegetables, garlic, onions, shallots, leeks and herbs such as chives. They help prevent DNA damage. Diallyl sulphides helps to lower bad cholesterol, are good for blood and circulation. Helps keep the heart and cardiovascular system healthy. They are also an anti-biotic and helps boost the immune system which is important for fat metabolism.

Amino Acids: — Acetyl L-Carnitine (ALC) inhibits the excessive release of Cortisol in response to stress and helps prevent the formation of belly fat due to stress and retards some aspects of the aging process.

BioFlavinoids- — Found in the white fleshy parts of citrus fruits just under the peel. Lemons, Oranges bioflavinoids and Grapefruits contain a compound that stimulates cellular mechanism that repair DNA according to Japanese scientist .

Coenzymes: — Vitamin B3 (Nicotinamide Adenine Dinucleotide) NADH, Coenzyme A and Co-Q10 facilitates the repair of DNA.

Enzyme Cofactors: — Alpha Lipoic Acid, DHLA (dihydrolipoic acid) aid in gene regulation.

Peptides: — Glutathione helps to activate enzymes that can help repair damaged DNA.

Phenolic Acids: — Ellagic Acid forms adducts with the body's endogenous DNA, blocking binding sites on the DNA of Cells that could otherwise be occupied by carcinogens or mutagens.

Polyphenols: — Apigenin,Epigallo-Catechin-Gallate (EGCG), Luteolin, Oligomeric

Plant Hormones Auxins: — plant phyto-hormones (DIM) Diindolylmethane and Indole-3-Carbinol reduces DNA damage and helps balance hormonal imbalance and the endocrine system.

Melatonin — prevents oxidative damage to the (mitochondrial) DNA.

<u>Proanthocyanidins</u> – Pycnogenol-from maritime pine or grape pip.

<u>Quinones:</u> – Coenzyme Q10

<u>Smart Drugs</u> – Idebenone studies show protective effects against excitatory amino acids, such as those found in MSG compounds as it guards against glutamate toxicity and is a protector of the myelin sheaths surrounding nerves and the brain.

<u>Other Food Substances That Help To Protect DNA:</u> – Folic Acid, EPA's RNA's, Inositol, Quercetin and Rutin. These are only some of the better known nutrients, keep in mind this information changes frequently as scientific research improves, new substances may be discovered daily; if you would like to see a more detailed list, please, refer to DNA researchers at major universities world-wide and in the United States, the ADA, the FDA or the CDC Centers for Disease Control. The bottom line is eat a healthy diet and live a healthy lifestyle.

Natural foods are loaded with nutrients and compliment a health lifestyle. Moderation is the key to eating anything. When we have a problem of excess weight, in order to reduce the weight we must eliminate more than we consume…. It is that simple. We must use up the energy of the foods we eat or our body will store the excess as fatty tissue deposits.

Our best source of nutrition is in the foods we eat. If you think about it, the nutrition that we get from plants are ready for absorption. If you plant a seed you get a plant that contains the nutrients you know that you will get from the particular plant, however, if you plant your vitamin supplement, nothing is going to grow. Food is the best source of nutrition but if you can't eat right, then taking nutritional supplements is a necessary step that is the second best choice. You can get most of these nutrients through a good multi-vitamin mineral as they are recommended on a daily basis to maintain good health and proper organ function.

THE BALANCE DIET & LIFESTYLE

What a healthy diet should consist of:

Water – flushes, hydrates, cleanses, nourishes and purifies the body and all its systems. We can only live approximately four days without water.

Fiber – Cleanses the digestive track helps the body metabolize fats

Vegetables – Provides high octane nutrition, essential nutrients and energy.

Enzymes – Required for almost all bodily functions, there are digestive and metabolic enzymes one helps break down food and to absorb nutrients and the other group helps in detoxification and activities of the organs and cells.

Anti-Oxidants – Protects the immune system and the body in a preventative way by preventing free radical damage.

Amino-Acids – are the building blocks of all healthy lean tissue and the end product of protein digestion. The effects of vitamins and minerals are affected by amino-acids therefore they are important in nutrient utilization.

Minerals – Every living thing on the planet has to have minerals. In the body minerals are the basis of the electrical impulses when mixed with the chemistry to generate the bio-electrical impulses that create energy production, growth and healing. Minerals are essential to promote proper utilization of vitamins and nutrients. There are bulk macro minerals and micro minerals or trace minerals.

Vitamins – are micronutrients that are needed to sustain life. There are water soluble and oil soluble micronutrients. Water soluble cannot be stored by the body and must be consumed on a daily basis.

Natural Food Supplements – are high in combination of important nutrients designed with specific health improving properties. When we can not eat all of the foods needed to provide the proper balanced nutrition on a daily basis food supplements are a natural alternative.

Herbs – herbs contain powerful nutrients that can help heal and restore the body. herbs help balance body, mind and spirit in physical, mental and spiritual ways. The use of herbs are common in most cultures and date back to the Romans, Egyptians, Persians, India, Native Americans, Myan and Peruvian cultures.

It is estimated that at least half of the population has at least one nutritional deficiency of at least one important nutrient due to eating an imbalanced or heavily processed diet that has very little nutritional value. The body goes into a form of starvation mode shutting down weight loss when we have nutritional deficiencies. The U.S. Food and Nutrition Board set a standard for the daily amounts of vitamins needed by a healthy adult. Their recommended daily allowance (RDA's) were the basis for the USRDA's approved by the U.S. Food and Drug Administration. These are the minimum daily requirements and one should not fall below this level of consumption in any weight loss plan or diet.

The Essentials

<u>Vitamins</u> – A, B1, B2, B3, B5, B6, B12, C, D, E, K, EFA's, Biotin, Choline, Folic Acid, Inositol, PABA, Bioflavonoids, Hesperidin and Rutin.

<u>Minerals</u> – Boron, Calcium, Chromium, Copper, Iodine, Iron, Magnesium, Manganese, Molybdenum, Potassium, Selenium, Vanadium and Zinc.

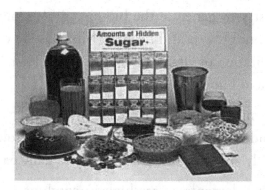

Avoid sugar and corn syrup which are sweeteners that are a major component in processed food, mainly because it is an abundant agricultural crop in America. Fifty-seven percent of our corn crop is used as animal feed. Five percent is manufactured into high fructose corn syrup. High fructose corn syrup is mixed in with many processed foods more often than sugar but is heavily used in the drink industry in particular in making soft drinks and soda. The consumption

THE BALANCE DIET & LIFESTYLE

of drinks containing high fructose corn syrup and soda is believed to be a major culprit in childhood obesity and diabetes.

READ FOOD LABELS THESE ARE FRENQUENTLY HIDDEN IN PROCESSED FOODS

Moderation is the key to eating anything. When we have a problem of excess weight, in order to reduce the weight we must eliminate more than we consume and use fat reserves. We must burn off the calories of the foods we eat to stop our body from storing excess fatty tissue deposits. It is that Simple. The diet is a very important aspect in weight loss. The body has to have essential nutrients on a daily basis in order to maintain good health and proper organ function. The body must have a balance of water, vitamins, enzymes, minerals, proteins, carbohydrates and fats to maintain good health.

THE TOP 3 FOODS YOU SHOULD NEVER EAT AND WHY?

1) Hydrogenated Fat-

It makes you fat! (A moment on the lips, 51 days on the hips) Hydrogenated fat was originally designed for livestock feed to grow beef faster.

It takes the body 51 days to metabolize one molecule! It interferes with metabolic processes can disrupt bio-chemistry. It may cause a biological transmutation into iron oxide 3 a toxic form of iron that binds with cholesterol and may form plaque in the arteries.

Eating it is the reason why men have 5-years less lifespan expectancy than women are. (Women can eliminate it threw menstrual cycle however after menopause the risk is equal among women and men)

2) White Sugar –

It turns to fat! It's hard to metabolize, it has to travel through the digestive process three times before the body can completely metabolize it. The body can biologically transmutate it into fat during metabolism. It is the most addicting substance on the planet. There are more sugar addicts than all alcoholics and drug addicts combined. The reason is this, sugar can also biologically transmutate into alcohol in the body. The

alcohol blocks all of the neurotransmitters in the brain causing cravings and withdrawl type symptoms. This may happen when there is an
underlying parasitic condition such as a yeast infection. The putrefying,
decaying matter of yeast type fungus, mixed with the sugar ferments into
alcohol making the body a human distillery. This is what makes us crave
sugar when we have an overgrowth of systemic candida or candidiasis.
The fungus may feed off sugar and make you crave sugar. However, the
alcohol withdrawal makes us crave it even more. Sugar addicts are bio-
logical-transmutated alcoholics. The fermentation occurs due to a similar process, like when making wine. The sugar and wine ferments and
creates alcohol. The alcohol is acidic, it damages the organs particularly
the pancreas, causing hypoglycemia that eventually leads to adult onset
diabetes. The resulting damage may affect the endocrine system and
organs. It may create all of the symptoms and ill health consequences
of Diabetes and Alcoholism. The progression is accelerated by the diet
and high sugar conversion to alcohol. When the body cannot eliminate
the alcohol through the kidneys, it evaporates through the skin causing
sweats and excessive thirst. All of the organs in the endocrine system are
eventually affected and function is lost or damaged. This may result in
adult onset disease and necrotic tissue formation.

3) White Flour-

It makes you fat! It converts into sugar and can be stored as fat. It is said to
be ten times more addicting than heroine is. It is bleached and refined; the
bleaching process is a known carcinogen. After it converts to sugar, it causes
the same reaction in the body as sugar and thus, may be stored as fat.

Eating junk does not satisfy the body or its needs. Ultimately, in order to lose
weight you have to feed the organs the essential nutrients required to maintain
their function and to maintain disease free health. Otherwise, the body will
experience uncontrollable cravings. For example, craving salt is usually a sign of
mineral deficiency, while craving sugar can be a sign of a hormonal imbalance
linked to many other reasons including blood sugar and pancreatic imbalance
such as hypoglycemia, parasitic infections or cravings may stem from simple
sugar addiction. Therefore, while losing weight you must receive proper nutri-

THE BALANCE DIET & LIFESTYLE

tion while simultaneously burning off more calories than you take in and by eliminating more waste than you consume.

Reasons To Practice Extreme Moderation When Eating Processed Foods

1) While losing weight, watch ALL condiments. Dressings, Sauces, Gravies they are loaded with calorie loaded additives.
2) Processed food items get the highest warning to avoid while loosing weight.
3) Red Alert: Watch for Hidden Fat, Sugar, refined flour and Salt in Processed Foods
4) They are usually high in the three foods you should never eat.
5) They should not be considered as Food. If you cannot put it in a "real" food category, do not eat it.
6) They are usually labeled "Junk Food"
7) They are processed, fortified, and artificial.
8) They are usually stripped of nutrients and artificially refortified. All the nutrients have been processed out and fortified back into the food.
9) They rob your body of enzymes needed to regulate proper metabolic function.
10) They actually age your body from depleting the enzymes & nutrient reserves.
11) They stress the body from the difficulty of trying so hard to digest the artificial additives that processed food contains.
12) They should have warning labels on the box for all of the health risk they pose from repetitious consumption.

If you eat three meals per day, you should eliminate at least three times per day to stay at a similar body weight. If you are loosing stored weight you must eliminate more than what is consumed in any given day. To achieve and maintain your ideal weight, a balance occurs in elimination and consumption. This balance is what allows you to have permanent results. There have been many diets designed with the hope of achieving permanent results, but without a whole person approach balance cannot be achieved. The diet is only the tip of the iceberg. By now, you have realized how successful weight management is imperative to adopting a wholistic lifestyle based on healthy living.

10 BALANCE DIET TIPS

1. Avoid heavily processed food items, especially, the "Whites". White Sugar, White Flour, White Sauces, Dressings and Gravies, these all tend to be high in Fat, Sugar or Gluten. Especially, hydrogenated fat, which can be converted in the body and stored as fat…Read labels to check for these and other chemicals hidden in foods. A general rule is that processed foods, stresses the body to un-process them in order for the body to metabolize them. The less natural, the harder it is for the body to digest, slowing the metabolic rate and metabolism down.

2. Eat one of the following concoctions prior to any meal it will help you to lose weight it will leave you feeling less hungry: Eat half an apple before each meal. Or eat two ounces of this mix: 1 of each small tomato cubed, small cubed Cucumber, Juice from ½ a lemon, 1 teaspoon fresh onion 1 tablespoon of Parmesan Cheese. Or a cup of cabbage soup seasoned with 1 tablespoon of olive oil. May add a tablespoon of plain yogurt, dill, or other fresh herbs or cold pressed olive oil to the cucumber salad or cabbage soup. Do not eat crackers or bread with these mixtures. Make meals from plenty of fresh fruits and vegetables because there is not one naturally occurring plant that contains saturated fat. Juicing is an option instead of eating. Eating raw or micro-biotic and embryonic foods also increases the metabolism because of the enzymes. When we over cook, we destroy the enzymes. Microwaving destroys enzymes, as well. So, not only are they saturated fat-free, when juiced, they are higher in energy rich nutrients and will speed up the metabolism, naturally. Do not microwave these foods it destroys the enzymes in the food, instead, steam if needed. Do not replace with store bought juices as the enzymes die usually within 15 minutes if not sealed and refrigerated. Even natural juices, the pasteurization process may kill enzymes. It is a sure product when you juice it yourself.

3. Do eat fiber rich foods. A whole grain, high in fiber and roughage, which helps the body to break down stored fats and cleanses the digestive tract for optimum digestion and elimination. Fiber-reduces cholesterol and fat in the body. A good high fiber diet makes a lot of sense and relieves the ill effects of stress. Fiber leaves you feeling fuller so it decreases the appetite. It cleanses the digestive tract. Stress causes more bile output and acid fiber can absorb it before it causes damage to the gallbladder, digestive tract and bowel.Soy is fiber rich plant protein and complex carbohydrate. However, read labels, avoid soy products with corn syrup or added sugars. Plain soy

protein may be added to juice recipes as well as other recipes. Studies show soy helps you lose weight by blocking storage of fat. Starchy foods such as brown or whole grain rice, corn or potatoes should be in moderation and never mixed with animal protein. Eat Protein rich veggies such as beans, seeds or nuts for protein and plant protein instead of fatty animal meats when possible. By properly combining your foods, you will get enough energizing fuel. Do not mix protein with starchy vegetables such as rice or potatoes or corn. However, do not mix these complex carbohydrates with animal proteins, to maximize your metabolism, eat these separately to aid in better digestion and allow enough time between consumption to ensure proper digestion.

4. Avoid the intake of saturated fats. Never eat Hydrogenated fat; it requires 51 days for the body to digest one molecule of hydrogenated fat. It is literally a moment on the lips a lifetime on the hips. Hydrogenated fat is found in snack foods, sauces and dressings. You will NOT loose weight while consuming this type of fat. Consuming this type of fat WILL make you fat. In addition, it is linked to shorting the lifespan and creating detrimental health effects and disease in humans. The expeller-pressed seed oils (also often called "vegetable oils"), such as soybean oil, have been added to western diets since World War II. Not only are these oils dominant in long chain fatty acids, but the way in which they are prepared and preserved lend to toxic *trans fatty acids* that modern research has shown is responsible for many health problems. These fatty acids have been altered from their original form by the refining process. Coconut oil on the other hand, is oil that has been a part of Asian diets for thousands of years, and has natural antioxidants that give it the longest shelf life of any plant oil. Traditional Asian diets have been typically free from most modern western diseases, such as obesity and heart disease Do eat vitamin F. Cold pressed Olive Oil or Walnut oil, in moderation, instead of Margarine and other altered fats. Use Lemon Juice and natural cheeses in moderation instead of salad dressings. A just as a tasty reminder, a rosemary twig in your olive oil and vinegar salad dressing adds fantastic flavor.

5. Take a multi-vitamin and mineral supplement and eat foods that are organically grown and that are in season. Do not take individual minerals it is better to take multi formulas because minerals work synergistically. Overdosing on a mineral may block the absorption of another mineral. This reduces the risk of growth hormones as well as chemicals used to

force out of season plants to produce crop out of season. Eat foods that are right for you blood chemistry type and your Dosha type, and eat colorfully, by mixing the color of your veggies and fruits you can ensure yourself that you are getting enough of all the vitamins and minerals that are essential. Taking supplements is very important however, there is no way a supplement alone can give you all of the nutrition necessary to sustain good health and proper organ function. There are over 250 nutrient compounds in an apple, and there are that many or more that are still unidentified. Fresh foods are imperative to good health.

6. Chew your food. In a controlled observation conducted in fast food restaurants revealed that 80 % of the subjects did not properly chew their food before swallowing. Mastication is imperative to trigger gastric enzymes and proper digestion responses. It is better to over chew than to under chew your food. Chewing your food breaks down the nutrient particles and activates better nutrient absorption, assimilation and utilization processes.

7. Listen to your body's natural signals. When you are eating and you belch or burp, this is a signal that you have filled the stomach to a degree, which it has expelled the layer of air that sits above the gastric juices. This is a good indication that you are approaching full. The exception is while drinking carbonated drinks that fizz and add air to the digestive track this is one of the reasons that the acids in carbonated sodas produce a negative impact on the digestive system not to mention they contain up to 17 teaspoons of sugar per 12 ounce serving and should be avoided during weight loss.

8. Do avoid sugary drinks, foods and alcoholic beverage when dieting. Sodas contain up to 12 teaspoons of white refined sugar, and sodium, which causes weight gain and bloating. Cakes and pies, are loaded with white flour and sugar, choose sugar-free/fat free deserts made with honey, raw sugar or splenda or still better yet fruit. If you must drink alcohol, limit your intake to one-half a small glass of wine per day and drink non-sugary wines, such as merlot, chardonnay, or cabernet sauvignon. It is recommended that alcohol be avoided while dieting.

9. Do drink herbal teas as much as you like, sip all day long on something this curbs your appetite. Use natural honey to sweeten, soymilk, or lemon. Only use caffeineated beverages in moderation and only use those earlier in the day. Dieters Teas and Weight loss teas are nice; the Ayurveda teas for your dosha type are ideal.

10. Do Drink Steam Distilled Water, eat right, and take multi-vitamin mineral supplement. You must drink distilled water; it breaks down and flushes fatty deposits from the body. Do drink no less than half your body's weight converted into ounces, while loosing weight. For an example, if your weight is 160 lbs, you will drink 80 ounces of steam distilled water daily.

Following these ten listed dieting tips it can help you to loose your excess weight. Weight loss starts when you make the food choices at the grocery store or market. Do not allow poor food choices in your shopping cart, much less your home. Remember, our eating habits are learned behaviors, save your children a struggle in their adult lives and allow the whole family a healthier diet menu, choose foods that are going to be healthier for the whole family.

Six Things Every Healthy Home Should Have In The Kitchen

There are six things that every healthy home should have in the kitchen for healthy food preparation. These six things will encourage you to prepare healthy meals and to cook them in a healthy manner. The brand name of these appliances that you choose is a personal choice. The six things are:

1. The Mind Body Juicer.
2. The Mind Body Food Processor.
3. The Mind Body Blender
4. The Mind Body Toaster Oven
5. The Mind Body Weight Loss Fat Buster Kitchen Grill.
6. The Mind Body Hot/Cold Water Dispenser

These kitchen appliances help you prepare healthy meals and should used and cleaned, daily to ensure that you are eating healthy well balanced meals. This also reduces the risk of blowing your diet as the nutrient rich foods that you will put though these machines in preparation of your meals will ensure that you are less likely to stray or crave junk food. The water dispenser will encourage you to drink more water and hot herbal teas. The blender will encourage drinking healthy mixed drinks and juices. The toaster often doesn't require as much power as a conventional oven and concentrates the heat for faster cook times; it also is healthier than the use of a microwave. Using a micro wave kills the enzymes in your food. You can pop whole sweet potatoes in the toaster oven or hot fruit cobblers. Fad diets do not work for very long. Appetite suppressants only work while you are taking them. The diet and diet aids are alright to jump start your weight loss but it is your healthier new lifestyle and outlook on the food you eat and the health choices you make that is going to keep the weight off permanently. It is important to observe what foods you tend to consume on a regular basis and seek healthy alternative options of the foods that sabotage your weight loss goals.

Weight Loss Recipes

Hot Vegetable Soup, Stew & Chili For The Soul
In the south, vegetables grow year round and there is always a pot of down home cooking. Try these southern recipes for weight loss. Mix all ingredients together and start on high, bring to a full rolling boil, reduce heat, cover with a lid and simmer until veggies are slightly soft. Cool and enjoy. These are low calorie, filling and satisfying to the appetite. Avoid fattening side items that can wreck your diet, such as crackers, cheese, sour cream or select non-fattening additions.

"Mind Body Magic Weight Loss Soup"

½ Head of Cabbage	1 Sweet Onion (chopped)
½ cup of chopped chives	1 Tablespoon of Naturally Iodized Celtic Sea Salt
2 sprigs of fresh Thyme or Parsley	3 quarts of distilled water
2 Tablespoons of Extra Virgin Olive Oil	1 Tablespoon of Cayenne Pepper (do not use Black Pepper, it clogs the liver)
4 Garlic Bulbs (medium-grated)	4 Red Potatoes (chopped)
5 Celery Stalks/Heart (chopped)	6 Carrots (chopped)

Alternatives – Replace peas or corn for the potatoes,
Replace the carrots with tomatoes
Replace chives with leeks or
Replace fresh fenugreek stalks for celery

Chicken Stew

1 Quart of Chicken Broth/Water	1 Free Range Chicken cooked and plucked off the bone
1 Pint of Corn or Mexi-Corn	1 Sweet Vidalia Onion, Finely chopped

THE BALANCE DIET & LIFESTYLE

1 Quart of Stewed Tomatoes

1 Pint of Baby Lima Beans (or beans of your choice)

½ C. each finely chopped Celery, red, yellow and green peppers

Sage, Bay Leaf, Salt, Pepper, 1 T. Olive Oil, A crushed garlic glove (to taste)

Mix All Ingredients and Boil Reduce Heat and Simmer Until Tender

Mind Body Chili

3½ lbs of Roma tomatoes

1 clove of garlic

½ sweet Vidalia onion

1 green bell pepper (chopped)

6 ounces of Red Kidney Beans

6 ounces of Red Pinto Beans

2 T. Chilli powder,

1 ½ pounds of Sautéed/browned meat

Add: spices & chilli pepper according to taste and level of heat desired. cook all ingredients on high bring to a boil reduce heat and cover. Allow mixture to simmer until all ingredients are soft. Fold in pre-cooked meat or soy.

Alternatives Vegetarian Optional– you may go vegetarian and add tofu or make your choice of ground, turkey, buffalo, ostrich, chicken, beef, kangaroo or alligator. Regardless of your selection, all should be free range, grass fed, organically grown without growth hormones.

Southern Bass Stir Fry

2 pound of Fish (de-boned bass or other white fish)

2. C.Broccoli

1-C. Bean Sprouts

1 C. Shredded Carrots

1 Sweet Vidalia Onion (Thick Chopped)

Bok-Choi Cabbage (Thick Chopped)

1-T. Olive Oil

Soy Sauce, Salt & Pepper To Taste

Wok all of the ingredients then add the fish & Soy sauce last

Mind Body Weight Loss Gazpacho

3½ pounds of Roma tomatoes	5 T of extra virgin olive oil
1 Can of spicy vegetable juice	1½ crushed garlic cloves
1 T sweet basil	½ yellow, ½ red and ½ green bell pepper (finely chopped)
½ sweet Vidalia onion (finely chopped)	

Blend all ingredients in a food processor.

Chill in bowl in refrigerator for two hours before serving. Serve cold.

Chives (garnish with fresh, chopped and sprinkled on top after soup is done)

Examples of Alternative Substitutes for Fattening Foods

Mayonnaise	Yogurt
American Cheese	Parmesan Cheese
Hamburger	Veggie Burger
Red Meat	Portobello Mushroom
Beef, Pork	Fish, Pheasant, Dear
Fries	Steamed Veggie Sticks
Potato Chips	Raw Veggie Sticks
Ranch Dressing	Lemon, Olive Oil or Herbs
Bread Wrap	Lettuce Wrap
White Bread	Sprouted or Whole Grain Bread
Flour Tortilla	Corn Tortilla
Processed Cereal	Cooked Oatmeal or Whole Grains
Soda Pop	Seltzer or Lemonade with honey or stevia
White Sugar	Honey, Stevia (in moderation)
Salt	Calcium/Magnesium/Vitamin C powder
Season Salt	Herb sprinkles
Black Pepper	Capsicum Powder
Iceberg lettuce	Leaf Lettuces
Hydrogenated Oil	Olive or Flax Oil

THE BALANCE DIET & LIFESTYLE
Hidden Calories in Food Preparation

It is important to pay close attention to the extra ingredients added during food preparation. This is usually where extra calories are coming from. It is definitely a major concern. Vegetable salads are low in calories. The calories and fat content greatly increase when adding cheese, salad dressing, croutons, meats. When you are preparing your salad and other foods be aware that calories add up when foods are fried or processed. This is usually from the addition of fats in the cooking process.

Hidden Sources That Increase Caloric Content in Salad Preparation

Food	Size	Calories
Lettuce	2 ounces	45
Onion	½ Cup	46
Garlic	½ Tablespoon	10
Carrots	½ Cup	40
Cauliflower	4 ounces	23
Tomato	½ Cup	38
Cucumber	½ Cup	39
Bell Pepper	½ Cup	40
Avocado	½ (small)	50

Food Additions

Parmesan	1 Tablespoon	20
Cheddar	½ ounce	60
Feta	1 Tablespoon	90
Egg	1 medium	77
Tuna in oil	¼ Cup	110 (drained)
Tuna in water	¼ Cup	80 (drained)
Boiled Shrimp	2 ounces	88
Sauté' Shrimp	2 ounces	140
Fried Shrimp	2 ounces	200
Smoked Oysters	3 ounces	90
Raw Oysters	3 ounces	50
Boiled Chicken	1 small breast	142
Grilled Chicken	1 small breast	190

Hidden Sources That Increase Caloric Content in Salad Preparation

Food	Size	Calories
Fried Chicken	1 small breast	218

Condiments

Lemon/Lime	¼ Cup	10
Olive Oil	1 Tablespoon	25
Red Vinegar	2 Tablespoons	23
Caesar Dressing	2 Tablespoons	180
Salsa	2 Tablespoons	15
Ranch	2 Tablespoons	195

Salad Toppers

Penne Pasta	⅔ Cup	200
Olives	2 Tablespoons	50
Croutons	8 medium	80
Corn Tortilla Chips	15 Chips	140
Crackers	3 Crackers	70
Macadamia Nuts	¼ Cup	190
Pistachio Nuts	¼ Cup	180
Sunflower Seeds	¼ Cup	185
Alfalfa Sprouts	½ Cup	20

Counting Calories

Alcoholic Beverages		Indian Food	
Pint of Beer	180	Lamb Tikka Marsala	235
Stout Beer	170	Chicken Korma	490
Lite Beer	100	Poppadums-2	45
Wine	85	Bombay Potatoes	200
Sherry	65	Bhaji (onion)	60
Vodka	55	Mint/Cucumber/Yogurt 2T	20

Bread Products		Chinese Food	
Biscotti	70	Bean Sprouts	90

Counting Calories

White Bread	84	Cashew Chicken	310
Whole Grain	79	Mongolian Beef	430
Biscuit	74	Fried Rice	250
Scone	190	Egg roll	190
Bun	190	Spring roll	180
Bagel	215	Fried Wanton (2 ounce)	150
Doughnut	205	Hot & Sour Soup	145
Danish	287	Egg Drop Soup	130

Spreads/Dip-1 Tablespoon		Meats	
Jam	60	Deer Vinison 6 oz.	290
Herbed Cream Cheese Spread	55	Bacon (slice)	65
Greek Taramosalata Caviar	90	Ham (slice)	50
Peanut Butter (Natural)	105	Turkey dog (low fat)	90
Olive Spread	25	Kebab (Lamb)	390
Sun-dried Tomato Pesto	85	Chicken Breast	340
Fruit Spread	30	Steak Ribeye 6 oz	420

DETOXIFICATION RECIPES FOR WEIGHT LOSS

Juicing is a low calorie, high energizing way to lose weight and cleanse the body of impurities while adding additional enzymes and essential nutrients. It is a good way to start a diet and purge, improve and increase metabolism. You will discover that lemon juice and cranberry juice is an important part of the mind body weight loss program because of their ability to cleanse the organ systems. Juicing is one of the healthiest food choices we can make. Juicing fresh organic veggies are very beneficial to the body in many ways. Fruits are a healthy part of every nutritious diet. However, fruits contain sugars that can sabotage your diet. Fruit is best consumed in moderation when juicing. It only takes a small slice of apple to add sweetness and taste.

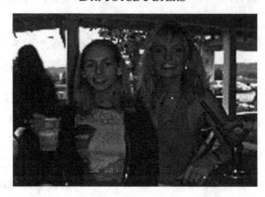

The maximum freshly juiced fruit juice serving is 1-3 ounces two times per day while the maximum vegetable juice serving is 10 ounces two times per day. The maximum recommended grass is ½ ounce two times a day because a shot of juiced wheat grass per day for seven days is equivalent to eating 450 pounds of vegetables for the nutrient benefit. Greens and Grasses are a natural source of calcium and magnesium. Calcium and magnesium are alkalizing buffers in the body that aid in protein digestion, biochemical processes and almost every other metabolic function in the body. A normal person should have no less than two servings of greens on a daily basis because greens contain chlorophyll which is a powerful detoxifying substance that is found in every living thing on the planet. The fiber in whole fruit slows the release of sugars down within the body. It is best to eat whole fruit with the fiber while dieting. Two fruits per day should be consumed two hours after or before the next scheduled meal. You may consume as many whole vegetables (in their natural state) as you like on a daily basis. In your juice program, keep fruits to a minimum. You can flush toxins, lose weight and build up the body all at the same time with a good juicing program. You can use alkaline juices to alkalize the body.

There are so many naturally occurring, health benefiting substances found in produce, that we have not to this day, identified all the nutrients and health giving substance in an apple, we still do not know all of the nutrient compounds and there is well over 200 known and identified. It is important for the juice to be fresh as well, store prepackaged juice is usually pasteurized as a preservative measure, this process kill a lot of the enzymes and nutrients needed for digestion. The enzymes give the food and our body energy. It is important to include fresh vegetation because you just cannot get the full health benefits by taking supplements alone. It is a good health investment to purchase a juicer and a food processor. Juicing provides the body with phyto-nutrients, anti-oxidants, minerals, vitamins, and enzymes. Grating nuts and seeds adds proteins to your juice mixers. Juicing is a low calorie, high energizing way to lose weight and cleanse the body of impurities. It is a good way to start a diet.

The juice recipes encourage detoxification of the body, cells and organ systems. Consume small quantities of the juices listed. Consume only 1-3 ounces per listed time schedule. It is recommended that one become accustomed to fasting using juice fasting and then move into water fasting, gradually. Do not over consume these juices, it may detox your body too fast and cause detox headache, nausea or vomiting. If you get any of these symptoms cease the fast until another time when you are stronger. If you get sick, do not give up, it is an indication that your body is very toxic. Eat something that is settling to your stomach and rest. You may continue the next day with better success and a slower toxic release. Prime the Liver at least once per week while dieting, after all the liver is the fat eliminator.

Water For Detoxification & Weight Loss

Most of the time, thirst is falsely mistaken as hunger. Most hunger pains are really dehydration. The drinking of pure water has more to do with health than the taking of any medicine, but not only drinking it but also bathing in it, steaming in it, cleansing ourselves inside and out of impurities will aid in weight loss. You may feel nauseated when you increase your water intake, as the body releases toxic buildup in the tissues as you begin increasing your water intake. The body will release stored reserves, which release other toxins simultaneously. Usually, nausea that occurs while drinking water is simply a sign of toxicity. If you become nauseated, do not give up, cease for the day and resume consuming your recommended daily consumption of water, the next day. As you slowly detoxify, the nausea will cease and your energy and sense of well-being will return. Water is of course one of the earths natural resources for which we cannot sustain life without. A good weight management practice is to drink or sip on water and low calorie sugar-free naturally decaffeinated herb teas up until an hour before scheduled meals. Do not drink before regular meals, as it will neutralize the layer of calcium that mixes with the hydrochloric acid and aids in digestion.

Dehydration is an enemy to your weight loss program. The body is more than 75% water. It only takes a decline of 1-2 percent of the body's water content to cause dehydration. When you are dehydrated, the endocrine system triggers a compensatory production of aldosterone, to cause the body tissues to retain water or cause water retention and water weight gain. It causes a puffy and bloated appearance making it hard to get the look of lean muscle definition. Do not allow yourself to become so thirsty that you feel dry mouth. (Referred to as cotton mouth) When this happens your body is actually reabsorbing toxic fluid from the bowl. Many mistake thirst as hunger. When you feel hungry, drink a glass of distilled water and wait a few minutes. If the hunger sensation is still present, eat a light natural snack, such as celery or half of an apple, depending on your craving at the time. If you are craving salty snack you need minerals if you are craving sugar it is blood sugar balance. Take a multi-vitamin supplement and drink more water. If you still feel hungry, then eat. Always keep in mind that drinking water throughout the day helps you feel full and decrease your desire to eat. Drinking water is one of the best ways to avoid food cravings and decrease your appetite. Drinking very cold water actually increases the fat burning effect. The body has to bring up the temperature of cold foods and drinks for digestion; this triggers a thermogenic effect in the body's fat reserves. The body needs water to burn calories and fat. Without adequate water intake, the body's fat deposits increase. Hidden dehydration may actually cause fat accumulation. Therefore, drinking water and other cleansing fluids increases fat metabolism.

Water Intake
Steam distilled water is the purest drinking water on the planet. No other water is as pure. Even the cleanest spring water and filtered water, may be contaminated or contain nitrates from spill off from cattle and other farms. These harmful substances along with unfiltered parasites and pesticides pose great health risk and are a present time a continued real threat to good health in our society from the creating of excess environmental pollutions in our environment. Steam distilled water is the safest form of water. It cleanses, purifies and neutralizes excess acids or alkaline, within the human body. Steam distilled water also, pulls out excess sugars, salts, flushes excess fats from the liver and purges the organ systems of toxins. Steam-distilled water is used in pharmaceutical preparations and sterile solutions. We also use it in irons to flush out heavy mineral deposits; therefore, it acts as a chelator person who is dieting to loose weight should drink half their weight called ounces in steam distilled water daily. This means if you weigh 120 pounds, you should drink 60 ounces of steam-distilled water daily.

That is 6-10 ounce glasses daily. Steam distilled water helps the body to eliminate excess fat. Steam distilled water will not leach minerals out of the body, unless the concentrations are imbalanced or in excess. Water is extremely beneficial for weight loss and renewed health.

Symptoms of a Healing Crisis

Sometimes when we start to cleanse our body deeply for the first time we may experience some discomfort in the form of detoxification signals. These signals are alerting you that your body is detoxing too fast or releasing toxins at a rapid rate. Instead of taking drugs to mask these symptoms you should rest, eat light foods, apply heat pad, or cold pack for headache. Taking drugs for the symptom will only prolong the detox process by driving the toxins back into the body. Hang in there and allow the toxins to come out. These symptoms will usually pass. If you feel that the symptoms are uncomfortable, contact your natural health care practitioner. If you feel that the detox symptoms are unbearable contact your doctor. But keep in mind that it takes at least eleven days into a fast for the body to release DDT and other pesticides. You may feel sick when you are actually gaining health. You may feel worse before you feel better but if you feel sick, stop the program you may be detoxifying too fast and have to switch to a more gradual method that's right for you. The best way to treat a healing crisis, is to prevent one. Going in the sauna for a week prior to the start is very beneficial in reducing detox symptoms. Be cautious of detoxing too fast as it may cause uncomfortable symptoms.

Detox Symptoms				
Headache	Nausea	Blurred Vision	Diarrhea	Cramping
Aches	Pain	Rash/Itching	Low grade fever	Chills
Sweats	Malaise	Weak	Lethargic	Sleepy

Day Two – Start Juicing!

Juices are detoxifying and should be consumed in very small quantities a few times per day. A shot of grasses such as, wheat grass, per day for one week is equivalent of eating 400 pounds of vegetables without adding a lot of calories. For fruits, one ounce is a starter dose, for vegetables, three ounces is the maximum dose. Even if you crave more the quantities should be kept small to avoid excess calories and sugars. Eat fruit whole, in juicing it is added in small quantity to add flavor. Do not burn yourself out by over-juicing in the start; this is a lifelong practice that needs to be followed on a daily basis. You can be creative and invent your own juice formulas, by switching the ingredients around to suit your individual taste.

The Balance Diet & Mind Body Weight Loss Cleansers

It is not recommended for those with blood sugar problems to do detox fast. For most people the broths are a more suitable approach. All broths and soups should be made with distilled water as it pulls out excess in the body. First, fast from 7:00 p.m. until 7 a.m. and drink one Liver Purge Juice Cocktail. Do not eat anything but drink as much steam distilled water as you wish until 10:00 a.m. and then start juicing the rest of the day. If you feel weak, nauseated or are a hypoglycemic, you may drink herb teas, fresh broth or bullion, puree of carrot-ginger soup or puree roasted tomato soup. Only consume what is drinkable without chewing. The soup should be puree and have no solid pieces. Drink 20 ounces of pure distilled water to flush out any excess residues from drinking these juice concoctions. Fatty residues can be re-absorbed if they are not flushed out of the body with 20 ounces of distilled water on a daily basis and promptly between 6 and 7 pm. Failure to follow this schedule will result in slowing down the weight loss process.

1st Day Organ Clearing Detox Regimen for Weight Loss

Kidney Liver Cleanse/7:00 a.m.
1 Gallon of Distilled Water (must be distilled)
Pour 40 ounces out of the Gallon
Add 20 Ounces of Fresh Squeezed Lemon Juice
Add 3 Ounces of Grade B Maple Syrup
Add 3 Ounces of Sorghum Molasses
Add 3 Ounces of Honey (preferably fall honey)
Add 4 Tablespoons of Epsom Salts

1st Day Organ Clearing Detox Regimen for Weight Loss

Drink this all day long until Bedtime then Drink:

Bedtime Gall Bladder-Liver Purge

Liver Purge Juice Cocktail Recipe

3 ounces of cold pressed virgin olive oil

A dash of cayenne pepper (skip if you have stomach problems)

The Juice of each – one medium Lemon and one stalk of Fennel

2 teaspoons of Epsom salt-diluted in 1 ounce of distilled water.

(do not eat or drink anything after consuming; go to bed for the night)

> Caution: do not do this organ flush if you have an acute gall bladder condition or on a day before colon hydrotherapy. A colonic may help two days prior to this flush and then two days after the flush. High-Colonics may be very beneficial if you are comfortable receiving them, it is strictly up to the individual.

The morning after:

Expect diarrhea chaff and gall stones to pass in the morning. Drink lots of water the day after and enjoy the following juice recipes and teas. Slowly add in light and natural foods such as salad greens, mellon and seedless berries. The following day you may add fish. Wait until the second day after the fast to add cheese, meat or bread back into the diet.

10:00 a.m./ Soothing Digestion Herb Tea's

You may enjoy a cup of herb tea an India Herbal Mint, Chamomile, Weight loss or Dieter's tea with lemon.

Noon/Lung-Blood & Kidney Veggie Juice Blend

Beet Root, Carrot, Cabbage, Celery, Dandelion, Fennel, Apple to sweeten

2:00/Immune System & Brain Herb Tea's

Energizing Booster Herb Tea, Ginseng, Gurana, Ginkgo, Peppermint, Echinacea, Eucalyptus, or Astralagas.

4:00/Fresh Energizing Veggie Juice

Dr. Joyce Peters

1st Day Organ Clearing Detox Regimen for Weight Loss
Wheat Grass, Alfalfa Sprouts, Cucumber, Spinach, Garlic, Radish, Carrots and Apple 6:00/Relaxing Chamomile Tea

Morning and Nightly Detoxifying Cleanser

1 medium lemon juiced and distilled water= 6 ounce cup – Drink a ½ of a cup of warm lemon water each night before bed, brush teeth and go to bed, leave the other ½ cup of lemon water for in the morning drink the other half and jump hard on your heels three times off the bottom step or stair to the floor on your heels to purge and release the illio-cecal valve and get the liver and lymph flowing for the day. Wait 30 minutes before eating breakfast.

Daily Lemon & Cranberry Cleanser

Start with a gallon jug of distilled water pour out your daily 20 ounce dose in a separate container. Mix 20 ounces of pure unsweetened cranberry juice with the juice of three lemons pour into the gallon jug and drink your calculated dose from the gallon of this concoction daily. Label the concoction "weight loss tonic" write this on the jug. This concoction will taste very tart because of the Malic and other acid content of the cranberries and the neutralizing effect of the lemon. Test your urine ph prior to using this flush, balance your ph before cranberry should you test acidic, you should not begin this flush prior to alkalizing your chemistry or alternate the cranberry with cucumber juice you will achieve better results and increase your metabolism of fats, carbohydrates and proteins by keeping your chemistry stable)

To determine your daily dose of cleanser:
1. Weigh yourself.
2. Divide your weight in half
3. Call the number ounces instead of pounds.

THE BALANCE DIET & LIFESTYLE

Distilled Water-Total body weight divided in half = daily water intake.

This is the least amount of ounces of water that you should consume on a daily basis according to your body weight. Next:

4. Subtract the 3 ounce (morning ½ cup of hot lemon water) and 3 ounce (½ cup hot lemon water bed-time) and the 20 ounces of distilled water from your total body weight.
5. Half of your body weight minus the 26 ounces is the amount of ounces of the Cranberry concoction that you should drink on a daily basis.
6. Your daily 20 ounces of distilled water intake should follow finishing off the daily dose of cranberry concoction between the hours of 6-8 pm.
7. No food should be consumed during this time or before drinking your 3 ounce lemon concoction before bed. You may drink a cup of herb tea, a cup of bullion or a cup of soup as long as it is drinkable and requires no utensils to drink 30 minutes after finishing the cranberry concoction or 30 minutes before consuming the 20 ounces of distilled water. No food after 6 pm.

JUICE CLEANSER RECIPES

Dr. Peters Pre-Weight Loss Liquid Detox Cleanse

A gallon of distilled water.
Pour 20 ounces of water out of the container.
Add 10 ounces of freshly squeezed lemon juice.
1 Tablespoons of sea salts
Cap the jug and shake until all of the salt dissolves
Add 3 ounces of fall honey (the bees produce honey on their own/no hormones)
Add 3 ounces of sorghum molasses (for calcium)
Add 3 ounces of grade B maple syrup (b-vitamins, potassium and nutrients)
Again, cap the jug and shake until everything dissolves
For each glass you drink add a pinch of cayenne pepper it adds a thermogenic effect that speeds the metabolism and encourages weight-loss
(skip the pepper if you have stomach problems)

Drink the following liquids:

> Drink herbal teas
> Drink steam distilled water
> Drink water with fresh lemon juice
> Drink metabolic cleanse drink mix
> Drink a protein drink mix at mid-day
> Drink herbal concoctions and tonics
> Drink vegetable juice (cold or heated)
> Drink fruit juices that aid weight loss such as mangosteen (1 oz a day)
> Drink freshly juiced juices (1-3 ounces per every 4 hours)
> Add herbal tinctures to purge organs and digestive tract.
> Drink water with fresh lemon juice daily
> Epsom salts in lemon water (to keep bowel evacuated)
> Add Letchin crystals to juice to offset mental fatigue and a detox headache.

The human body is over 80% water. Utilize your mind body power, with a black magic marker; write a positive affirmation for your water. Use one of these phrases or similar words and write them on the plastic gallon jug of distilled water that you pour your daily 20 ounces from.

"Fat Eliminating Water"	"Weight Loss Water"	"Detoxifying Water"
"Slenderizing Tonic"	"Sliming Potion"	"Fat Free"

Nightly Lemon Water Concoction   3 ounces (must be drank nightly before sleep)
Evening Pure Distilled Water   20 ounces(must be consumed 6-8pm)
                                  23 ounces (total to be consumed after 6 pm)

Example:

A 180 pound person would consume 90 ounces of water on a daily basis on the Mind Body Weight Loss Program. The water based concoctions are 70 ounces of the recommended daily water intake. Therefore, you would subtract the 70 ounces from the 90 ounces and have 20 ounces of water to drink for the remainder of the evening before 8 p.m. to flush out fatty residues.

> 90 ounces (daily recommended water intake for a180 lb person.)
> -20 ounces (daily mandatory/minimum pure water consumption
> =70 ounces (daily recommended water based concoctions)

THE BALANCE DIET & LIFESTYLE

    70 ounces (daily water based concoctions)

    -3 ounces (morning lemon water)

    -<u>3 ounces </u>(nightly lemon water)

    =64 ounces (total daily cranberry/water based juice concoction)

    3 ounces (upon arising) Morning Lemon water-

    +64 ounces (before 6 pm) Cranberry Concoction-

    <u>+ 3 ounces</u> (before bed) Nightly Lemon water-

    =70 ounces (total daily water based juice concoctions)

    70 ounces (total daily water based juice concoctions)

    +20 ounces (mandatory daily distilled water)

    =90 ounces (daily recommended water intake for 180 lb. Person)

The 6 ounces of lemon concoction always stays the same. The cranberry concoction varies depending on the dieter's body weight and tolerance for the acid. Pure distilled water must be consumed after drinking the cranberry concoction, on a daily basis with out additives of any kind to rinse out residues of the juice water cleanses and therefore stays the same for everyone, no less than two ten ounce glasses per evening while on the concoctions. The pure distilled water must be drank before 8 pm to allow the kidneys time to void before sleep and to allow approximately an hour before drinking the final 3 ounce, lemon water concoction before sleep.

Additional Water or Fluid Intake

There are many forms of super hydrating clustered water formulas on the market some are better than others and there are imprinted waters that are frequency enhanced and structured waters that have medicinal qualities all provide healthy benefits and are better for preserving health than drinking other drinks. I prefer to do a deep cleanse before using this so that toxins are not driven deeper into the tissues. Always remember never to drink fluids 30 minutes prior to a meal. However, when taking digestive enzymes take them 30 minutes before a meal with a sip of water. You may drink additional drinks such as herb teas, fresh juices, and additional water earlier in the day as long as you consume your recommended juice concoctions before 6pm and the 20 ounces of distilled water between 6pm-8pm. In the evening the only exception is herbal teas and they should be consumed after 8:30 pm and before 9 pm. Allow 30 minutes after drinking tea to drink the 3 ounces of lemon water. Always brush teeth before going to bed to neutralize acids from your teeth and rinse with distilled water this also, prepares you to check your ph in the morning before eating or drinking anything else, upon arising and helps to eliminate incorrect ph readings.

Nightly Meditation: Focus your intent for weight loss, feel your desire and passion build up within your whole body as you desire to achieve your weight loss goal. Visualize yourself thin, see your clothes, your activity, and a happy smile on your face. As you drift off to sleep imagine the pristine, pure distilled water flushing out fatty residues from your body and digestive track just as though you were rinsing out a sink. Imagine all the fat residues going down the drain and out of your body. Imagine your body shrinking as the fat deposits are rinsed from your body as you loose all of your excess weight.

Organ Cleansing Juice Recipes

Rotate once a week between these cleansing and detoxifying blends. The fresher the juice the more nutrients and enzymes that it contains. Fresh juice is always recommended as the enzymes die quickly once juiced. For vegetables three ounces is the maximum juice for each of these recipes and One ounce of the concentrated herb juices are the maximum dose.

Bowel Cleanser Juice Cocktail
Prune, Cabbage, Spinach, Celery, and Garlic Juice. (1 Tablespoon of Castor Oil)

Lung/Respiratory Juicer
Cabbage, Beet-root, peppermint leaves (raw cabbage contains an enzyme which guards against lung cancer)

Anti-Viral/Anti-Parasitic Juicer
Mango, Black Walnut, Pau'dArco Tea, Apple

Liver Cleanser
Cilantro, Coriander, Milk Thistle, Alfalfa Sprouts, Dandelion, Apple

THE BALANCE DIET & LIFESTYLE

Kidney/Bladder Cleanser
Lemon, Watermelon, Cranberry, Fennel, Dandelion, Hibiscus, Red Clover Blossom, Parsley, Dog Grass, Blue Vervain, Greater Celandine, Buchu Leaves

Cellulite Buster
Unsweetened cranberry juice, a pinch of cayenne and distilled water

Lymphatic Cleanser
Unsweetened cranberry juice, Distilled water, Echinacea, Goldenseal

Pop-eye Energy Booster
Wheat Grass, Spinach, Tea Leaf, Apple

Night Cap/Night Shade Plant Juice Cocktail
Potato or Sweet Potato or Eggplant or Tomato (not recommended for arthritics)

Extra Juice Blends
Fruit juice blends release sugar into the blood stream very quickly and should be used in moderation, one to three ounces maximum serving per four-hour period allowing time for digestion which is usually three ounces only, twice a day. Vegetable juice blends are longer lasting and tend to satisfy the appetite better without adding sugary calories. Adjust your juicer to keep as much pulp and fiber in the juice blend as possible.

Fresh Fruit Juicer
Apples, Pears, Grapes, Papaya, Mango, Banana, Fresh Coconut milk.

Northern Berry Juicer/Anytime
Strawberries, Blueberries, Raspberries, Cherries, Plums, Black Berries

Sunny Citrus Juicer/Breakfast
Oranges, Grapefruit, Cumquats, Tangerines, Tangelos, Pineapple

Southern Juicer/Anytime
Peaches, Nectarines, Plums, Muscatine's, Scuppernongs, Grapes, Apples, Persimmons

Soul Food Juicer
Sweet Potato, Cucumber and Peas

Polish Juicer
Cabbage, Dill, Garlic, Cucumber

Oriental Food Juicer
Bock-Choi, Bean Sprouts, Carrots, Snow Peas

Native American Food Juicer
Corn/Maize, Squash, cucumber

California/Florida Juicer
Oranges, Tangerine, Lime, Grapefruit

Hawaiian Juicer
Pineapple, Banana, Papaya

Caribbean Juicer
Lime, Coconut Milk, Mango, Passion fruit

New Zealand Juicer
Kiwi, Apples, Mecca Honey

Australian Juicer
Eucalyptus, Grapes, Apples, Pears, Honey

Mellon Juicer
Watermelon, Cantaloupe, Honey Dew

European Juicer
Apples, Pears, Grapes

Smoothie Suggestions:
You can make your juice recipes into delicious meals. However, watch the calories while your adding these delicious additions to your juice recipes.

Add spices such as vanilla, nutmeg or cinnamon to create more flavor variety. Add liquid herbal tinctures or freshly juiced herbs for added medicinal and nutrient value. Add soy, whey powder or ground nuts for texture and protein. Add ground flax seed for fiber and additional cleansing benefits. Add banana or yogurt for smoothie texture or a scoop of fat free/sugar free ice cream or homemade soy-cream. You can even make your own healthy frozen yogurt or soy cream at home using organic soymilk or yogurt, stevia or splenda, natural vanilla extract. It taste like snow cream and it makes an excellent breakfast shake when mixed with a nutrient rich drink mixes that are organically grown and that contain no GMO's (genetically modified organisms). Enzymes aid digestion and absorption of nutrients. Freeze dried, enzyme rich, additions include Super Blue Green Algae. Fresh enzyme additions are Barley Greens, and all Sprouts, All are nourishing and make good cleansing Smoothie/Shake additions. Mellon's contain only 15 calories per 5 ounces on average. Melons are high in anti-oxidants, carotenoids that alkalize and assist the kidneys in homeostasis.

Mellon Shake and Meal Replacement

8 ounces of mellon (of your choice)   1 cup of soy milk (sugar free)
4 tablespoons of protein powder   1 cup of ice
1 shot of wheat grass

mix and blend in blender until smooth.

Coconut Mango Smoothie Meal Replacement

1 small Mango (cored)   ¼ cup of grated Coconut
¼ cup of unsweetened Coconut Milk   ½ medium lime
4 t. of plain protein or soy powder   1 cup of ice
1 shot of wheat grass

blend all ingredients blend in blender until smooth.

Berry Cooler and Digestive Enhancer

4 ounces of blueberries, raspberries or   ½ cup of plain liquid kefir cultures (or
strawberries   yogurt)
4 tablespoons of protein powder   ½ cup soymilk (sugar free)
1 cup of ice

blend in blender until smooth.

Banana Smoothie

1 large ripe banana   1 cup of liquid kefir cultures (or yogurt)
4 tablespoons of protein powder   1 teaspoon of carob flavoring extract.
1 cup of ice

Pineapple Fat Metabolizer Smoothie

5 ounces of fresh Pineapple   1 cup of plain liquid kefir (or yogurt)

3 tablespoons of protein powder   ¼ teaspoon of nutmeg

1 cup of ice

mix and blend in blender until smooth.

Tips: Add Flax Seeds or nuts for protein. Add fresh pineapple to every recipe as it contains bromelain an enzyme that aids in protein digestion when mixed with this fruit enzyme.

Options:May add a teaspoon of honey to taste.

May omit the ice and serve over ice instead of blending with ice.

Food Color Therapy

When it seems difficult to know what food is good for you. An easy way to get a broad-spectrum of balanced nutrients is to eat a colorful array of vegetables, fruits and protein. Balance the colors. Just as research studies indicate with other primates, humans need to be able to acquire healthy sources of calories and nutrients from the environment to sustain a healthy disease free life.

Healthy Food Facts

Fresh growing plant foods get their color by the nutrients, which they contain.

For millions of years humans lived successfully in good health by eating fish and fowl, the leaves, roots, and the fruit of plants. It is a natural system that is hard to improve upon. Since the processing of natural foods, disease has become more increasingly prominent. Make sure your diet has a wide array of colors.

Mind Body Balancers & Cleansers

Lose weight as you balance your energy centers with the colors of the rainbow. Juice fruits and veggies of the same color together. Sprinkle in Ayurvedic spices to balance. Adjust the color to each chakara drink one ounce of juice for each chakara, separately, on the hour through out the day. Meditate as you sip on the juices individually. Imagine the cleansing and restorative powers of the juice as it trickles into your system. Visualize the juice purging away, excess weight, darkness, impurities fat and energy blocks in the associated chakara and organ systems. Concentrate on cleansing and clearing the pathways of perception in

THE BALANCE DIET & LIFESTYLE

your mind and body. Let your spirit soar and delve into the collective conscious of the universe. Use this technique often to renew your energies.

Green

Cucumber	Broccoli	Asparagus	Olive	Green Tea
Herbs	Spinach	Lettuces	Apple	Collard
Kiwi	Honey Dew	Cabbage	Field Greens	Mustard

Yellow (contain small amounts of essential fatty acids)

| Squash | Lemons | Yellow peppers | Yellow onions | Mango |
| Bananas | Apple | Chamomile Tea | Corn | |

Brown

| Almonds | Nuts | Nuts | Oatmeal | Soy |
| Bulgur Wheat | Kasha | Whole Grains | Brown Rice | Teas-Herbal |

Black

| Flaxseeds | Grapes | Black Berries | Mushrooms | Hemp seeds |
| Walnut | Black Cherries | | | |

Blue

| Blueberry | Grapes | Blue Indian corn | Water |

Red

| Strawberry | Tomato | Potato | Watermelon | Grapes |
| Pomegranate | Apple | Raspberry | Cranberry | Red Pepper |

Purple

| Eggplant | Grapes | Radishes | Turnip | Cabbage |
| Mulberries | Boysenberry | Marion berry | | |

Orange

| Apricots | Carrot | Sweet Potato | Caneloupe | Oranges |
| Cumquats | Tangerine | Tangelo | Pumpkin | Papaya |

White

| Cauliflower | Onion | Grapes | Potato | Turnip |
| Mushrooms | | | | |

Rebuild Adrenals High Stress Diet

The adrenal glands regulate the stress hormones. When we get an adrenal hormone response the body burns off 500mg of vitamin C, instantly. The Adrenal diet should consist of foods high in vitamin C. You should get your vitamin C from natural food sources and not an ascorbic acid supplement which can make a negative acidifying effect on the chemistry.

Foods High in Vitamin C are Good for Adrenal Stress

Tangelos	Apples	Tomatoes	Peppers	Red Potatoes
Citrus	Oranges	Lemons	Grapefruit	

Enhanced Liver Function Diet

The liver regulates fat metabolism and cholesterol levels. If you have liver problems you will need to reduce fatty foods, heat processed oils & saturated fats that the liver cannot process. Therefore, the toxic, taxed or weak liver will need more fresh fruits and vegetables in the proper combination. Some vegetables are naturally high in biological sulfur. The liver has to have sulfur to produce the enzymes required to metabolize fats, detoxify solid waste toxins and to carry out other functions, as well.

Healthy Liver-Sulfur Containing Cruciferous Vegetables & Others As Listed

Sweet Potatoes	Artichoke	Alfalfa Sprouts	Avocado	Beets
Collard Greens	Turnips	Rutabagas	Turnip	Mustard Greens
Milk Thistle	Dandelion	Garlic	Onions	Peppers
Broccoli	Cabbage	Bok Choy	Radicchio	Radishes
Brussels Sprouts				

Ovaries & Male Glands Need Good Fats or Vitamin E & F

The Ovaries are sensitive to growth hormones in commercially grown livestock and meat. Men need omega 3's to balance testosterone. Also, the reproductive system is sensitive to environmental toxins which convert to estrogen excess and a build up of fat around the hips and thighs.

Fish	Mackerel	Salmon	Herring	Shrimp
Poultry	Olives/Olive Oil	Eggs	Coconut	Avocados

CHAPTER 6

Weight Loss For All Age Groups & Body Types

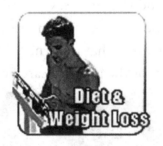

A WEIGHT CONTROL LIFESTYLE WILL VARY FROM PERSON TO PERSON and will change overtime depending on age and health status. The BMI or body mass index is a general one size fits all scale based on height and weight. Frame structure is not considered in this method of body measurement. Small framed individuals will commonly weight less than this scale and larger framed individuals will tend to weigh more and still be in a range that is healthy and acceptable. It is important not to judge your total self worth by your appearance or your weight. It is important to consider that being overweight is unhealthy in many more ways than physically.

Healthy Individual Weight

Each unique individual has many aspects that have contributed to their weight condition. This is an important consideration, in designing a successful weight loss menu. A person may eat according to their chemistry, health status, age and individual preferences. A balanced chemistry ensures the bodies ability to to properly metabolize a combination fats, carbohydrates and proteins. Our personalities, eating habits and matters of the mind fully develop between birth and five.

Most people acquire a taste for foods that they enjoy and that they adopt as comfort foods and develop bad eating habits. A very high percentage of the population are addicted to the refined white flour and sugar in processed foods. Weight loss occurs only when a reduced calorie diet is followed on a consistent daily basis and when sabotaging foods and behaviors are eliminated from the diet. Weight loss is maintained only when exercise and healthier lifestyles are adopted. Healthy alternative food options and modified eating behaviors must be implemented to insure permanent success. Avoidance of yo-yo dieting must be obtained to eliminate the risk of failure in achieving permanent weight loss goals. It is important to read the section on Learned Behavior Modification when dealing with children and weight loss. Our eating habits and subconscious personalities about food are developed between birth and age five. Suggestibility is how children learn. Information that is learned through suggestibility is usually learned from the mother, or the primary caregiver.

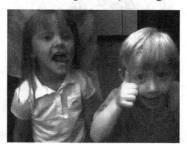

Healthy Weight Control Tips For Children

Overweight and obesity is the biggest problem in children's health, today. Approximately forty percent of all school aged children are overweight. Weight problems begin at birth. A healthy lifestyle is important starting with the first introduced foods. Infants learn eating behaviors by observed example from our caregivers. Infants are often overfed excess calories and the calories in formu-

THE BALANCE DIET & LIFESTYLE

las are no comparison to the balanced nutrition in a mothers breast milk. If a baby becomes accustomed to feeling bloated and overly fed on formula, it sets the stage for overeating. If an infant becomes fat, chances are that it will grow though an overweight childhood and become an obese adult.If a child weights more than 10% over average weight for a child their age they are considered overweight, if they weigh over 20% they are considered obese. It is important to avoid addicting or habit forming foods from birth, such as refined sugar and white flour which are typical ingredients for junk food.

Be conscious of what you teach your children about food and food choices. Be conscious of what your parents and other influential adults teach your children about food. Be aware that your children's babysitters and care givers will have an impact on how your child thinks and believes about food by example through learned behaviors. Be aware that it is not necessary to always clean your plate. Do not force your children to eat. Allow them to decide when they are full. Children have been noted to literally stuff their food such as peas, corn and other food up their nose and in their ears to try to do something to get the food in their body that their parent is demanding they eat. There is a happy medium to this junk food dilemma but teaching your child healthy choices start at birth. The first table foods should be a healthy well balanced diet. Childhood obesity is becoming rampant, today with all the fast food advertisements, which target children that are generally, high in fats and sugars. If you think about our food choices for children, you can clearly see why. Cheeseburgers, pizza, fries, pop tarts, sugary cereals, candy, and cookies.

Our holidays are bombarded with cakes for Birthdays, Candy for Halloween, Easter, Christmas, Valentines, and etcetera. Moderation and preparing healthy food alternatives are important. The problem is this. How many kids are in your child's class? Someone could have a birthday everyday or has a birthday every day, someone in class at school, church, dance recitals, athletic teams, and even with the divorce rate and extended family increases the chance with added step brothers or sisters. This makes consumption of sugary foods in moderation an unlikely scenario.Change has to be made. Children must be made aware of the fact that "Refined – Sugar" is the most addicting substance on the planet and that excess sugar is converted to fat and stored in the body contributing to weight gain, obesity, and other illnesses. We should view refined-sugar as the habit forming substance that it is. Children deserve to be and should be warned that refined-sugar is an addicting substance. Most food suggestibility is instilled in the child when the caregiver delivers the first foods in the baby's mouth at a deep subconscious level. Who and how this initially occurs will affect eating behaviors and begins the cycle of learned behaviors about food.

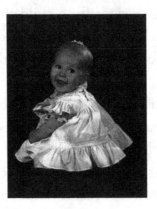

Infant Feeding Tips for the Caregiver

Schedule a meal-times regimen for the baby according to its pediatrician.

Trust that the baby innately knows when it hungry and when it is full

The baby will adjust to regimens and feeding times.

The baby will cry and let you know if it is hungry, wet or sleepy.

Trust the baby, the baby knows what it is feeling.

It is important not to encourage the baby to take just one more bite.

It is important to stop feeding if the baby turns its head or shakes its head no.

It is important not to allow the baby to gorge.

It is important to listen to the babies burp cue.

Allow the baby to stop eating when it obviously doesn't want any more food.

Never have the baby to finish off the whole jar of baby food just because there is a little more left in the jar.

Children instinctively, tell the truth about everything.

Why would a child say they are not hungry if they are hungry?

If the baby has a tendency to over-eat or is gaining weight too rapidly take it to its pediatrician for an evaluation, immediately.

If you are concerned about malnutrition, give the baby a liquid vitamin supplement that is recommended by a health care provider.

Take the baby for regular health care check ups.

THE BALANCE DIET & LIFESTYLE

When children see their parents become upset with them not eating and eat only for their parent's approval. On the flip side children have been noted to eat paper in class from the lunch schedule being too long after the breakfast or too early from the end of the school day. Other situations to consider, is forced supplementation. When children begin throwing their vitamins in a corner, houseplants, under the mattress or hiding them anywhere to keep from taking a handful of vitamins in the morning you are overwhelming them.

Tips For Parents

Avoid allowing children to choose and eat unhealthy foods.

Accept responsibility for being a parent who values good nutrition.

Helps your child make healthy food choices.

Take action. Change and make healthy food choices for your kids when they don't for themselves

Acknowledge your own learned eating behaviors that may cause a bad influence on your kids.

Avoid excess weight are and don't teach your kids to repeat the same nutritional mistakes that you have made in the past.

Teach healthy eating and healthy lifestyle habits to your children from birth.

Set an example to your children by eating healthy, exercising and taking nutritional supplements.

Focus on teaching your children healthier eating habits.

Teach your kids about how junk food choices resulted in the "Mass Epidemic" of Weight Gain and Obesity

Encourage children to avoid vending machine foods, snacks and sodas.

Keep quick healthy foods on hand because many times when children are hungry junk foods are the only option that is available.

Healthy foods are not usually found in vending machines.

Pack snacks for your children such as Apple and oranges.

Demand better quality fast food, even if it is more expensive.

Realize that by doing organic foods, you are practicing a form of preventative medicine, and it is worth the investment in your health and the health of your family.

Start gently exercising babies from birth by taking a baby yoga class.

Have a daily exercise routine for children before they start school.

Children need to know from the beginning of life that refined-sugar can be just as bad for your health and as addicting as some drugs are. Children should be informed that people do if fact develop "sugar addictions" and that even though sugar may taste good, too much is bad for them and after consuming refined sugars people tend to crave it and become addicted to it.

Fast food advertisements tempt children with free playground area's or with a free toy surprise for kids with their meals. According to Time magazines special issue, overcoming obesity in America, thirteen billion dollars are spent annually on food advertisements for kids and the article estimated that for every hour a child watches television the obesity risk rise by six percent. The incentives vary from a free toy in the box of cereal or caramelized popcorn to Collectable stickers or toy movie character. This encourages children to go back for more sacks of junk food just collect to the whole set of characters. The children's "Kid's Meal" food market consists of artificial colored and sugared cereals, pop-tarts, sweets and sugary drinks. The toy, gift or play area's are fine, the menu is the problem. Whom do we hold accountable? Our children are becoming sugar and junk food addicts from the time they are able to take their first bite.

Children's Primary Fitness and Health Concerns

15% of children between 6 and 19 are overweight
1 in 6 children are headed for obesity.
Each year, there are additional increases of children that are becoming overweight.

Healthy Solution

☺ If a child is over the age of six and under the age of 19. Health camps for children, which focus on developing a healthy lifestyle, proper diet and nutrition, and exercise are beneficial to children of all ages.

Forget Childhood Myths

The eating habits that we develop begin at birth. The programming of children's eating habits occurs all through the developmental years up until school aged. Usually by the age of five our personality is already developed. Quite often inaccurate information is taught to children in this age group, regarding food. This information affects our food choices all through life. Eating habits start at birth and develop as the personality develops. It is important to be aware of how we

THE BALANCE DIET & LIFESTYLE

were programmed as children and how as parents that we are programming our own children and influencing other children to eat around us. As parents or caregivers, it is as important to have an example from the whole family as a unit. The mother as the usual primary caregiver has the most influence. The father is the paternal, strong, male side of the personality and can offer the infant a strong sense of direction. If a child has an overweight parent it increases the risk of the child being overweight by forty percent and if both parents are overweight the risk of being over weight rises to eighty percent. If you do not want an overweight child do not be an overweight parent. The male parent role model is important to encourage the physical and psychological growth, direction, exercise, sports, teamwork and sense of strength and independence. The mother is the nurturing caring side of the personality she is important to teach feminine qualities, care giving, gentleness, love and emotional direction. There are many more aspects to the parental role model and siblings, babysitters and others in the child's environment affect the child's development as well.

One of the most common problems in weight loss, is false learned behaviors from childhood that are unconsciously imbedded in our subconscious mind. These thoughts and false beliefs are constantly unconsciously driving our behavior and choices. If you recall ever hearing these phrases, it is important to replace these false eating cues with truths.

Typical Childhood Brainwashing
"You better eat or you are going to starve to death".
"It is rude not to clean your plate".
"Hurry up and eat your food before it gets cold".
"You can not go out and play until you eat all of your dinner".
"If you are good, we will go get ice cream afterwards"
"You get what you are served like everyone else, you eat what the rest of us are eating."
"This is what we all are eating you should, just eat it, too."
"If you don't eat your dinner you can't have a desert"

Take a moment to think of the consequences of these statements. They all encourage the development of over eating habits. As a mental exercise, think of each statement and analysis all of the negative repercussions of believing these false statements. In the eyes of a child care givers are gods. As children we depend on our care givers to teach us the right information and as children we accept everything that we are told as the absolute truth. We have to acknowledge inaccurate information and move beyond it to make behavior modification and positive growth changes. For an adult, freedom of choice selection is one of the most pleasurable aspects of eating out at a restaurant; everyone chooses what they like to eat. Children should have alternate food options. Start them early; let them know up front, as you are teaching and raising them that as they grow they can grow a strong healthy body by practicing moderation. A single bite of something is o.k. But overindulgence, can make them sick later in life.

Teach children the extreme importance of their diet in relation to their health; stop being conscious about nutrition and the importance of a healthy nutrient rich, well balanced diet. It may take persistence to get your child to accept a new vegetable. It takes approximately 10 introductions to get a child to accept a new vegetable so don't give up too soon. Juice fresh veggies for babies, toddlers and small children. If you start them out early it is normal to them, and they love it. It is important to use organically grown produce. Even if it cost a little more it is worth paying the extra money to buy it because the quality and cost difference is worth more than the accumulative health consequences of the toxic other option. You are paying for the health of your children and your family. You are paying extra for the prevention of disease and illness while maintaining good health. As children are developing, it is important to recognize that examples of eating and exercise. Stressful interaction between caregiver and child over food, is deeply imbedded in the subconscious mind and has lasting effects. These are the means that we receive information to develop our lifestyle, learned eating habits and behaviors.

PARENTAL MIND BODY WEIGHT LOSS TIPS FOR HEALTHY CHILDREN

1) Unite together and be effective leaders for children that you have influence over. Start feeding toddlers health foods, only. Stick together in keeping the family healthy. It takes team work.
2) Set a eating time regimen. Have meal and snack schedules.
3) Do not ever delay the schedule or regimen for more than thirty minutes.
4) If a child will not eat, do not give them heavy between meal snacks.
5) Give them water to drink and explain that they will have to wait until the next scheduled meal.

THE BALANCE DIET & LIFESTYLE

6) Make children wait until the next scheduled meal or snack. They will usually eat at the next meal and will be more acclimated to eat at scheduled times.

7) Do not teach children that it is bad behavior not to eat.

8) Do not force children to eat. Put the healthy food on the plate and if needed help them eat. Allow children choices in food selection.

9) Do not create stressful situations around food selection and consumption.

10) Do not make children feel guilty, different or bad just because they do not want what the other children are eating.

The National Centers for Health Statistics and National Centers for Disease control and prevention studies show that there were dramatic increases in childhood obesity in the age group of 6 to11 years of age from 1988-1994. These were almost double ratios as compared to the childhood obesity rates between 1976-1980. Even more astounding are the statistics that compared to the rate of obesity in 6 to 11 year old children from 1971-1974. The obesity ratio has tripled from 1974 to 1994 in just twenty years. This is an indication of the seriousness of the weight problem at hand. The ratio of obesity can be an indication of what the future health status will be in the development of weight related and adult onset diseases. Studies show that major factors in the increase of childhood obesity run parallel to the increase in the number of hours that the individual child spends on average watching television, home videos and DVD's or playing video games. This means that, by far, when children are less physically active at playtime the result is an increase in weight gain and obesity. It is important for children to exercise even more so than in the past with the introduction and increase of nutrient poor, fast foods into the diet. The increase in childhood sedentary lifestyle could possibly be from a lack of energy from mass consumption of nutrient deficient processed or fast foods. The message is clear; we have to offer our kids healthy fun alternatives. Teach your children the great benefits of healthy eating and physical exercise through rhymes and stories. You may find the Mind Body Health Programs Children's books helpful in teaching your children to stay healthy and physically active. Start teaching your children healthy living practices and exercises at birth when they are still infants. Take a yoga for babies class with your infant. Be an example do your exercises with them by walking them in their stroller, getting faster as they grow, jogging and doing your exercise while they watch you and learn as they grow. Watch fitness shows on television or invest in yoga and home fitness videos such as the Mind Body Exercise video/DVD and Mind Body Yoga video/DVD. As they grow, allow them to do the exercises with you. Toddlers love this, and it is the best time to show them by example the importance of exercise. The cutest thing I ever saw in my life was my baby daughter doing leg lifts in a diaper. This proved to me that children mimic the behavior of their parents as she was copying me while I was doing my morning workout and counting out the sets in baby talk. It still gives me a good laugh and when you see your baby exercise, it will give you a good feeling, too. Teach your children to exercise when they are very young it will stay with them a lifetime.

As they grow you can sign them up in dance class or sports depending on their preference but the sooner you get them involved in a physical activity the better.

If you are a more of an outdoor type person, Start taking hikes, bush walking, bike riding or repelling. Water, snow or jet skiing. All activity is good. The more natural the better, it teaches our children not only to exercise for fitness but to enjoy and appreciate the beauty of our planet and the importance to be in synchronization with our surrounding natural environment. It teaches them to observe the natural beauty of life. It pulls them away from mechanical distractions, it takes them out of our computerized, televised, synthetic world and back in touch with the real world and helps them to synchronize and keep in touch with their own unique and individual inner self and their place in the natural environment. It is so easy to sit on the couch, grab a quick snack from the fridge and sit for hours sedentary eating snacking and watching TV. It is important to get our children away from this pattern. Teach them that when we are outdoors, hiking up a mountain, also allows us time to think our deepest thoughts and to feel our deepest feelings. You most likely wont be eating all day while you are participating in outdoor activities. By being active, you are burning calories and converting stored fat into energy. The result is a lean, strong, healthy body. Exercise helps children to grow a strong body. Exercise helps the body had better metabolize the foods that you eat. Exercise allows the body to use stored fat, allowing the body to produce energy from it. With less weight from accumulated fat, you have more energy. With the proper diet, you can avoid future accumulation of stored fat.

PARENTS OATH:
"I take responsibility in teaching my youngster(s) to
eat healthy foods."

Parental Mantras:
I teach my child(ren) to eat for the right reasons.
I create a peaceful, pleasant environment for family meal times.
I allow my child(ren) freedom of choice.
I set my eating habits and behaviors as an example to my child(ren).
I encourage healthy snacking in my home environment.
I buy foods that are healthy for my family.

As a parent and caregiver, it is a good practice to do a meditation to get in touch with what it is like to be a child, again. Through a meditation, go back to your own inner child. See your inner child growing and learning to eat the foods to help it grow up healthy. Give your inner child the unconditional love it has always wanted and the love it needs. Give your inner-child permission to make its own food choices. Love your inner child and tell the child within that "No one can ruin your life unless you allow them to" Tell the child within that it is o.k to reach a slender weight" the inner child needs to know that it does not have to eat for the wrong reasons and that it should only eat for nourishment when it is truly hungry.

Pre-Teen Weight Control
Every stage of development is important in a child's life. We relate to all the stages of our development in forming our self-image and self esteem. The pre-teen stage of development is most crucial as we are developing our reason logic and decision making skills from ages 10-12 years of age. In my twelve years of working with children's health issues from a mind body perspective, I have concluded that helping the pre-teenager to understand their own thoughts and feelings can help them succeed in developing a healthy teen experience without going through a wreck less or over-indulgent teen experience, without junking out on junk food and even alcohol or drugs. If we teach our pre-teens how to cope with meditation and calming foods, herbs teas and natural substances, it

gives them more of a image of self – care with a true appreciation for preserving their mind and body without the use of drugs and alcohol as they realize that healthier alternatives can give them a natural feeling of peace and harmony as their growing bodies change. This approach helps the pre-teen to become more aware of self during a stage of development that tends to be focused on their peers and gaining peer acceptance.

The mind body approach to pre-teen well being can help the pre-teen to succeed in social settings with ease, including the high peer pressure school setting. Teaching pre-teens how to become balanced in their own mind and body can be of great emotional benefit at a time when emotions are most sensitive while the pre teen seeks approval and acceptance amongst their peers. Being content with one's self is the first step in being content with others. The pre-teen stage of development is crucial as in this stage the pre-teen learns to feel connected with others in their own age group. When a pre-teen feels disconnected he/she may turn inward or to food for comfort. Pre-teens need structure and guidance as they are developing the ability to have inner structure and self control. Pre teens are extremely sensitive to judgment and being labeled good or bad.

Each child is innately good, they only need confirmation that they are making the best place for themselves in society. Mind Body Medicine teaches the pre-teen that we are all one and one for all and these concepts help a pre-teen feel more connected to their peers that seeking to be the extroverted "cool" one in class or by introverting and shutting themselves off from their peers during this stage of development. The pre teen needs to recognize that everyone has similar feelings in this stage of growth and that each person, including themselves have special talents and gifts that are to be recognized and cultivated as an individual but that it is what we share with each other that makes their group of peers, better as a whole, that is most important.

Autonomy is important but, being part of the group is just as important and makes them very special, too, as being connected to a group is what it takes to form a healthy and balanced society. Once this is realized then the pre-teen can work on becoming their personal best for a lifetime. Pre-teens begin to notice the differences in the shapes sizes and colors of their peers. When children feel that they vary, too, differently than others it can affect the way their fundamental personality, behavior and temperament develops even though these are

THE BALANCE DIET & LIFESTYLE

often biologically based and have certain observable aspects in earlier life. An individuals characteristics mature over time according to life's experiences and in various different situations. Developing flexibility while maintaining structure and order teaches the pre-teen self-control and allows the pre-teen to learn as an individual how to do things in moderation which is crucial to healthy living and weight control.

Teenage Weight Control

Around age 13 , hormones are changing dramatically within the body. Puberty is a natural stage of growth and change which transitions a child into a young adult. Growth is a natural phenomenon for this stage of development in life. Some parts of the body may grow more quickly than other parts. The body shape can appear unbalanced and awkward at times during this growth state. Children need to be counseled and reassured that they are going through growth changes naturally and normally. Effective teen counseling begins at the pre-teen stage. Let them know that their body is changing and things may seem a little awkward but are that what they are feeling and experiencing is perfectly normal. It is important to keep a positive feeling of acceptance in the social and family structure during this transition of growth. Sometimes, teenagers feel self-conscious of the changes that are occurring in their bodies.

Self esteem can be greatly affected during this stage. Encourage children to stay physically active in sports and activities to build lean healthy muscle and to burn off excess physical energy. It is important to prevent fat gain during these hormonal changes. A study of the U.S.D.A. showed that 1 in 4 teenagers is overweight to the point that it puts them at serious health risk later on in life even if they slim down as adults the study shows increased risk of cancer, heart attack stroke and other health problems from being an overweight teen. However, it is important to reassure a teenager that their body is growing and that growth at their age is a natural and necessary process.

Sometimes, teenagers get their roll models from magazines, peer pressure or movies. Teenagers want to mimic models, stars and their peers. Keeping up with popular or current fashion, style, trends and image are important aspects of the teenage growth phase as these things connect them to their generation. Individuality and self esteem are important for a successful future. Let them know that 100% of magazine models are photo's are retouched in some way, to make them look perfect for the magazine ads. We do not have to look like a magazine model to be beautiful, healthy and happy.

Eating disorders can become an issue with teenagers. Self assurance and healthy self esteem is important in raising a healthy teenager. Common eating disorders are anorexia nervosa and bulimia. These behaviors usually begin in the teenage years when peer pressure is at its peak. the general belief is that magazine advertisements feature perfect bodies. In actuality, super models generally appear under nourished. The teenage population strives more than any other age group in "fitting in". Give your teen publications on healthy living and take your teen to mind body groups or camps. Teach your teen to recognize that their teen idol is human but that teen idols are glamorized for marketing reasons. Discuss with your teen about the marketing of teen idols are meant to play into the teen psyche to pressure teens to copy the image, and that it actually encourages teens to follow the market trends in fashion, it only becomes unhealthy if moderation isn't exercised or if you find yourself becoming fixated on trying to achieve an image of a super model or super athlete image. We should consume food to sustain life and nourish the body of its essential nutrient needs. Unfortunately, our culture has encouraged a lifestyle of gluttony or the extreme opposite anorexia and bulimia. All of the variations stem from psychological causes. The mind aspect has to be dealt with before the body will respond. It is important to be able to control behaviors and maintain a healthy, normal body weight. Normal size is based on genetics and individual body structure. It is important to practice moderation in all you consume. Some times this requires the advice of a professional counselor. If you feel you may have a disorder or if someone has mentioned that they believe you may have a disorder and your eating habits are adversely affecting your health it is time to seek professional help.

Women Weight Control In Child Bearing Years

In late puberty and early adult hood, there are many hormonal changes that are occurring in the growing body. Organs, which produce the hormones that increase fertility, take precedence within the endocrine system. The body and mind work together as one, in times of stressful changes, the body does not know if you are going through famine or a false starvation mode response. The female body compensates to prepare for pregnancy.

THE BALANCE DIET & LIFESTYLE

In females, at the approach of childbearing years, the hips naturally broaden, additional accumulated fat is gained and the breasts enlarge to prepare for a successful pregnancy and delivery during the reproductive stage of life. This is nature's way of ensuring the survival of the species. This occurs because the body cannot distinguish between physiological stress and psychological stress. In males, the shoulders broaden and manly features develop such as muscle mass, physical strength and endurance increase to prepare to protect the female and his offspring. During this time it is usual that extra fat accumulation occurs. This is nature's way of ensuring survival of the species. This is also the reason that it is normal for a woman to carry more body fat than males during the reproductive stage of development. Recognize that you will instinctually want to put on more weight for these reproductive reasons and avoid the following behaviors.

Behaviors to Avoid
> Stress Overload-taking on too many overwhelming burdens.
> Career Burnout or Exhaustion-not enough R&R/rest and relax.
> Increased fast food and on the go junk food consumption.
> Using caffeine and sugar to keep going instead of rest.
> Physical inactivity-sitting behind desk and computer all day sedentary lifestyle-napping with youngsters, all work no play.
> Poor Diet – Starving then bingeing.
> Eating because you are at home with children, watching soap-operas and eating bon-bons. Go out for physical exercise, daily.

There are special considerations in the hormonal and bio-chemical section of this book to aid in better understanding of the changes the body goes through in relation to accumulations of body fat. Physical activity come natural and is needed by the male and female during this active stage of life. When we become imbalanced during this stage with sedentary job or lifestyle fat accumulation occurs easily. See the section on exercise, biochemistry and bio-hormonal imbalance for more information and illustrations.

Avoiding the Middle Aged Spread
As we age and hormones decline, digestion and energy levels tend to decline, this can lead to weight gain. As we approach mid life hormone production be-

gins to decline and the organs which regulate metabolic and reproductive rates, usually slow down. Dealing with the middle age spread is not always easy. This may trigger the development of body fat as the endocrine system and hormones are affected. The metabolism of carbohydrates depends on the pancreas ability to regulate blood sugar levels. The pancreas must have chromium and vanadium to release a steady stream of insulin hormone. Without these two nutrients, blood sugar levels are unstable. The long-term deficiency of these two nutrients may be the first stage of the development of adult onset diabetes. The other glands that slow usually are the thyroid and the stomach and digestive system but all of the glands and organs in the endocrine system are affected. Exercise is imperative to slow the progression of the aging process and in order to keep and maintain lean muscle from turning into flab.

Two thirds of adults are overweight in the United States.
Half of the overweight population are actually obese.

If we allow ourselves to lose our muscle tone the tissue becomes flabby, sagging and hanging loosely on the bone structure causing the aged appearance. If we suffer from bone shrinkage or loss, it compounds the aged look. We can suffer bone loss from acidosis or having a chemistry that is too acidic because the body is self-healing, if there are not enough calcium buffers to alkalize acid excess, the body will pull the calcium from bone and joints. There are over a quarter of a million types of calcium. Some regulate chemistry; some regulate bone and muscle mass. See the chapter on hormonal imbalance for more information and picture illustrations. Deficiency may occur from an imbalanced chemistry, not from lack of nutrient in the diet.

According to biological ionization, the ph stability point for chromium and vanadium is 5.8-6.0 therefore, it is imperative to have a balanced chemistry and especially in mid-life to properly metabolize carbohydrates. As hormones are naturally declining within the endocrine system, nutritional support is necessary to optimize the function of the system. Nutritional support is needed however, should the chemistry be imbalanced, the essential nutrients may not be absorbed, assimilated and utilized by the organ if the ph is imbalanced. It is as important to monitor your chemistry and eat the proper balance of alkaline and acid foods as it is to limit the intake of sugars, fats and salts in order to loose weight and keep it off permanently. The liver has to have biological sulfur to

THE BALANCE DIET & LIFESTYLE

produce the 500,000 enzymes a day just to regulate normal metabolic functions. Good liver health is essential to loose weight, metabolize fats, maintain healthy cholesterol levels and eliminate solid waste toxins from the body. See the section on chemistry for further information.

To achieve and maintain successful permanent weight loss, it is important to have a lifelong plan, this means make weight management a lifestyle. It is important to avoid feeling deprived. However, moderation is the key even when making healthier portions keeping the calorie count down is still the key. It is therefore important to learn and adopt the behavior that smaller, healthier portions can satisfy you completely. Instead of having a portion, that is really enough for four or five people. Allow yourself to be satisfied with the normal portion. Know at that moment that you will eat again later after your body has had a chance to digest what you have just consumed.

People On-The-Go Diet

If you are one of those people who are always on the go, have a tight lunch schedule or tend to eat at fast food restaurants, this is a few fast food tips. First of all, eat more foods containing vitamin C and B to offset your stress. Look at the menu at any fast food restaurant and you will quickly see that most items are loaded with fat and excess calories. Be cautious when eating at these establishments, look for the Lite menu at fast food restaurants and food and desert bars. Food bars are another place to exercise caution. No one should eat all they can eat…no one needs a double slab of meat on a cheese burger stacked between two white bread buns with greasy fries and a sugary drink. The improper mixtures of foods, are the real problem. There is a chemistry to weight loss and food combining. There are hidden culprits of this nature that are linked to the epidemic of weight problems.

Fast food restaurants call these "combo-meals" because they are a combination of everything all in one. We cannot properly digest all of these things at once in the digestive system because it processes and digest these foods differently. The body uses certain elements to process proteins and certain things to process carbohydrates. The body digest proteins one way and carbohydrates another way. Dining in these types of places is only acceptable when you choose from the lighter healthier menu and avoid combo deals. Combine your food properly.

Food bars are fine if you watch the caloric intake, the choices you make and always select the healthier food items and a normal size portion. Moderation is the main issue. Dining in all you can eat or fast food restaurants should not be practiced on a daily or regular basis unless, they have a special menu focused for the individual managing their weight or offer a lite-menu. It is important to keep positive mental outlook and high self esteem during this transition phase. Life does not end at mid-life and some say that life is just getting good at this stage.

The Real Man Diet

Being overweight is one of the main culprits that affects a man's strength and endurance. One of the most popular diets that I have ever written is for men and has been the topic of many media interviews. I named it "The Real Man Diet" because it consists of real foods that contain nutrients that are important in strengthening the male body and the special hormonal chemistry of males. Managing your weight as a man and staying physically and sexually active will help keep you healthy, strong and confident and will make the difference in quality of your health for the rest of your life. It is important to always eat a well balanced diet and avoid excess calories. Men who eat a heavy meat and potatoes diet or who drink beer and eat chips an junk while watching the game, will inevitably end up with the "beer belly" as men tend to gain around the waistline. You can maintain a very attractive physique and ensnare her senses with this high performance diet, especially designed for men. It has long been said that the way to a man's heart is through his stomach and new research indicates that it may be true in more ways than one. Therefore, if it's good for the man, it is also going to be good for the one who is lucky enough to be the partner in his life or at least it is guaranteed to make them smile and more. Based on studies at Berkley University, some foods indicate that they can enhance physical strength and endurance as well as enhance the sex drive. Outside the study, other foods which contain certain nutrients, such as protein, which contains the amino acid "Arginine" is shown to be a powerful muscle builder, this amino acid is known to increase performance, stamina and blood flow delivering oxygen and nutrients to key muscles when needed most which can be good for sustaining strength and endurance during any physical activity or exercise.

Do you want know what the foods of stamina and seduction are? The foods that are really good for male stamina and virility are common foods containing: Zinc, Vitamin C, Vitamin E and Beta Carotene. Examples of these foods

THE BALANCE DIET & LIFESTYLE

are Oysters, Grapes, Strawberries and Oranges have Vitamin C or zinc. Nuts, Almonds, Broccoli & Fish have Vitamin E and Magnesium. Spinach, Carrots & Sweet Potatoes contains Beta Carotene. Research studies show that, good forms of protein provide branched chain amino for sustained endurance. Branched chain amino acids are used as an energy source during physical activity and exercise.

Protein helps stimulate the release of anabolic hormones that promote muscle formation. Combined with physical exercise, the result is increased lean body mass and decreased fat mass. Arginine plays a key role in stimulating release of anabolic hormones that promote muscle formation. Arginine is recognized as a semi-essential amino acid for good health although it is readily synthesized from ornithine. Protein is a good provider of energy, but, all of these foods can help in a strong and powerful way to increase male stamina and virility. Good nutrition is important, but the man's lifestyle is important, too. Care of the "Body" is important in addition to what you eat. It is important to stay physically fit by getting regular exercise, manage stress and chronic illnesses in a healthy way, if you are a smoker you should quit smoking and cut back on alcohol in addition to learning to eat and drink in moderation. There is also the Mind component practice positive thinking and develop healthy relationships, as emotional factors can effect performance, too. All of these "Mind Body" factors can play a role in male performance and are linked to sexual dysfunction. Medical treatments are also available but doctors confirm that diet and lifestyle is powerful in the prevention of performance problems. The key component is to eat a healthy well balanced diet, exercise, eat normal portion sizes, exercise, stay physically fit and active, and indulge in a feast of romance stimulating foods that are sure to sustain divine energy for the two of you to do the Tango and much, much, more. And lastly, enjoy a glass of wine instead of heavy alcohol, put out the cigarette and light a candle instead as you train your mind and body to learn to relax and enjoy intimacy without substances and stimulants other than what is found in food. These are just a few tips from my "Real Man Diet" that can help you manage your weight and help to change your health for the better.

Nutrition for Athletes & To Prevent Age Related Muscle Wasting.
One of the best foods for athletes and for prevention of the loss of muscle mass as we age, is protein. Arginine an amino acid found in many forms of protein, may

play a key role in muscle formation, reduction of physiological stress, and in helping to maintain a strong and healthy immune system. However, taking L-Arginine without L-lycine can trigger dormant viruses, therefore, taking a multi-amino supplement is a better choice. The number one, muscle building food for Athletes is Protein which contain amino-acids. Protein helps increase strength, endurance and your ability to utilize oxygen thus helping you sustain high-intensity exercise for a longer period. Numerous studies in world-class Olympic athletes have documented these effects. Protein should be increased in training diets and proteins are excellent for energy. Caution should be used to increase the protein intake without adding animal sources. Therefore, vegetable proteins such as soy, beans, nuts, whole grains and fish are the best choices. Proteins such as beef & chicken produce acid ash residues which in excess, contribute to unhealthy acid imbalances in the body, and therefore, should be balanced with alkalizing carbohydrates and eaten in moderation. Extra protein is necessary for athletes, however, since protein increases acid levels in the chemistry, high urea's and heavy uric acid concentrations have been linked to deaths in active athletes. Urea's are the undigested proteins within the body. A sign of high urea's in the body are unusual or pronounced deep wrinkles in the forehead area another symptom is feeling fatigued when you wake up in the morning. With all the high protein training food supplements on the market one must be aware of these warning signs to reduce risk of toxic urea levels. Periodically, one should give the body a rest from the hard digestion of these high protein food supplements and allow the body adequate intervals of alkalizing to off set any imbalance that may be occurring within the body.

Geriatric Weight Management

In men and women, after menopause and andropause many people give up at battling the bulge and think that it is natural to become old, tired and fat. Even thought the body has a tendency to develop more fat tissue as the hormones decline. It is not true that there is nothing that we can to to slow down the aging processes and enjoy being physically fit for life. Keeping a positive and youthful outlook is the first step. Exercise helps to prevent muscle loss and also decreases the risk of the occurrence of atrophy. The metabolic rate and energy flow tends to slow down unless preventative interventions are made. When the body begins to age at an accelerated rate, it is important to keep active to keep your body fat index in a healthy range. The best thing to slow down aging is to keep active and exercise to keep fat accumulation down and

THE BALANCE DIET & LIFESTYLE

to stimulate an increase in the metabolic rate.

Dehydration is the enemy in an aging body. Connective tissues become less flexible as we age due to dehydration and improper nutrient utilization problems. It is important to eat a well balanced diet and to take food supplements. It is important to balance out the caloric intake with the activity level. As the activity level usually decreases with age our caloric intake should be reduced as well because we do not need as many calories as we did in our active youth. Light flexibility training is important. Stretching and yoga is ideal to maintain muscle tone and flexibility, for the elderly and can reduce the risk of muscle strain or sprain. Brisk walking is recommended three to five times weekly. And light weight bearing exercises are important not only to maintain muscle tonicity but to help new bone growth and as a preventative to fracture as it aids and building strong bones. Light weight exercises, such as the Mind Body Exercise program are ideal for geriatric and elderly. Swimming and water aerobics are excellent exercises, as the weight bearing stress is minimized in the water and it takes pressure off of the joints reducing pain and damage to the joints, muscles and ligaments while burning off calories and strengthening the muscles.

Weight Management Tips for the Aging

Eat early and eat often throughout the day. Eat healthy and smaller portions. Snack on carrots, celery sticks, an apple.

Chew your food carefully, deliberately and slowly. It stimulates digestion produces enzymes and bile to help you absorb nutrients better and feel fuller longer.

Always stretch the muscles lightly and thoroughly before exercise to avoid injury. Join a yoga class or water aerobics class for increased flexibility

Time your exercise regimen where you are not out in heat of mid-day hours to reduce risk of heat stroke.

Exercise in the cooler times of the day, morning preferably and avoid over exertion.

Keep your exercise regimen on a schedule.

Start slowly and increase your activity level over time to reduce the risk of injury.

Stay physically active and mentally motivated to preserve your physical health.

CHAPTER 7

Hidden Imbalances & The Chemistry of Weight Loss

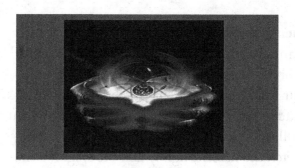

THE CHEMISTRY CONTAINS THE CONSTITUENTS TO MAINTAIN BALANCE WITHIN THE body. If there is an imbalance in the chemistry, there is usually a hormonal balance as well. The signals that regulate homeostasis, internal balance, may become mixed due to compensating efforts of the body to generate something that it is missing that is required for the body to function properly. Sometimes the body may send hunger signals that may be a false hunger signal. These signals may cause cravings if the body is lacking something that is essential to regulate proper function. When this happens the body begins to compensate. The signals may be false. You may get a hunger signal when it is really thirst or a craving for salt or ice because your body needs minerals. These false signals may cause other symptoms or send a signal from some other organ when the imbalance isn't a hunger for food but something that a particular food may contain.

The Importance of Balanced Chemistry for Weight Loss

The body is an amazing self-healing organism that is constantly striving to maintain balance in the chemistry and organ systems. An example of this incredible phenomenon is when the body overheats or becomes too cold. The body sweats to restore the correct temperature when it becomes overheated. When the body is cold it shivers to create friction or heat to bring the temperature back to homeostasis. When the body is balanced and all bodily systems are functioning properly, this is called homeostasis. The stomach is part of a compensating organ system called the endocrine system, this system contains organs that are linked together to produce all the hormones in the body.

Malfunctioning or dysfunctional organs in this system may be the link to a series of hidden hormonal imbalances that may not be in a disease state, but may fluctuate randomly and cause mixed-up signals. Another culprit may be synthetic neuro-transmitters which have been suspected to produce false hunger signals. One culprit may be artificial flavor enhancers that trick the brain to think it is receiving something that it is not. If you have weight gain in certain areas of the body it may be due to imbalances in the organs that regulate the metabolism in those areas of the body.

If you have distinctive weight gain in particular areas of the body which fall into weight gain in any of these distinct patterns, you most likely have a bio-hormonal imbalance which may have stemmed from a bio-chemical imbalance which created a nutritional deficiency of essential nutrients to these organ systems. Your chemistry is very important for proper digestion and metabolism in weight loss and management and this single aspect, alone, may be the reason of past failures in weight loss attempts. The state of health known as Homeostasis is where everything in the body is balanced and functioning in a perfectly normal manner. In Homeostasis, all organ functions are at maximum level of efficiency. The body is able to utilize the nutrient fuel it receives and is able to make. According to biological ionization of the chemistry has to be, 6.3-6.6 ph in order for the body to absorb and assimilate all the nutrients that are essential to human health and proper organ function to remain in Homeostasis.

If you have either one of these body shapes, you should see your physician before beginning any new diet or exercise program. To balance your body type, read the chemistry of weight loss chapter and the sections on bio-chemical and bio-hormonal imbalances, the importance of homeostasis and healthy diet for the individual organ systems and body types.

Body Shape Type A   Body Shape Type B   Body Shape Type C

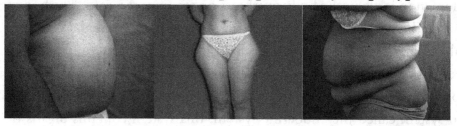

Body Shape May Reveal The Cause Of Your Weight Gain

There are three individual body types that can easily be identified by the way you gain weight. These types are a result from imbalances within the chemistry which are creating dysfunction in the organ systems. However weight gain of this magnitude may be serious to your health and increase the risk of disease.

A) Liver/Pancreas – Apple shape/Pot Belly
B) Ovary/Hypothalamus – Pear shape/Thunder Thighs/ Big Hips
C) Adrenal/Thyroid/Pituitary-Balloon Shape/Weight Gain All Over

In this chapter, I will explain how homeostasis is sometimes lost and how to correct imbalances in the chemistry to restore the functions of the organ systems.

In Homeostasis, the body is able to utilize the nutrient fuel it receives and is able to balance the chemistry and manufacture enzymes, hormones to keep the body in a maximum level of function and health. Dr. Reams also discovered that each nutrient has a ph stability point and certain essential nutrients are less stable than others are in an imbalanced chemistry. In an imbalanced chemistry can interfere with the proper absorption, assimilation and utilization of nutrients. The first nutrient that is affected by an imbalance in chemistry is Iodine. Iodine is the least stable of all essential nutrients. In addition, Iodine is the master nutrient of thyroid function. Imbalances that create proper iodine absorption, assimilation and utilization affects the metabolism and therefore can lead to weight gain. Imbalances in body chemistry may be the cause of past failures in weight loss attempts. The line down the middle of the chart represents Homeostasis, it is where everything in the body is balanced and functioning in a perfectly normal manner. In Homeostasis, all organ functions are at maximum level of efficiency. This chart is an illustration of nutrient biological ionization the state of homeostasis needed to absorb nutrients.

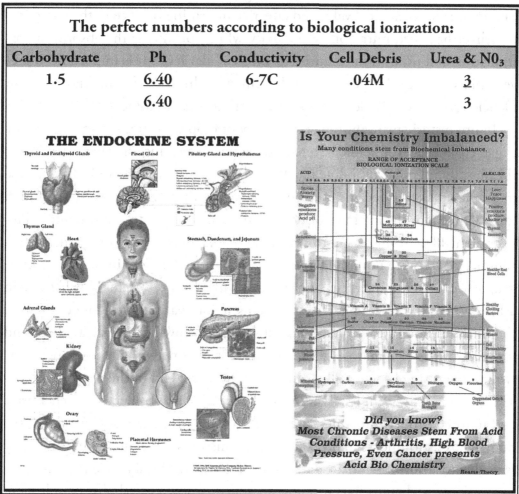

The perfect numbers according to biological ionization:				
Carbohydrate	Ph	Conductivity	Cell Debris	Urea & NO$_3$
1.5	6.40	6-7C	.04M	3
	6.40			3

Years ago Dr. Carey Reams, who earned a PhD in Biophysics and Biochemistry, used his knowledge to create a biochemical profile for a person's individual chemistry to detect imbalances early on before they actually developed into disease. It was discovered through Dr. Reams research that the energy that food produces in the body is a different from the caloric energy value of food. The balance of both energy calculations is equally important in human health and nutrition and is often time overlooked. He named this process biological ionization, and according to Dr. Reams, it is very important for the chemistry to be in a range of optimum iodine absorption, assimilation and utilization by the thyroid, the gland that regulates metabolism, therefore, in permanent weight loss and weight management it is important that your chemistry is balanced. There are others who have continued researching Dr. Reams work, those of us who continue to explore his work have discovered amazing revelations in our own research and find increasingly that it is valid and effective in brining balance to the chemistry to deliver balanced nutrition to the body while optimizing the absorption, assimilation and utilization of nutrients on a cellular level. It is important to prevent Bio-Chemical Induced Organ Dysfunction In Weight Gain and Nutrient Deficiency Links to Biological Ionization of Nutrients Homeostasis

In pre-historic man, during famine or poor crop conditions, starvation mode triggered a release of acidic adrenal hormones decreasing the chemistry below the ph stability point of iodine blocking absorption to the thyroid, the decrease in Iodine uptake slowed the metabolism to allow survival of the species through long winter months in times of decreased fresh food sources and famine. Pre-historic man ate from season to season. The alkalizing vegetation of the spring, summer & fall were not available for consumption therefore in winter months, acid ash producing meat protein was consumed more often. This extra acid ash, as well as the acidifying effects of being in "starvation/stress mode" lowered the ph just enough to block iodine absorption, slowing the metabolism and allowing prehistoric man to go longer periods of time without food. After the winter, the spring brought alkalizing vegetation, the end of the natural fast and a reduction in stress and starvation response, which re-balanced the chemistry and restored proper function. Understanding the primitive mechanisms of the body helps us to understand that If the chemistry is imbalanced, and the body is unable to absorb, assimilate and utilize all of the essential nutrients, this alone can push the body into starvation mode, shutting down metabolism resulting in perpetual weight gain. The body uses specific nutrients to metabolize fats and convert sugars into energy but if these nutrients are not being properly absorbed and delivered to the fat metabolizing organs it causes an imbalance. The essential nutrients are required to carry out metabolism and the body will instead manufacture and store fats from the excess calories. Live food has a higher energetic frequency pattern than processed food and digestion varies greatly between types of foods.

Parasitic Infections in Bio-Chemical Imbalances

Yeast and fungal infections are common and may become systemic within the body. A fungal condition may be hidden for years and can not only disrupt homeostasis they can cause intense sugar cravings and may be an underlying cause of yo-yo dieting. It can also be the cause of an acidic bio-chemical imbalance that affects the absorption of the nutrients needed by the body to metabolize carbohydrates, fats, and proteins. Research is inconclusive on the full nutritional value of hyponically -grown fruits, vegetables and produce and some experts believe that they lack all of the nutrition that natural grown crops absorb from the soil and may even have detrimental effects on human health and immunity. The threat of dangerous micro-organisms in our food supply is always a risk-factor in commercially grown produce and livestock. The fact remains that the typical American diet is affecting the health status of our society as a whole. Declining nutritional quality means lowered immunity and less resistance to disease. Recent recalls on food such as spinach, oysters and seafood are an increasing risk that presents as potentially harmful affecters of health. These types of micro organisms affect our health and metabolism for longer than just the initial acute stage of infection. They can sometimes cause permanent damage, organ dysfunction and impairment. We already know by the surveillance reports of food borne illnesses report by the center of disease control reports that there are viruses and bacterial infections that can be transmitted by food-born micro organisms is a major health concern, of these diseases are transmitted by infected food handlers. The most common food born organisms are Campylobacter, Hepatitis A, Giardia, Calicivirus, Botulism and Salmonella and all of them can make us sick but, what is more shocking in these reports are that there are more unidentifiable micro-organisms than identifiable ones. Many new or unidentified viral forms that are plaguing our health or are mutating on a daily basis at the rate of over 9,000 per year on average. These parasites cause detriment to our health and organs, the organs that regulate metabolism. Parasites in livestock cause diseases such as mad cow disease. People that have been exposed to this are banned as blood donors for the long term affects are lingering. These are only a few of the hidden culprits to be addressed in effective ways for the purpose of restoring our health and to regain our immunity and resistance to disease.

Our immune system and eliminative organs are imperative to weight loss. The weight issue has hidden culprits that must be dealt with and parasites are major culprits in the many hidden causes of imbalance, disease and weight gain. This is not the only cause, or the primary cause just one dynamic in piecing the puzzle together to find the solution to the weight epidemic. The good news is, there are things that you can do to protect yourself from some of these body snatchers but we are not sure of how to stop noroviruses because foods can become contaminated at the source or the point of service and can be spread by water, direct person contact, airborne or in human body fluids and recontamination persist despite disinfections measures. One thing is certain; is for each of us to make a group effort to become more pro-active in our own health care before these disasters occurs on a grand-scale. We need more educational programs that teach our youth prevention, weight maintenance and healthy lifestyle practices. History has a tendency to repeat itself, lives are being lost on a daily basis let us not wait for a health disaster to occur as it did in ancient civilizations, not necessarily from parasites, but Obesity. Protein and acid waste debris from parasitic conditions, excretions and parasitic die-off, produce imbalances in body chemistry from the excess acid ash residues excreted from parasitic waste which may lower the ph and may destroy the molecular structure of a nutrient or block the absorption, assimilation and utilization of essential nutrients. In particular, the resulting acid imbalance may affect iodine uptake to the thyroid due to biological ionization of an essential nutrient. Without the essential nutrients required for maintaining an optimum metabolic rate, slow the metabolism slows and weight gain increases. Iodine has a ph stability point of 6.2 –6.6 and is the least stable of all nutrients. Therefore, the thyroid is the first organ affected by bio-chemical imbalance. The thyroid requires iodine to produce metabolic hormones which regulate metabolism the destruction of iodine by bio-chemical imbalance is certain if a systemic parasitic condition is present. Parasites must be effectively eliminated to ensure the proper ph required to absorb, assimilate, and utilize all of the essential nutrients required for proper organ function and in maintaining a healthy chemistry that assist in maximizing the metabolism of fats, carbohydrates and proteins. Parasitic cleansing is imperative in maintaining healthy and stable blood sugar levels. It is important to eliminate all sources that are creating cravings for sugar and simple carbohydrates and therefore sugar-feeding parasites must be eliminated. It is necessary to frequently detoxify, cleanse, balance the internal body chemistry and balance the mental and physical body on a regular basis. This can be achieved by utilizing a holistic approach to healthcare with natural treatment options. It is important to utilize a holistic approach to optimize the state of health.

Probiotics are beneficial for replenishing friendly intestinal flora you can take these in supplement form or get good bacteria from the diet by eating foods such as kefir, miso, sauerkraut, yogurt, buttermilk, cheese and fermented foods. Diatomaceous earth in a form suitable for human consumption is a good anti-parasitic agent as it kills parasites by forming a crystalline substance in the parasites intestines similar to glass. Taking garlic supplements and drinking herb teas on a regular basis is beneficial to protect against parasites and taking herbs such as Pau d' Arco is another helpful way and preventative step in reducing your risk of getting a parasitic, viral or bacterial infection.

Natural Parasite Expeller Garlic Relish

1 Fresh Bunch	Chopped Parsley
½ Cup	Chopped Garlic (finely)
1 T.	Vinegar
1 T.	Natural Sea Salt
¼ Cup	Olive Oil (cold pressed)
1 T.	Pau d' Arco Tea (loose)

Preparation:Finely Chop and Mix (parsley, garlic, vinegar, pau d' arco and salt.)
1. Add oil to cover ingredients. Stir
2. Cover and store in refrigerator.

HORMONAL IMBALANCES & ORGAN DYSFUNCTION

One of the biggest culprits in weight gain is hidden hormonal imbalances and the resulting organ dysfunction affecting the metabolism and eliminative organ systems and lowering their ability to properly metabolize and eliminate excess fat in the body. The body chemistry affects the hormonal system as it is the imbalance in the chemistry that interrupts the absorption of the essential nutrients that the endocrine system needs to maintain good health and proper organ function. When a hormone producing organ becomes depleted of the essential nutrients that it needs to produce hormones, the organ becomes dysfunctional and may eventually lead to disease. The metabolic effects of thyroid hormone are imperative to good metabolism. If the thyroid function slows down, the metabolism slows down and we gain weight because the imbalance affects fat metabolism. Other metabolic functions affected are Glucid synthesis: glycerin, water and electrolyte metabolism resulting in hypothyroidism & edemas. Many organs and glands are part of the endocrine system and there are many imbalances and endocrine disorders and that affect disease and weight gain including obesity.

Homonal Imbalances

 Linked to Poor Nutrient Utilization of the Organs in the Endocrine System. Hormones are produced by the Endocrine system. They are manufactured in the glands, organs and tissues of the endocrine system. Hormones are released into the blood stream and carried to all cells. They stimulate cells to increase or to decrease their activity or to secrete another precursor hormone. The hormones are the communication signals within the body that trigger metabolism, digestion, elimination, growth, sexual activity and stress response. What may be considered normal hormone values may actually be low for an individual who is normally at the high end of the value ratio. This may create a slowed metabolism if the individual was naturally on the high side of normal and now are on the low side of normal, this is not enough to call the decrease in function, a disease, but it is still low for that individual and may contribute to weight gain and the onset of disease.

It is important to consider that everything, which we consume, because it produces an acid or alkaline ash residue as the body breaks it down and metabolizes it. Very few things, that we consume, are neutral in ph. This is a very important factor to consider because the ph affects the function of the organs that produce hormones. Most of these artificial substances previously mentioned, produce acids in the body, which may eventually disturb our ph and homeostatic balance within the body. This may contribute to bio-chemical and bio-hormonal imbalance in the body. It only makes sense to keep your food consumption of artificial substances at a minimum level. In addition, eat as natural as possible when loosing weight to allow the body to spend all of the enzymes breaking down old stored fats and maintaining maximum metabolism of the natural foods you consume. This will give the liver a break and allow it to

THE BALANCE DIET & LIFESTYLE

get to the process of regulating stored fat. Utilizing and metabolizing the stored fat for energy instead of using everything, it produces to try to figure out how to make these unidentifiable substances into something it can recognize, digest and eliminate. As you can see, it is very difficult for the body to digest anything that has been chemically synthesized or overly processed. The first step in balancing bio-chemical, bi-hormonal or metabolic imbalances within the body is to cleanse.

Tips for Restoring Balance in the Chemistry and Hormonal Health

1) Internal Detoxification Cleanses – a metabolic, hepatic or liver cleanse and kidney cleanse and a colon cleanse – is very important herbal formulas work well because they are natural. All decaying matter produces putrefaction toxins and create a zenobiotic or cadavering effect in the body. It is important to flush poorly digested foods & fecal matter from the body. Colonics cleanse the colon.

2) Hydration & Purification-Drinking only steam distilled water during the intial excretory organ flush and kidney cleanse.

3) Healthy Diet A change in diet – avoids additives as much as possible and eats as natural as possible. Eat a healthy well balanced diet, and alkalize with your foods if you are acidic. Avoid herbicides and pesticides they biologically transmutate into estrogen excess.

4) Maintenance Cleansing – while loosing weight going through this liver detoxing process and should be done periodically on a regular basis, based on the state of the diet.

5) PH Balancing-Check morning urine ph to make sure chemistry is in the 6-3-6.6 range Ideal ph is 6.4 if your ph is below 6.3 you are acid and should alkalize to maximize nutrient absorption. Adjust your ph by eating alkalizing foods or juice and take a supplement designed to keep the chemistry in this range. Ph paper can be purchased at most pharmacies, health food stores or you may ask your doctor.

6) Immune System Support – Boosting the immune system can decrease our risk of infectious illnesses, viruses, parasites, fungus and bacteria all of which rob our body of nutrients and decrease our energy and quality of health. We have to eliminate all possible risk and keep our energy at an optimum level to loose weight. Formulas with transfer factors or colostrum, which increase our natural killer cell production, beta-1, 3-D-glucan stimulate immunity and herbs such as

Echinacea, goldenseal, Pau d'arco, astralagus, Reshii mushroom and elderberry are good to take at the change of season will boost immunity. Furthermore, many amino acids will help strengthen the immune system.

Iodine is the first nutrient affected by biochemical imbalances and is the least stable of all essential nutrients to biochemical changes in the body. Therefore, the thyroid is the most sensitive to biochemical imbalance and without adequate uptake and absorption can lead to thyroid dysfunction and slowed metabolism resulting in weight gain.

The Negative Effects of Toxins and Heavy Metals

The most common reasons for toxicity induced Organ Dysfunction is hidden environmental factors such as consumption of heavy metals and other toxic substances. The biggest scare is the mercury found in fish Our body was not originally designed to metabolize all of the artificial chemicals that we are exposed to in the world, today. With all of the herbicides, pesticides, artificial preservatives, flavor enhancers, food colors, dyes and all of the other processed food additives. It is averaged that each American consumes over ten pounds yearly of these artificial substances, not to mention medications and other chemical substances. Residues of some of these chemicals biologically transmutate into estrogens estrogen is the female hormone that encourages fat tissue and breast growth. Estrogens are like apples, there are many varieties. In particular estridiol is a dangerous form of estrogen that increases the risk of some cancers. However, phyto-estrogens as found in unprocessed organically grown soy, can compete out the dangerous estrogens for good estrogens at the hormone receptor site. There are over 2000 receptor sites on a cell. At least 500 need to remain open to allow an exchange of information to the mitochondria, the energy factory of the cell and to take in nutrients and excrete waste. Toxins can build up in the tissues and cause prolonged negative effects in the body. Many mysterious symptoms are due to hidden causes that we have no test to detect. Anything that we consume or take into our bodies that are not natural is going to cause some problems or an imbalance with the metabolism.

A prime example of biological transmutation is how the body metabolizes hydrogenated fat found in most snack foods. Hydrogenated fat is made by heating the fat molecule up to temperatures exceeding 750 degrees Fahrenheit and infusing an atom of hydrogen into the fat molecule. Now, there is no way the human body can heat up to this temperature to break down that molecular structure, so, it pulls enzymes from the liver to break down it's composition in order to metabolize it. It takes the human body over 50 days to metabolize one molecule of hydrogenated fat. It does so by biologically transmutation hydrogenated fat in to Iron Oxide 3. A toxic form of iron that can interfere with all sorts of metabolic functions. Iron oxide 3 has been proven to increase the risk of strokes. The consumption of hydrogenated fats and the body's biological transmutation into Iron Oxide 3 is one of the main reasons that men have a shorter lifespan expectancy than women. Women have a menstrual cycle, which help their bodies to eliminate it from their system on a monthly basis. However, women who have stopped menstruating or have had hysterectomies have shown to be of equal risk of stokes as men with the consumption of hydrogenated fats. Hydrogenated fat should be viewed in this manner by a dieter "A moment on the lips, at least 50 days on the hips". Hydrogenated fat is listed as one of the 10 foods that should never be consumed. Hydrogenated fat should not be considered as a food source due to its contribution to weight gain and ill health effects. Chelation therapy and enzymes are of great benefit in the elimination of heavy metals and some wellness centers offer hydrogen peroxide drip therapy.

The metabolism regulates weight gain. The human body is designed to metabolize, natural foods grown in nature. Anything else is recognized by the body as a foreign toxin and many scientists believe that biological transmutations occur from the body trying to make a toxin into something it can digest and eliminate. If the body doesn't recognize a substance because it is man made, it will try to change it into something natural that it can recognize or metabolize. It is believed that just as the body can make some nutrients that the body can change some substances into other substances to eliminate them from the system by altering the molecular structure enough to digest and metabolize it as something else in order to eliminate it. This is why some scientist believe that pesticides affect a rise in (FSH) follicle stimulating hormone and estridiol levels which appear to be associated with a higher risk of some types of cancers and may also affect fertility.

Balancing Process

Eliminating toxins and rebalancing the system requires patience and dedication because it is a process that takes time. Maintaining bio-chemical balance can be simple. However, rebalancing or restoring the body to homeostasis and the body's natural ability to heal itself should be part of a healthy lifestyle. Imbalances in the chemistry, trigger bio-hormonal imbalance. Success may depend on how many adult onset disease states have developed and how much damage has already resulted from the chronicity of the condition.

Overweight people are out of balance. Obese people tend to have a decreased sensitivity to catecholamines-which induce lipolysis. Other documented causes include hormonal endocrine factors such as hypothyroidism, hypercortisolism and hypo-pituitarism. It is necessary to detoxify and cleanse to keep balanced chemistry. We should cleanse, build and support the whole system on a regular basis. Regular cleansing is the only way to prevent these types of imbalances.

Hormones affect metabolism, the thyroid hormones are the main regulators of metabolism, any excess of hormone or foreign substance which may mimic a hormone, poses a threat to metabolism and weight control. Hydrogenated fat is only one example. The body pulls enzymes from the liver to break down the molecular structure of any foreign or molecularly altered substance these substances usually produce toxins and acids in the body. The liver could use those enzymes for other functions and therefore this stresses the liver. It is the organ, which breaks down of our solid waste toxins to be eliminated from the body, including excess fats and cholesterol. The repetitive daily consumption of hydrogenated fat not only causes rapid weight gain and is thought to biologically transmutate into iron oxide 3 which is said to be the reason why men have a five year less lifespan expectancy than women who may eliminate it through menstruation, because it is a toxic form of iron similar to rust, which binds with cholesterol to form plaque in arteries and blockages in the body. There are over a quarter of a million different types of calcium transmutations. Calcium acts as a buffer in the body. The body uses calcium for many functions and in particular to keep the chemistry in balance, alkalizes acid excess, and maintain homeostasis, the body's optimum self-healing state. If there is not enough free calcium in the diet, the body will pull calcium from bone to alkalize the acid excess or to digest acid ash residues from an acid diet. All meat protein produces acid ash residues. This takes more alkalizing agents and calcium to digest. Calcium's vary in ph

THE BALANCE DIET & LIFESTYLE

from 12.0 to 6.6 and may be used in balancing the body chemistry. However, the biological ionization, ph stability point of most calcium's are 5.8-7.2 in other words, the chemistry must be 5.8-7.2 for the human body to absorb, assimilate and utilize calcium at an optimum level and to maintain homeostasis.

Effective Rebalancing Program Components
1) Correction of bio-chemical and bio-hormonal imbalances.
2) Implementing therapies that cleanse and detoxify the body, reduce congestion, help drain the excretory systems, while increasing resistance and immunity by cleansing, supporting and building up the immune system and nutrient content in the blood .
3) Increase physical strength and removal of metabolic waste by exercise and fitness programs.
4) Achieve permanent results with behavior and lifestyle modifications.
5) Consuming a healthy diet consisting of properly digested food items rich in enzymes, which reduces acid build up and purification from undigested foods.

Over five percent of the mineral content of the body is Potassium. Potassium is an important alkalizing element. We should consume food high in potassium on daily basis, avocado, sweet potatoes and bananas are high in potassium. Potassium does most of the work in alkalizing the chemistry. It helps waste pass out of the body, in the kidney it acts as a diuretic to flush out acid metabolic waste and helps regulate the water balance in the body and homeostasis. Dandelion tea is high in potassium, sodium and chloride all are necessary electrolytes to maintain homeostasis.

Bio-Chemical and Bio-Hormonal Problems & Solutions

Problem & Solution
It is important to recognize the hidden sources that may create IMBALANCE in the body. Take action to correct imbalances due to hidden imbalance or toxicity factors CONSIDER AND CORRECT imbalance to achieve WEIGHT CONTROL.

DR. JOYCE PETERS

Solution:

1) It is recommended that you see your doctor for help with testing and Treatment of these types of imbalances.2) Recognition that cleansing and detoxification are a necessary and mandatory part of any effective health care and weight management plan.3) It is necessary to balance and stabilizing hormones, organs and glands.

CHAPTER 8

Emotional or Stress Related Weight Gain

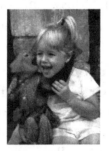

Get The Stress Monkey Off Your Back!

It is believed that stress and negative emotions are the main culprits in most health conditions including weight gain and obesity. Many view stress as an unavoidable monkey on their back, but there are many ways to adopt a stress management lifestyle. Many people claim to overeat when stressed or use food as a comfort to cope with stressful situations. Our society seems to be living in a race for life. It seems that most people are too rushed to eat slowly, and chew their food properly. Being overworked, Stress and Negative Emotions Lead to Fatigue and Exhaustion. When we live a "High Stress" life, we have over active adrenal gland function which can produce an acid bio-chemistry leading to metabolic, biochemical and bio hormonal imbalances. Stress, negative emotions, fatigue and exhaustion in combination creates adrenal burnout. The centers of disease control issued a report that over 75% of all visits to primary care physicians are related to stress or anxiety in some form. Stress depletes the body and has acidifying effects that can affect health in many ways that is why Stress is known as the "Silent Killer". Many over-eaters are "Stress-Eaters" or "Emotional Eaters" and the stress condition must be address to ensure successful permanent weight loss and weight control. Stress wears on our emotions and on our Body, Mind and Spirit.

The Emotional Eater

Sometimes people eat to stuff back stress and repressed emotions. It is important to recognize this pattern and take healthy measures to overcome this type of eating to ensure weight loss success. Get rid of the psychological garbage and all unwanted, unneeded or false beliefs that you have been hoarding. This negative psychological garbage is crap that clogs up the metabolism of the healthy mind body connection needed for weight loss. And like crap it needs to be eliminated and flushed away. Live your life for you, it is your life.

Tips For Developing Healthy Emotions

Allow yourself to feel a sense of acceptance and approval. Self love is important to permanently achieve your weight loss goals and dreams. Release all thoughts of yourself that are stressing, weak and ineffective. Visualize yourself as emotionally strong, destressed and effective in obtaining your weight loss goals.

Release the stress and emotional attachment to fear, worry or anxiety of how others perceive you.

Emotions are powerful. Do not fear your emotions. Emotions channeled appropriately are your power.

Establish a firm emotional grounding. Feel your feelings as they occur. Express your thoughts and feelings as they arise.

Don't bottle up your stress, inside. Do not stuff your emotions down with food or stuff your emotions back to deal with them later. From a metaphysical perspective, putting your emotions on the back burner, can manifest as the physical symptom of back pain, a hindrance to

THE BALANCE DIET & LIFESTYLE

your exercise program. Exercise feeling your emotions.

Holding on to angry emotions or frustrations can show up as layers of protection in the form of fatty bulges. It also is exhausting keeping angry emotions held back inside. When we feel attacked we go into defense mode, animals in the wild puff up their coats to look bigger, we put on fat layers and toughen up our skin so to speak. This protective layer of fat is a defense from hurts from the past, the past cant come back to hurt you, let it go and let go of your false need for an additional protective shield in the form of fat layers.

Be assertive in troubled relationships, not aggressive when standing up for your needs, desires and rights in a relationship while at the same time be respectful of the rights and needs of others. This golden rule will help to prevent emotional hurts or guilt which will reduce the risk of emotional eating in emotional eaters. If you are breaking off a relationship with someone who has hurt you, this doesn't mean telling them all of your negative thoughts toward them, that will cause guilt, it is not your place. You may be tempted to say you are an insensitive, lying, cheat refrain from such negative communications they will only cause adrenal responses and create imbalances in your chemistry, just say, "you have hurt me in a way that I can not continue this relationship" then end the conversation and move forward with your life without the negative relationship. You cannot resolve your hurt by saying things that hurt others.

Observe improper means of protecting your emotions. Improperly used verbal or physical defenses that are ineffectively used to protect ourselves emotionally can weigh us down and stress our relationships with others. When we build barriers in our personal relationships it can lead to the build up of protective walls that block intimacy and create unsatisfying relationships. Emotional eating is common in this situation as the person uses food for the emotional comfort that is lacking in their personal relationships.

Use open, honest and positive communication and constructive critisim. This is effective communication from the heart. You cannot heal your life by hurting others. practice the golden rule, "Do unto others as you would have them do unto you" create a life filled with healthy emotions, sweetness and joy. Positive emotions create positive changes in body chemistry and reduce the need for emotional eating in emotional eaters.

Recognize that we cannot change the world around us but we can control how we react or respond to it. We can create happiness, peace, love and harmony in our world or we can create unhappiness. Happiness is a pleasurable emotion that we need to fill our lives with as much as possible. Happiness is also a state of mind, a choice, and a decision. No one has the power to ruin or wreck your life unless you allow them to.

The Negative Effects of Stress

Stress wears us down and can create decreased metabolism and immunity. In addition it can trigger other auto-immune responses. As society has evolved into the high stress competitive communities that the rate of auto-immune disorders have risen. All of the stresses in the body leave us at a point that we are too tired to enjoy the simple beauty and health in life as it was intended and it triggers our defense mechanisms which affect metabolism.

Stress is another hidden culprit in weight gain, because, there are unmistakable patterns that show up in health that are clearly caused by stress. Often these patterns can be seen before obesity disease states are set in motion, requiring medication or surgery. Weight control and prevention can help the human body's defenses against the development of obesity related/stress related illnesses. Most of us were not born with an adult onset disease but we may have the hereditary factors that put us at risk of developing an adult onset disease.

Stress is usually one of the major culprits in the development of adult onset diseases. However, we usually do not develop "Adult Onset" conditions until adulthood. "The middle age spread" tends to trigger some adult onset diseases, therefore, keeping your weight under control is a benefit to the prevention of disease and the stress of dealing with a medical condition. What changes in our body to "trigger" the onset of adult onset disease? As our lives become increasingly fast paced, the magnitude of stress-related health problems is growing at an equally alarming pace. Stress uses more nutrients especially vitamin C and B-complex and the depletion can lead to lowered immunity. Every time your body has an adrenal hormone response, your body burns up at least 500 mg. of vitamin C. In cases of stress, the body needs more than the usual daily-recommended allowance of essential nutrients. In addition, when cutting calories to lose weight, more nutrient supplements are needed as well. To reduce stress, add nutrients through dietary supplementation while reducing food intake while on a weight loss program. It is important to take a good multi nutritional supplement while dieting and to keep in mind. However, read the section in this book on body chemistry because if the body chemistry is imbalanced, the body cannot absorb nutrients as well as it needs to. Each nutrient has a ph stability point and if the nutrient is in a imbalanced body chemistry that is outside of the range of the ph stability point, the nutrients molecular structure is dissolved rendering the nutrient useless. Therefore, the nutrient cannot be absorbed and it is passed through the body without being absorbed. If you have stress, it is important to have your chemistry checked to make sure that your dietary supplements are not just "expensive urine" as the old adage goes. In other words, the acidifying effects of stress can destroy the properties of nutrients rendering them ineffective and may block the absorption of nutrients. Acids are corrosive. Alkalizing diets, which tend to contain more enzymes can help with this problem but you can over alkalize to, so there has to be balance in all dieting approaches. Many dried herbs tend to be alkalizing and have enzymes and vitamins and minerals as well as other botanical agents that tend to have positive effects on the body and some such as Kava, Passion Flower, Valerian and St.Johns Wort, help with stress. What this means is that Stress is a contributing factor in weight gain and is also, one of the leading causes of death and obesity. Stress is directly linked to weight gain and as a contributing factor to coronary artery disease, respiratory disorders, cirrhosis of the liver, cancer and accidental death.

Acidifying Effects of Stress & Fatigue on the Body Chemistry and Endocrine System Contributing to Weight Gain

The National Safety Council estimates that 1 million employees are absent on an average workday because of stress-related problems. Meaning stress can make you immobile and perpetually inactive which leads to a sedentary lifestyle that is detrimental to weight control. Over 89% of Americans report experiencing some level of ongoing or chronic stress. Even more people experience fatigue on some level. In relation to obesity and overweight conditions. People tend to eat for energy when they are tired or fatigued. Exhaustion is a major culprit in weight gain due to the stress hormones that are released within the body.

Chronic fatigue or long-term stress can cause weight gain due to the consumption of foods that give the body quick energy that are usually high in calories which convert into stored fat.
Fatigue and Stress in combination can lead to exhaustion.
Exhaustion can cause the release of stress hormones associated with weight gain and other conditions or disease states.
Stress and Fatigue are not a friend to weight management

The number one method of treating stress related and anxiety disorders are pre-scription drug medications. However, lifestyle awareness and making the neces-sary changes to eliminate the circumstances that are creating stress or fatigue is the best way to eliminate the detrimental effects of stress and fatigue. Adopting a healthier lifestyle, which avoids fatigue and stresses as much as possible, is the one true answer. There are several natural and complimentary fatigue and stress relieving medicines. There are also nutritional supplements that can be integrated into your stress management program. Safely and effectively such as, Vitamin C, Valerian Root, Passiflora, Passion Flower, Kava (where legal) and St. Johns Wort, just to mention a few of the basics. These aid the body, with less side effects and dependency risk than traditional medicines, which can in some cases lead to weight gain and bloating from toxic side effects. According to the infamous Pulitzer prize winner, scientist and researcher, Linus Pauling, each time our body has the adrenal hormone response, the body burns up 500 mgs. of vitamin C. Vitamin C is very important to high stressed individuals. Dr. Pauling was infamous and is still very highly regarded for his mega dosing of vitamin C and cancer research. However, Dr. Pauling and his wife both died of cancer. The original research tested natural vitamin c. Natural vitamin C ap-parently has a higher efficacy within the body in comparison to synthetic forms such as ascorbic acid. Ultimately, It is important to seek advice from a profes-sional on which natural remedies will be best for you.

Stress is more so an indication that one has become out of balance with main-taining a hectic lifestyle without providing a means for rest of the body, mind & spirit to recuperate. Response to Reaction is out of synchronicity. Eventually too much stress leads to burn out or depletion in some form. The Adrenals produce the fight or flight hormone, the survival hormone, which triggers a starvation mode response. It is through research on biological ionization, that when the body chemistry is altered from homeostasis in the 6.3-6.6 ph. that the iodine uptake and utilization is impaired by bio-chemical-imbalances, leaving the thyroid deficient of essential iodine absorption and assimilation. Thus affecting the decrease metabolism and metabolic function of the body. Long-term stress can lead to weight gain and slow metabolism because of this correlation.

It is believed that the acidifying effects of stress and negative emotions and thought patterns contribute to bio-chemical imbalance in the body, disrupting the absorption of other essential nutrients that affect normal functioning of other glands or organs of the endocrine system which can lead to bio-hormonal imbalances. The pituitary gland is the master gland of the endocrine system. The pituitary gland is behind the eyes in the brain and is connected to how we look upon the world. It responds to how we perceive and react to the environment that we are in. When we are stressed by our outside environment, the body automatically turns its energy into external survival mode. When we turn our energies to the outside world to protection and survival mode, we simultaneously turn on our outward survival instincts and turn off our inner healing energies. How we respond to our environment has an impact on our inner physical healing in the organ systems. Since, the endocrine system is a "compensatory system". This may lead to a cascade of imbalances that over time may trigger adult onset diseases and other serious illnesses.

Three Ways Stress Affects the Mind & Body

1) Stress robs blood from the digestive and eliminative organs to send it to the extremities for quick physical energy to escape danger and to prepare to fight or flee. When we are threatened, our body goes into storage mode, because stress signals the body that it is a time to preserve resources not a time to be eliminating them. Therefore, weight loss cannot occur because no blood flow to the intestines slows elimination and metabolism processes and decreases waste removal increases fat storage.

2) Stress affects immunity. The Immune system shuts down to focus resistance to any outside attack, robbing the thymus gland and immune system the nutrients it needs to produce inside protection against, bacteria, viruses, fungus and other parasitic invaders. Stress lowers our resistance to disease.

3) Stress takes the blood away from the brain disrupts thinking, reasoning is decreased. Blood is shifted from the front brain to the back brain

when under stress. Boxers override their brain energies and direct them to the physical body. After repetitively forcing the mind and body to do this so many times, boxers may eventually seem to have no common sense because continually diverting their intellect to develop super physical function at the expense of "brain-muscle". If we override our true hunger signals we eventually desensitize our natural instincts to control hunger.

The body is self-healing, the body will try to repair damage from the imbalance. Acid is corrosive and will cause damage. Just like battery acid will burn a hole in fabric and stomach acid can dissolve a nail. The body will use buffers to alkalize the imbalance, pulling calcium from bone to alkalize. Kidneys need alkalizing agents to regulate homeostasis. The whole body is a balance of chemistry, hormones and proper signaling. Stress can create such an imbalance that it must be treated holistically. Pills & Supplements alone are not the solution.

Balance the Mind & Body to Reduce Stress

Balance in both Mind and Body is the Medicine that is essential to treating this aspect of health.

One must manage their stress and fatigue to achieve permanent weight loss.

Find the source causes of stress and fatigue and eliminate them.

Develop healthier new behaviors in dealing with and managing the stress and fatigue.

If we just take a pill to do the job, eventually, the body will burn out again it is only a matter of time.

Avoid stress, anxiety & negative emotions to reduce fatigue and exhaustion.

Create a stress free life, one that you enjoy.

Meditation, Yoga, exercise, healthy lifestyle, balancing therapies, are all a means of stress management, but it is essential to get to the deepest source of the stress or fatigue problem and either eliminate the source or organize a healthy effective treatment plan which addresses and deals with the source of your stress. The first step is to become aware of your stressors.

THE BALANCE DIET & LIFESTYLE

THE TYPES OF STRESS

External stress   These are stresses outside of the body. Environmental influences which are out of our control, which creates intense anxiety or discomfort. Also, adverse physical conditions or stressful psychological environments. An example is when we are in a natural disaster such as a hurricane, earthquake, tornado or flood.

Internal stress   These are internally induced stresses such as negative emotions or can be a result of fears, physical and psychological beliefs or behaviors. An example is intensely worrying about an upsetting event that may or may not occur. Where you repetitiously imagine a bad situation and the negative outcome if it were to actually occur. An example would be taking a flight during a high terrorist alert and imagining a terrorist hi-jacking your plane and the worst-case scenario that may or may not occur and the negative outcome.

Behavior Determines the Outcome Result On Health

Stress reaction   Is our own behavior and how we react to stress. This involves the effects on all bodily systems, physically, mentally, emotionally, and psychologically. Our perceived resulting outcome. The stress response involves all body systems .The cardiovascular, heart and blood pressure, the immune system, the respiratory system and rate of breathing, the digestive system, the eyes, ears and other sensory organs. All systems react to defend against the perceived danger. Our level of fear affects this factor. It is important to address our own fear factors to reduce our negative reactions to stressors. Learning not to over-react to stress can be a beneficial behavior modification tool.

Stress Over Reaction

Think of our intial instinctual reaction to fire. If we are caught in a burning building our initial reaction may be to freak out and loose control, run or flee. However, we know how important it is to remain calm and follow a structured escape route plan. If your clothes are on fire you stop, drop and roll, but the intial stress response is flight. Sometimes when the fight or flight mechanisms kick in we may have the urge to over react and want to take flight or flee the perceived danger. As we know this is the wrong thing to do if our clothes are on fire, it will only fuel the flame. The same scenario occurs with starvation mode response, when we are stressed or fatigued we may have urges to overeat this fuels the weight gaining process. We have to mentally overcome these urges by understanding how our body is over-reacting to the stress or fatigue and control those urges effectively. The psychological response to stress affects every physiological system in the body. The fight or flight mechanism prepares us for every stressful emotion. The brain or hypothalamus, produces a flood of peptides and neuo-peptides that provide the means to survive the stressful situation these heighten reaction responses. These autonomic responses affect the sympathetic and parasympathetic nervous system, the body mind and spirit as well as every organ system to prepare to fight or flee.

Over Reaction Intervention Tips

Acknowledge when you are feeling the discomfort or stressed feeling.
Take your mental focus away from the stressful emotion.
Focus on your spirit, bring in a feeling of love direct your attentions to your heart.
Remember a previous stress free, joyful or fun experience.
Ask your mind, spirit and heart for the quickest and best possible solution and for the most proper response to the stressful situation.
Trust and heed the advice that you receive from your higher self.
Feel the positive result from the previous steps enjoy the relief from properly handling your stress in a positive manner.
Avoid the urge to eat during and immediately after the stressful situation. When you do eat focus on enjoying the meal as nourishment for your body not as a stress reliever, clear your mind completely of the stressful situation before eating.
Self acceptance and Self love. Pat yourself on the back for the good manner you handled your stress.

THE BALANCE DIET & LIFESTYLE

Stress Level Evaluation Quiz for Weight Control

This is a stress test. If you are experiencing high stress levels, as it is imperative to good health and weight loss to get your stress under control to prevent the false starvation mode response. Life is constantly full of challenges and experiences that can be stressful to us. Just remember each experience occurs for a reason. It is part of our individual journey to learn the lessons of our experiences. However, we can make changes to decrease our stress and the negative health consequences of the stress we endure. Again, conscious awareness is our first line of defense against stress. This test is designed to help us become more consciously aware of what stresses in our lives that may be making us overweight and ill.

Stress Quiz

What do you feel is a stressor to you?

Do you tend to eat more when under stress?

Did you experience a major life crisis before a period of marked weight gain?

Do you feel stress has contributed to your weight gain?

Is your stress level mild, moderate or intense?

What, in your opinion, is the cause of your stress?

Have you experienced a separation or death of a close friend?

Have you experienced a break up or divorce of a partner or spouse?

Have you or a close friend or relative experienced a disease or illness?

Have you increased your responsibility at work or home?

Have you moved?

Have you changed jobs?

Are you a "stress eater"?

Do you use food as a comfort or relief from Stress?

Do you have a satisfying personal life?

Have you suffered a tragic event?

Are you happy with your current life situation?

Have you or a loved one been involved in an accident?

Stress Quiz

Are you unhappy with love and relationships?

Do you exercise or have a hobby/sport?

Are unaccomplished dreams or goals as constant source of worry for you?

Do people annoy you or are you involved in a conflict?

Are you adding additions to the family?

Stress Quiz Totals

Number of yes answers   Number of no answers

_____   _____

Stress can cause weight gain. It is highly recommended that each individual look for the true source of their stress and find ways to diffuse or eliminate the root source of the stress. It is important to the health of our Body Mind and Spirit to find a healthy outlet to diffuse or eliminate the stress instead of internalizing it. that may slowly grow into disease. In addition, prevent the perpetual deterioration of health. For tips on developing a stress free lifestyle, see the Life Balance Pyramid in the Maintenance section of this book.

Avoiding The Stress of Self Neglect and Self Avoidance

Take care of your self, your health and your needs. Many times we find our self carrying the burden of a lot of other people and forget to time to take time out for ourselves. Taking on the burdens of other people is tiring. We all have responsibilities, but what we often tend to do is take care of responsibilities at the expense of our own health or exercise time. A lot times we are looking out for the needs of others but it is important to take time out to look after ourselves. When we take time out for ourselves, we become stronger and more effective in our daily lives. We all need time to rest and recharge our energy; it makes us more effective in taking care of the needs of others in the end. It does not mean that you are selfish or lazy; we must do this to stay healthy. We can also become quite resentful if we do not take time for ourselves and for doing the things that we enjoy out of life building stress and repressed anger, which eat away at our health, emotions and mental health. In reverse, some people use the excuse of being so busy taking care of others and responsibility that they don't have time to take care of themselves because they don't want to take a deep look into their selves and prefer focusing their attentions on others as an excuse not to make the changes necessary to make a positive life change. Sometimes this is because the person doesn't want to be the leader to bring about change in the system or family because someone else is usually the leader in the system. Sometimes, we attract people to ourselves who may have something wrong with them and we focus on fixing what is wrong with them rather than fixing what is wrong with ourselves because it is painful to see our own shortcomings and it is easier to fix someone else rather than fixing ourselves. This can lead to suppressed anger issues. It is important to feel our emotions and find healthy solutions in developing a healthy lifestyle.

Suppressed anger builds up like a pressure cooker inside us. Repressing angry feelings and emotions is exhausting and requires a lot of energy to hold it inside ourselves. This energy can be used to exercise and to do the things that we really want to do. Sometimes we feel like it is too late to try to reach the goals and dreams of our youth. Never give up on the dreams of your youth. You can still get out and do the things you really want to do if you are willing to put the effort and energy into it. You will have to work at it but nothing is as rewarding as staying true to your inner-self. Working on your own personal goals and dreams keeps us in a healthy state of growth. You can achieve happiness living a life that your only working on the dreams of others.

Excuses People Use To Neglect Their Weight & Health

> I am stressed out and I do not have time to take care of me. (Myself)
> I am too busy to eat healthy; I only have time for fast food.
> Caffeine and sugar keeps me going, I cannot function without it.
> I am working too many hours & am too tired to exercise when I come home.
> I walk a lot and am active enough at work.
> I get enough exercise at work. I do not need to exercise.
> I have to run errands and take the kids or relatives places.
> I have sickness/I am not able
> I have no place to go exercise.

The blood vessels shift the blood to the extremities to allow the body the fuel to have extra fuel to fight or take flight. Therefore, long term stress can lead to disease due to chronic starvation of internal organs being deprived of essential nutrients to perform their function. In particular, obesity, diabetes, high blood pressure, high cholesterol, heart disease, lowered immunity; inflammatory illnesses, metabolic disorders, female and male reproductive and or sexual dysfunctions, Stomach & digestive disorders, kidney problems, and even cancer can be triggered by stress conditions. It is clear, however, that the body cannot comparatively distinguish between psychological and physiological stress. The body has the same response to psychological and physiological stress. Stress can and does trigger the survival mode responses as well as the starvation mode responses which may lead to weight gain and obesity. Stress is acidifying to the human body, too much acid or acidosis can and does affect nutrient uptake, absorption, assimilation and utilization. Acid does affect the body's ability to utilize essential nutrients and acid does destroy the properties of nutrients. Some nutrients are less stable in acid, in particular, Iodine is the first nutrient affected, and Iodine is the master nutrient for the Thyroid function. Thyroid function regulates metabolism. The Thyroid is part of the compensatory endocrine system; a decrease in its function can affect the function of other glands and organs in the system, resulting in a perpetuating imbalance of bio-chemical and bio-hormonal balance with in the body chemistry.

The Metaphysical Psychology of Stress

Many times physical ailments manifest when we are too busy to take a look at what is really bothering us in our life. Take time and make the effort to change when it is time for change before the subconscious start sending you warning signs. Usually the subconscious will give us little warnings that show up as discomfort or illness within our body. If left unresolved, it can show up as big warnings, accidents or serious injury. It is the subconscious minds way of saying take care of this before it is too late. If you are constantly misplacing things what is out of place in your life. If you are constantly loosing your glasses, what do you not want to see in your life. If you are constantly sick, ask your self what you are really sick of. If you have a sick stomach all the time, What is in your life that you just cannot stomach anymore? If you are stiff and don't feel like exercising what are you not being flexible about, maybe it is that your schedule is too stiff to suit you. If your knees or feet hurt, ask yourself if you are happy with the direction you are taking in your life. If your shoulders hurt, what burdens are too heavy to carry on your shoulders. If your neck hurts, what are you sticking your neck out for?

THE BALANCE DIET & LIFESTYLE

Negative Thoughts Create Stress

I want to enjoy life but circumstances will not allow me to
I want to have fun but no one likes to do the things that I enjoy with me
I want to do things for me but I have to do things for others
I give my all of my time pleasing others instead of pleasing my self
I wanted to live my life for me and I am living it for them.

Do not allow your life to become so busy and hectic that you start avoiding the things that you need and that are a necessity for you to stay happy, healthy and fit. Avoid life overload and burn out. Sometimes, people's lives become so hectic they tune out their real needs, thoughts, emotions and signals of pending illness. When we neglect our needs and fall into a pattern of self-avoidance, we are in survival mode constantly. We are walking around with an overload of message units and none of them are pertaining to improving health or quality of life. People tend to become unhappy when all the joy is stripped out of their life. We have to work at staying happy and meeting our own needs. We are much easier to get along with others when we take care of ourselves, emotionally, mentally and physically. Trying to please others and never pleasing your self is not healthy. This is a prescription for defeat. Allowing this pattern to develop in your life is a form of self-sabotaging behavior. It is best to pace yourself, take care of the most important things in life and create a healthy balance between, work, rest and play. When you are not overworked, you will find that you actually enjoy your exercise and fitness program and that it is easier for you to do. It will become like "childs-play", fun & easy. When you make the change and inform others of the change, allow time for the change to occur. However, stick to your new schedule and you may even notice that everything in your life becomes a joy when you balance your activities to a less stressful system. In life, "take time to stop and smell the roses along the way".

Break the Pattern of Self-Avoidance

Have a discussion with loved ones or co-workers and ask for their encouragement and support in your weight loss and healthy new lifestyle. Devise a plan to loose the excess weight and to create the image that you desire and life and the health that you want.
Practice open honest communication. Feel your emotions do not suppress them.

Do not neglect or avoid your own needs.

Have an accountability partner, one who can help you stick to your plan.

Asses your relationships and correct the ones that are not healthy for you.

Life is not going to get better until you decide to make the change.

The transition will occur if you choose to make your life better.

There is no time like the present; each day has a new beginning, start today.

Negative Self Talk and Suppressed Angry Emotions

Oftentimes negative emotions are hidden because we stuff them back instead of dealing with uncomfortable feelings. These are the two unhealthiest things you can do because it poisons your life. The healthiest thing you can do in this situation is always find the positive in every situation to feel your anger and let it go instead of changing your positive nature into a negative one. Even though you may feel that others negatively influenced you and that influence contributed to your weight gain, release all negative emotions. Be proactive. Stop blaming everyone else and take your life back into your own hands. Accept responsibility of your decisions and actions. Above all, keep your thoughts positive they are a reflection of the life you create. Negative self-talk can be very destructive. "Words can heal or words can kill". According to Dr. Candice Perth, the discoverer of peptides, the hypothalamus will actually produce and release more peptides into the body, that correlate with the thoughts coming from the brain, that actually changes the body according to our thoughts.

Self-Talk

Do not talk to yourself in a negative way. Sometimes we forget this simple fact. Avoid looking in the mirror and thinking negative self-talk such as:

"My life is a constant stress"
"My stomach is fat"
"My thighs are flabby"
"I am out of shape"
"I hate this life"

THE BALANCE DIET & LIFESTYLE

Instead, look in the mirror and tell yourself these types of things everyday:

"I enjoy the wonderful life I have created"

"I am doing good and sticking to my healthy lifestyle"

"I am looking good"

"I love you"

"I am slim"

"I am beautiful"

Write the positive words on your body so that you don't forget. Also, write the positive words on your mirror so you see it each morning as begin to create and start your day.

Self Realization Statement

"No one has the power to ruin your life unless you give them the power to do so".

Mind-Body Tips for "Stress Eaters"

If you find your self eating in times of stress you are a stress eater. The following suggestions can help resolve your reasons for "stress eating".

Identify your stress eating patterns and devise an emergency action plan.

Prepare an elimination food menu of things that you tend to "stress eat" and remove them from your house, do not purchase them for others in the household.

Avoid eating in excess of normal meals and snacks when feeling stressed.

Use stress relieving herbs and specially formulated stress supplements to give the body extra nourishment and support for stress.

Avoid refined sugar and flour combinations such as cookies, cake and ice cream.

Eat scheduled meals to avoid temptation to binge.

Practice Behavior Modification Mantras, Meditations

Practice Yoga and do the "Mind Body Stretches" to relieve tension and stress.

Get a massage to help ease the stress and tension.

Do things to help yourself feel satisfied in other ways than eating.

Recognize your emotional needs and do not use food as a substitute.

Go outside, take a walk, and breathe the fresh air fill yourself with other things than food.

Go to the gym; exercise at least 30 minutes everyday. Do the "Mind Body Weight Loss Exercises".

Consume most of your calories before 6 pm and do not eat refined carbohydrates after 6 pm.

Sleep and Rest when needed instead of eating to reduce the stress and fatigue from lack of sleep.

Give and receive supportive hugs and love with your friends and loved ones.

Make love with your partner; release your sexual tension and stress in healthy ways.

Identify and eliminate the source of your stress and avoid over eating during decision-making time.

Do not use food as a stress relieving tranquilizer or painkiller during stressful times and experiences.

Express your stresses to your stressors in a healthy manner.

If your stress is related to a person, practice open honest communication to achieve support and understanding.

Avoid or eliminate when possible stressful situations and encounters.

Many people have incredible difficulty in managing their stress. Stress is detrimental to health and robs life of its simple joys.

If you are experiencing overwhelming stress, instead of resorting to self-destructive relief, seek stress management counseling as soon as possible. Many people resort to drugs or alcohol to manage their stress. Improper substance use is self-abusive behavior. These substances are acid forming, which create imbalance within the body. Long-term mismanagement of stress is just as bad as substance use. The negative effects of negative emotions resulting from stress degrade the quality of health over time. Healthy stress management is imperative for weight management and in maintaining good health and quality of life. Do not allow yourself to fall into the bottomless pit of a stress trap or resort to substance abuse. Cope with stress by making eliminative lifestyle adjustments. However, If you suffer long periods when you feel unmotivated, see your doctor. You may be suffering clinical depression. Do not put off seeking help if you cannot motivate yourself to start living a healthier lifestyle. The MBWLP Behavior Modification therapy helps but is not intended to replace medical advice.

Portable Therapeutic
Stess-Reduction Device

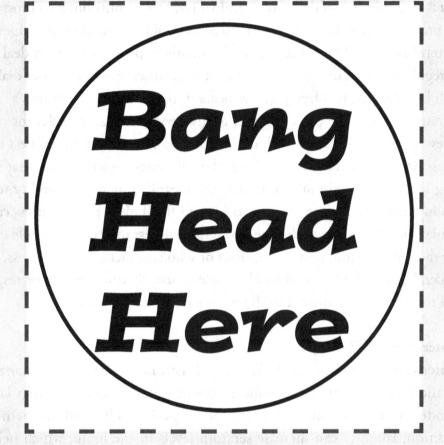

Instructions:

1. Live a balanced lifestyle to reduce stress.
2. Alternatively, Hang Device on Wall or Brick Building.
3. Follow The Directions As Indicated In The Above Circle.
4. Repeat Step 3 until Relief is Achieved or Until Consciousness is Lost.
5. If Consciousness Is Lost, Cease Stress Reduction Therapy.
6. If consciousness is regained Repeat until relief is achieved.

Disclaimer: This is just a joke. As you can see, Step 1 is the only acceptable option for stress management. Please, do not attempt to try any of the other steps 2-6 as this may be hazardous to your health, not to mention that it could cause a terrific headache and even worse damage. Living a balanced lifestyle is the number one choice, plus, it's less painful and can reduce stress more effectively.

Stress is nothing to joke about, Stress is a Real Killer! Stress causes disease and weight gain. Balanced living is the key. Einstein is quoted as saying the definition of insanity is repeating the same thing over and expecting a different outcome. Identify and stop your stress patterns. Stress can become a habit, if you get stuck in a mindset of daily stress and worry. Stress contributes to most high blood pressure and is the sole cause of 40 percent of hypertension cases. Elevated cholesterol and blood fats-occurs most frequently in people who must deal with stress regularly and it increases their risk of heart disease. Adult –onset diabetes or high blood sugar, this frequently appears in the mid-40's sometimes as a delayed response after the cause is gone. Many people eat as an outlet for stress. Very few people under stress will lose weight. People seldom do the best thing for stress which is exercise. Persons with these illnesses commonly say that stress is a big factor. Low resistance Stress usually means greater vulnerability to the common viruses that cause illnesses, colds and flu. This is because stress causes particular blood proteins to decline and serious illness may result. People under stress who have inflammatory conditions or who contract a serious illness, such as cancer, kidney disease, or stomach problems usually don't recover or respond as well to treatment compared to those who are relatively stress-free.

Laughter as Stress Therapy

Laughter can be the best medicine or at least one of the best in managing stress and in preventing stress induced weight gain. Studies show that laughter produces brain chemicals that indicate a positive effect in biochemistry. In addition, laughter can increase seratoin levels in the brain, which help us to lose weight. The Positive health effects of Laughter have been documented in laboratory test. Before and after blood samples taken after patients experienced laughter from watching a funny movie, listening to comedian or just by reflecting on fond memories can create a positive change in the chemistry and an increase in seratoin. The hormone that we produce when we are in love that also helps us lose weight. This is a good reason to laugh a lot. Go see a live comedy show to keep your fat burning Seratonin on the rise. Laughter can be the best medicine for weight loss. Spend time with fun friends and people that make you laugh often, to achieve a happier lifestyle and especially, while losing weight.

Hatha-Yoga is a form of yoga, which involves deep belly laughter as a meditative practice. Forcing your self to laugh out loudly. Doing this can be quite humorous especially if you can coerce a friend to try it with you. I bet the neighbors will wonder what your up to. All you do is this; while sitting in yoga pose; think of something that is really funny. Start with a chuckle and raise your laughter into a crescendo, allow your laughter to build into a roaring laughter, then, keep your laughter going as long as possible and allow it to gradually exhaust you and subside. The effects are amazing. In addition, it is a fun exercise. Deep belly laughter works every muscle in your body and face.

CHAPTER 9

The Mind Body Exercise Program

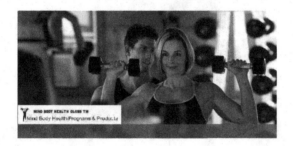

EXERCISE IS YOUR BEST FRIEND IN WEIGHT LOSS. IF THERE is anything close to a magic pill for weight loss, it is exercise. Studies show that regular physical activity may prevent a genetic predisposition to overweight or obesity. Exercise is an important part of a healthy lifestyle that can help save your quality of life and health. Studies also, show that strength training boosts your metabolism and helps to build lean muscle. Two pounds of muscle can burn off ten pounds of fat in a year. Therefore, gaining five pounds of muscle, through weight bearing exercises, can help you burn off up to an additional 25 pounds per year because muscle uses more calories for fuel. If you do not increase caloric intake, and you increase physical activity the body will tap into and burn stored fat for energy and provide fuel to build muscle. Fast walking can burn fat and encourage weight loss, too, by adding 10,000 steps to your daily walking routine. Pedometers are a small electronic devise that count the number of steps you take, they are the best way to track how many steps that you are walking in a day. Pedometers can be found in most fitness centers or online at http://www.shop.mindbodyhealthprograms.com

What are Mind Body Exercises?
Chi Gong, Yoga, Tai Chi and The Mind Body Exercise Program are exercise regimens that work the Mind and Body at the same time and are based on types of ancient health practices or martial arts which are great Mind Body Exercises to practice. These systems involve movement through specific stylized postures and gestures that are practiced with regulated deep breathing and in addition to holding and releasing precise poses. These practices improve the Mind Body Connection and have been used in cultures around the world as a key part of healthy living practices. The Mind Body Exercise Program by Mind Body Health Programs, are 3 Mind Body Exercises that tighten and tone every major muscle group, that can be done in just 10 minutes twice daily almost anywhere, so there is no excuse, not to exercise.

What To Do When You Hit The Wall?
When you hit a weight loss wall add "Mind Body Exercise" and wellness spa therapies to your life, in addition to walking no less than 5,000 steps daily, adding up to 10,000 steps to help jump-start your weight loss, again. Once it restarts you may taper off, again.

Tip When Starting A New Active Lifestyle and Exercise Regimen
Taking an Idebenone supplement may ease the transition of adopting a healthier new diet and lifestyle because it protects against the effects of cellular hypoxia that may occur after exercise. Especially, in people who are out of shape that are beginning a new exercise program and who are changing their physical activity while trying to get back in shape. Therefore, it is great for helping sedentary people or so called "couch-potatoes" in getting back into an exercise routine. It is an anti-aging compound that can help lessen feeling mentally fatigued while

on a diet or detox program. It helps information transfer across the corpus-cal-losum, into the learning centers of the brain improving balance between the left and right brain hemispheres making behavior modification easier. Therefore, It may help ease the transition between lifestyle changes and enhance the mind body connection.

Exercise Tip For Men

The two exercises that enhance the appearance of the male physique most are push-up's and sit-up's. Men should start out doing 10 of each and work their way up to 50 each day adding more as strength and endurance is gained.

If you feel that you don't have the physical strength and energy to exercise, that is a false belief, but you can start with breathing and stretching and walk-ing, these are the most common mind body exercises. Most everyone is capable of a living a lifestyle that includes some form of exercise. Exercise does not have to be strenuous to be beneficial.

The number one exercise fact is:

"Physical activity is needed to lose weight, stay slim, physically fit and healthy".

Studies show that short sessions of exercise are effective and that several short ses-sions are just as good a one long session of exercise. Most adults should get a mini-mum of 30 minutes of moderate physical activity and children should get an hour of moderate exercise daily. Regular exercise burns stored body fat and improves overall physical fitness. It also, helps reduce stress, improves digestion and elimina-tion, increases endurance and energy levels, promotes lean body mass.

American Exercise Fact:

Less than one-third of adults in the United States are currently getting the rec-ommended amount of physical activity to stay healthy, physically fit and trim.

> **Exercise Rule #1** – "Never allow yourself to fall into the sedentary category!"

Don't be discouraged about exercise; If you are one of those people who has ever exercised hard on a weight loss program and lost weight, but, then mysteriously stopped losing weight and became stuck, there was a hidden cause. Your metabolism kicked into primitive survival mode. The primal stress instinct tricked your body into thinking you were in war and famine and shut down your metabolism to protect you and your immune system from the stress. When this happens it causes some people to give up because they don't understand why they stopped losing weight. Exercise is important in weight loss and in weight management. If you diet without adequate exercise, oftentimes, you will experience a phase of weight loss of ten pounds followed by a phase where you hit a wall and can not loose any more weight. This wall is known at the base metabolic rate set point. When this occurs, when you have reached your memorized fat storage, which is not necessarily the healthiest level of fat storage.

If you have ever felt that exercise did not help you lose weight in the past and now find it hard to find the motivation to exercise again because you experienced "hitting the wall" on your last diet and gave up because you didn't quite understand the mechanisms of your body. Don't give up, this time, you can over ride your set point if you hit a wall in weight loss. To restart your fat burning and weight loss increase your calories of healthy protein and good fats a little and increase exercise and activity level, until weight loss resumes. This tricks the body's fat set point to lower and it is the only solution known to help you break away from the programmed fat set point and establish a new one. Exercise will recalibrate your set point and jumpstart the metabolic rate to continue the weight loss process. When you hit that wall and feel like you are not losing weight, increase your exercise, it will quickly help you to break through that wall and help you to continue losing your excess weight.

Mind Body Exercise Improves Emotional and Mental Health

Exercise has a positive effect on brain function and mood.
Exercise increases the mental faculties as it increases circulation, blood flow, nutrients and oxygen to the brain while increasing waste removal.
Exercise increases our ability to multi-task, ignore distractions, and respond and react quickly.
Exercise increases neurotransmitters.
Exercise gives you an "oxygen high" and neurons function better when they get oxygen.
Exercise increases alertness and mental energy.

Fire Breathing

Start with a breathing exercise. Fire Breathing or the Breath of Fire is a mind body practice that is used in yoga. It is a great breathing exercise for increasing your metabolism. This continuous rapid diaphragmatic breathing technique rejuvenates and energizes you. It can be through the nostrils or mouth. Breaths should be controlled to ensure evenness of the inhalation and exhalation. You may become dizzy the first time or you may get an "oxygen high". With practice, you will master the technique over time. This is a very detoxifying breathing exercise and it helps balance your chemistry because every time you exhale, you release carbonic acid which helps maintain homeostasis. Begin by sitting in Yoga pose. Fill your lungs with four deep breaths and as you exhale release all tension form your mind body and spirit. Then quicken the pace of your inhale and exhale cycles as quickly and evenly as possible. The rhythmic cycles should resemble a see-saw in evenness of rhythm, pumping the oxygen in and out of the lungs at an equal pace. Keep in mind a soft and tranquil pace while achieving this balance until you reach a state of euphoria. Build up you time and gradually increase to longer periods of fire breathing over time. To create the results you desire simply become more active. Believe in your self! You can do it! Nothing is impossible.

The Health Benefits of Physical Exercise
Loss of excess body fat & weight
Helps to burn stored fat into beautiful radiant energy
Increased and improved digestion
Decreases harmful stress
Increase in energy, decreases fatigue
Improvement of moods and sense of well-being
Increased total blood volume and nutrient assimilation
The muscles including the heart are strengthened
The risk of high cholesterol is decreased, increased HDL
Positive changes in body composition and muscle tone
Stimulates the excretion of toxins and metabolic waste
Improvement of bone density
Improves self image, self confidence
Increased sense of peace in mind, body & spirit
Increased productivity and endurance

THE BALANCE DIET & LIFESTYLE
Increased oxygen uptake to the cells, organs, brain and body
Improvement of overall physiological & psychological fitness
Increased Libido
Increase chance of longevity

THE CHOICE IS YOURS… While losing weight, a good slogan to remember is "You have to use it, to lose it".

Consequences A Lifestyle Lacking Exercise:
Accumulation of fat and excess weight
Increase in cellulite in women
Increase in apple and pear shaped physique
Decrease in hour-glass and trapezoid physique
Increased risk of muscle atrophy & disease
Increase in infertility, Decreased Libido
Decrease in self-esteem
Increase in depression
Increase in fatigue, decrease in energy
Increase risk of cancer, diabetes, heart attack, and strokes
Increase risk of injury
Increase in stress
Increase in shortness of breath
Increase risk of early death

According to the American College of Sports Medicine, every adult should exercise a minimum of 30 minutes of moderate intensity exercises on a daily basis to maintain healthy weight, good health, proper posture and muscle tone.

Recognize these important exercise facts:
Recognize that exercise accountability can help keep you motivated and on track with your weight management goals.
Recognize that any exercise is better than no exercise at all.
Recognize that exercise in the morning speeds up metabolism all day
Recognize that exercise is necessary part of any weight management program.
Recognize that exercise improves the body physically and psychologically.
Recognize that exercise makes you look and feel great.

Recognize that exercise is one of the best ways to stay youthful.
Recognize that exercise gives you the physical endurance and strength
to stay active.

You should believe in yourself and your abilities to exercise regularly because
you were born a winner. You are probably stronger than you think. In fact,
you won the first race of your life because you were the strongest and the fastest of all of your competitors. This race was the race of life. As your father
released you as a sperm with thousands of your potential siblings you were the
fastest swimmer of them all, as you swam up stream in seminal fluid search-
ing for the holy-grail golden egg you had the innate intelligence to be the
strongest and most intelligent sperm to penetrate the ovum first. Once you
bored through that cell membrane you crossed the finish line into the egg
where your cell memory allowed you to grow into the beautiful baby human
that you were born as. This fact alone should give you the faith to believe in
yourself, your strength, your determination to succeed and your ability to succeed was already established since day one. If you body was powerful enough
to win that race you are powerful enough to do anything in this life that you
allow your mind to do.

You were born and still are an exceptionally strong and powerful being. Post
a reminder picture of a physically fit mentor or yourself when you were at your
most physically fit peak. Post these pictures on your refrigerator door, in your
car, on your bathroom mirror and on your front door so that you see it each day
before you start your day and each night before you go to bed. Remind yourself
constantly of how you want to look and feel. This is a mental exercise. Physical
exercise is important to your weight loss and permanent weight management. It
is an important part of the balanced lifestyle. Before beginning any new exercise
program, always see your doctor for medical clearance. Seek advice from your
physician if you are pregnant or nursing before beginning any exercise program.
There are many types of exercise, which target specific results.

Tips for exercise success:
Choose an exercise that you enjoy and that you can do on a daily basis
without skipping.
Know and accept that exercise is a mandatory part of staying slender
and physically fit.

THE BALANCE DIET & LIFESTYLE

Know that being active is the only way to achieve physical fitness and how important it is to get in the habit of being more active.
Join a gym, exercise or yoga class.

Exercise Commitment

If you cannot join a gym, make a commitment to yourself to stick to your personal exercise routine.
Recruit a reliable, dependable and accountable neighbor or friend as your exercise partner.
Have a weekly accountability meeting with your exercise partner to monitor your weekly results.
If your accountability partner is allowing you to slide without opposition, select a new partner.

"Mind-Body One-Step Miracle Exercises"

This powerfully effective exercise program that was designed to be a quick, effective and easy way to tighten and tone your entire body, while working every major muscle group. The Mind-Body Exercise Program targets "problem areas" with minimum stress to the joints and body. The Mind-Body Miracle Exercises consist of three ten-minute exercise routines that target all the major muscle groups in the body. These are designed to be safe and effective for healthy individuals. However, proper positioning is imperative to avoid strain and injury. It is recommended to seek counsel from your doctor or a qualified fitness trainer to insure proper form and positioning.

Exercise Caution: Avoid injury, always stretch, warm up and cool down. Do not bend your neck or back or apply pressure to the back of the head this keep the neck straight at all times during all of these exercises. Keep your toes straight ahead to reduce knee and plantar stress. If you notice any discomfort, stop. exercising and correct positioning before resuming any exercise. As with any exercise routine see your doctor for medical clearance before starting any new exercise routine. A fitness trainer may help to ensure proper positioning and help to maximize the effects of your exercise routine and help you avoid injury. Drink plenty of water to flush out lactic acid and reduce soreness from exercise.

Calculate your Light Aerobic and Maximum fat burning heart rate:

To calculate your specific fat burning light-aerobic heart rates, simply subtract your age from 170, this will give you your peak fat burning light-aerobic heart rate, to determine your fat burning light-aerobic heart rate subtract your age from 160 to calculate you maximum light-aerobic fat burning heart rate subtract your age from 170. To calculate your full capacity cardiovascular maximum aerobic heart rate subtract your age by 220. The maximum cardiovascular heart rate is not necessary for weight loss purposes and in fact can block fat metabolism if your heart rate exceeds your maximum-light aerobic fat burning heart rate, which is lower than your maximum full exertion cardiovascular aerobic heart rate. The least technical and most simple thing to remember is to keep your heart rate between 120 and 150 beats per minute to burn stored fat.

				Aerobic Max
Minimum & Maximum Light-Aerobic Fat Burning Heart Rate Ratios				
Heart Rate:	160	170	180	220
Age:	− 35	− 35	− 35	− 35
	125	135	145	195

MIND BODY DAILY STRETCH ROUTINE

Start by stretching to warm up the muscle groups and proper form and positioning is important to avoid strain or injury.

1) Start by standing feet shoulder width apart arms to the side and breathe in as you extend your arms into the air and exhale lowering your arms back down to your sides and release and relax your muscle tension and stress from your mind, body & spirit. Repeat 3 times.

2) Clasp your hands together and place them behind your neck. Gently bring your elbows together as you drop your head down. Feel the gentle stretch in your upper back. Open your elbows and arch your upper back forward, as you fully open up your chest up arching your middle back open to the universe and tilt your head upwards toward the heavens, breathe in all the energies of the universe as you inhale the breathe of life deep into your lungs. Feel the gentle stretch in your

THE BALANCE DIET & LIFESTYLE

upper back and diaphragm. Squeeze the shoulder blades toward each other, hold three seconds, exhale and release.

3) Bring one arm at a time above your head and bend at the waist reaching the opposite direction into the sky as you stretch and elongate your body as if you were growing toward the sky, tips the toe on the same side to deepen the side posture stretch. Switch sides and repeat the same procedure. Repeat 3 times.

4) Rotate your pelvis in a circular motion clockwise while adjusting your knees and loosening your joints in the lower back and extremities. Repeat the same motion counter-clockwise. Repeat 3 times.

5) Spread your legs and fold your upper body forward toward the earth as you bring your arms over your head and touch the ground. Raise the upper body up toward the sky bringing yourself up to a standing position with legs apart and arms apart in the air. Repeat 3 times.

6) With feet still apart and facing forward, twisting from your waist line twist your upper body to the right and hold for 3 seconds and then switch sides and twist your upper body to the left and hold for 3 seconds. Repeat 3 times.

7) Bring your feet together and stretch your shoulders and upper back by doing shoulder shrugs and rotations. Rotate the shoulders in a forward motion and a reverse rotation motion three times. Repeat 3 times.

8) Twist your upper body. Shake you lower body and legs and jiggle them vigorously to loosen up all the muscles in your lower body next jiggle your arms and upper body vigorously to loosen up all the muscles in your upper body. Jiggle the whole body together and and get the circulation going and the energy flowing. You are now ready to begin your Mind Body Exercise Routine. You may do either the morning or evening exercise routine of your choice, it is better if you rotate the routines to keep your exercise routine balanced. However, you must do at least one routine daily to loose weight. It is preferable that you do both. You will increase your rate and speed of weight loss by doing both and increase your fat and calorie burning potential.

The Mind-Body 30-Minute Morning Lite-Aerobic Exercise Routine

Aerobic exercise is like a magic anti-aging pill that slims your body quickly and beautifully. When doing the "Fast Walk-Jog" keep your heart rate between 120 and 150 to keep your body in the fat burning mode. Be careful not to over exert yourself or go into your maximum full aerobic state because it will stop your fat burning process. If you feel weak, faint or dizzy cease exercise immediately and resume at a slower pace after you feel better. Drink plenty of water during exercise.

Fast Walk-Jog

Begin by walking slow and steady for two minutes; gradually walk as fast as you can without running. At the eight minute mark, add a jog step into your walking pace, never allow the heart to go over 150, stay in fat burning mode, keep doing this up until the twelve minute mark. At the twelve minute mark, slow your pace back down to 120 beats per minute for two minutes, slow down to a fast walk for two minutes and then cool down by walking the last two minutes of exercise.

Cardio-Jumping Jacks

Begin by doing light and easy jumping jacks, jump up bringing your hands over your head while spreading your feet apart in the jump. Next, jump back with your feet together bringing your arms back down to your side. Do this for four minutes then as you continue on the four-minute mark add the following movement on the down jumping jack. On the down, bend your knees going into a squat and pulling your arms down to the front of your body bending your arms at the elbow while you clench your fist and pull them down to your sides as you squeeze and tighten the muscles in your arms, chest, shoulders and upper body. Do this until the four minute mark and resume doing light jumping jacks for the cool down. Stretch the body and shake-out tight muscles to relax the body after your workout.

The Mind-Body 30-Minute Night Time Anaerobic Exercise Routine

After becoming familiar with your regular exercise routine, you may add weight for the additional effect of weight bearing exercise. This will increase your results and the effect of the exercises. Adding weights to your exercise routine, quickly reduces body fat, adds more muscle definition and helps the body tone while producing lean muscle mass and bone. For quicker results, you may add weight to your routine by using wrist and ankle weights or dumb bells according to your strength. Start with the lowest weight and gradually work your way up to higher weights. These exercises are beneficial in conditioning the major muscle groups.

THE BALANCE DIET & LIFESTYLE

It is recommended for weight loss to do a daily minimum of 3 sets of 10 repetitions and gradually build up to 3 sets of 20 repetitions over time. The amount of repetitions vary depending on the age and fragility of the individual.

Older and frailer individuals should start with one set of 10 repetitions, and gradually work up to three sets of 10. Healthy beginners should do 1 set of 15 repetitions and work their way up to 3 sets of 15 Healthy Individuals should do no less than 3 sets of 20 repetitions and work their way into more until the point of fatigue. The first step is to choose the exercise that is right for you, according to your health and abilities. You should exercise a minimum of 30-45 minutes 3 to 5 times per week. In order to burn stored fat we have to reach a target heart rate of 120 beats per minute and not exceed 150 beats per minute in order for our exercise to burn stored fat. If we exceed this rate, the fat burning process shuts down. Avoid pushing yourself too hard during the work out because exceeding the "fat burning heart rate" will sabotage the fat burning action of the body by exceeding the fat burning zone.

Calories Burned Based on 30 Minutes of Activity

Based on a 30 minute time frame:
Weight Training-burns off between 160-200 calories depending on the exercise.
Walking – at 4 miles per hour burns 240 calories.
Brisk Walking – at 5 miles per hour burns 290 calories.
Jogging – at 6 miles per hour burns 316 calories.
Running – at 7 miles per hour burns 400 calories.
Cycling – at 10 miles per hour burns 200 calories.
Step Aerobics – burns approximately 300 calories.
Fast Swimming – burns off 300 calories
Kick-Boxing-400 calories.
Fast Dancing-350 calories
Moderate Ballet Dancing-290 calories
Slow Dancing – 175 calories
Sexual Activity – 100-400 calories (varies greatly depending on several factors)

It is very important during weight loss, to exercise at least 30 minutes to an hour daily. Swimming is a very good exercise for weight loss and is a form of resistance exercise. Walking, Jogging or Running are all excellent forms of exercise for weight loss and is one of the most slimming of all exercises.

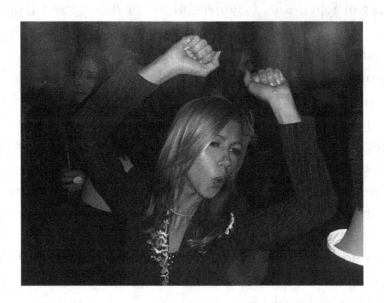

Dance

A timeless and fun activity that makes a great exercise is dance. Pick an activity that you truly enjoy doing, take a dance class. Don't be afraid to try something new. If you want to be inspired by dance go see River Dance. No one expects you to be as talented as Dancing with the stars or Michael Flatley, the Irish Lord of the Dance. But the fact is dance classes are fun and there is a wide array available from salsa, hip-hop, disco, tango, swing or even clogging choose the style that you are most comfortable with. Any dance that keeps your feet moving and gets your circulation going will work.

Get your dancing shoes on! Do it for fitness and do it for fun. You can do it alone or do it in groups so therefore; it is inspiring and offers group support which is very motivating. Dancing burns off a lot of calories slims the body beautifully and lifts the spirit. To avoid injury, a professional dance instructor or personal fitness trainer can help design a program that is right for you. Personal fitness trainers are not just for the rich, famous, they can help you design an individualized personal fitness program that is right for you, and it is worth the investment.

While exercising keep in mind how the body works to produce fuel for energy during exercise, during endurance activity, is that nitrogen is removed from the branched chain amino acids and converted to alanine. Alanine is then transported though the blood stream, from the muscle to the liver where it is converted to glucose. The liver then returns glucose back into the muscle in effort to supply the energy to fuel and increase power and performance. Glutamine and Arginine are considered essential during metabolic stress. Glutamine is the primary carrier of nitrogen to skeletal muscle and other tissues. It boosts protein synthesis, helps buffer lactic acid buildup that occurs during exercising. It also reduces central nervous system fatigue. Several studies have shown that the arginine plays a key role in stimulating the release of anabolic hormones that promote muscle formation. It is also a precursor to nitric oxide, which promote healthy blood vessels. These amino acids are important in the building, the growth and recovery of the muscle. You can get these amino's in balanced form from consuming protein.

Body Mass and Weight Index Chart

Body mass index, or BMI, is a term known to most people. However, it is the measurement of choice for many physicians and researchers studying obesity. BMI uses a mathematical formula that takes into account both a person's height and Weight. BMI equals a person's weight in kilograms divided by Height in meters squared. (BMI=kg/m2). A slight variance is acceptable for hereditary compensation for the very thin or larger boned people.

A BMI of 22-27 is normal for people age 45-54
A BMI of 23-28 is normal for people age55-65
A BMI of up to 29 is normal for people over 65.
According to the BMI scale
Healthy weight – BMI from 18.5 up to 25
Overweight-BMI from 25 up to 30
Obese – BMI 30 or Higher-Clinically overweight

Healthy Cosmetic BMI Range, weight gains can carry health risk for adults.		
Height	Weight	BMI Range
4'10	91-117	18-20 BMI

Healthy Cosmetic BMI Range, weight gains can carry health risk for adults.		
5'	102-117	19-22 BMI
5'5	119-137	20-23 BMI
6'	148-170	18-24 BMI
6'4	156-204	21-25 BMI

THE MIND BODY AFTER EXERCISE YOGA FLEXIBILITY WARM UP & COOL DOWN

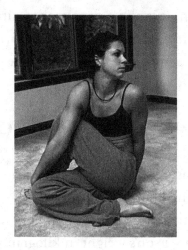

Mind Body Yoga Program

Yoga originated as a integral part of Mind Body Medicine as it is a major aspect in Ayurvedic and Yogic living practices. Yoga is also a form of strength training as most poses allow you to hold the muscle in one pose and then assume a different pose that allows the previous muscle to relax before going back into the first pose. Yoga tightens and tones the skin after weight loss. Yoga soothes the Mind, Body and Spirit. Yoga allows you to focus on what you intend to achieve in a meditative way during each yoga session. Yoga internalizes an awareness of good posture, health and healing in your daily life. Yoga helps you to find your center, focus your mind in your body and breathe each moment in deeply and teaches you present mind consciousness. During yoga you concentrate on the present moment and push away thoughts of the past and future. During your complete yoga session you will remain in a meditative healing state of mind and focus on your breathing throughout your whole yoga session.

THE BALANCE DIET & LIFESTYLE

Yoga is a healing practice with many great health benefits. Yoga really helps to tone the muscle and can be an important part of your weight loss program. The optimal level of obtainable flexibility though the practice of yoga is determined by individual factors. The longer you practice yoga the more accumulated results can be seen. Yoga is good for most everyone. The exercise intensity level is of mild discomfort and can be incorporated into your weight loss exercise program 2-3 days per week. There are yoga classes that you can enroll in to practice in a group. There are many types of Yoga; most of them are excellent for weight loss and weight management. Some particular poses work very well in slimming problem areas. Yoga is effective against stubborn cellulite. Yoga is an excellent alternative form of healing that is very suited to the needs of thyroid patients. For beginners, yoga's gentle stretching and emphasis on breathing can be done by almost anyone, and reaps immediate rewards in terms of energy, reduction of stress levels, flexibility and reduction of muscle and joint stiffness, and much more in terms of peace of mind and general harmony. Practicing yoga is an excellent way to tone muscles, eliminate aches and pains, dramatically reduce stress, increase oxygen and help breathing. While I have also tried to do aerobic exercise, I have found that I look forward to yoga unlike aerobics! And very quickly have very rapid results from practicing even a few times a week. For me, and for many others, yoga is much more than exercise it is brings the mind, body, and spirit into balance. I would recommend finding a good yoga class if you can, but you can also start with a home video such as the Mind Body Weight Loss Yoga Video. Yoga as an exercise increases flexibility. Flexibility refers to the range of motion or joint mobility. Yoga is excellent to help stretch and lengthen the muscle. It is important for any training program to include stretching because it warms up the muscles to help prevent injury. Yoga is useful in increasing flexibility to the spine and can help you maintain youthful mobility. As we age it is common for our body to develop a decrease in flexibility or hypo mobility due to a decrease in activity. If we make it a habit to practice yoga on a regular basis, we can maintain the flexibility of our youth. Yoga helps to prevent shortening of muscle tendons that are a result from inactivity, muscular asymmetry, age and disease. The regular practice of yoga can be considered as prevention from sprain/strain and hyperextension type injury because Yoga increases flexibility in healthy muscle and ligament tonus and improves joint flexibility.

Yoga Preparation and Stretches

Caution: receive a medical clearance before performing any exercise program. Always seek proper Asana positions by a certified yoga instructor to avoid injury.

While sitting in yoga pose, in a open-legged sitting position, bring soles of feet together, rest your wrist on your legs, arms open, shoulders straight, maintain good posture and relax your body and mind. Focus your mind and attentions on your breathing focus and concentration of your intent. Focus on what you intend to achieve in each yoga session. Internalize an awareness of good posture, health and healing in your daily life. Find your center, focus your mind in your body and breathe this moment in deeply as you concentrate on the present moment and push away thoughts of the past and future. During your complete yoga session remain in this meditative healing state of mind and focus on your breathing throughout your whole yoga session.

On the floor, in the yoga pose, place right hand on left knee as you twist your torso and gently stretch your mid-lower back. Hold three seconds, rotate and switch sides and repeat.

Clasp your hands together and place them behind your neck. Gently bring your elbows together as you drop your head down. Feel the gentle stretch in your upper back. Open your elbows and arch your upper back forward, as you fully open up your chest up arching your middle back open to the universe and tilt your head upwards toward the heavens, breathe in all the energies of the universe as you inhale the breathe of life deep into your lungs. Feel the gentle stretch in your upper back and diaphragm. Squeeze the shoulder blades toward each other, hold three seconds, exhale and release.

Laying flat on your back bringing your knees to the right or left side on the opposite side, turn your neck to the opposite side of your lower trunk. Feel the gentle stretch down your sides and into your lower back switch sides and repeat.

Laying flat on your back, bring your knees into your chest, fold your arms around your knees and squeeze your legs into your chest.

Laying in fetal pose on your back. Arch your body upwards onto your shoulders and extend your legs, touching your toes to the floor over your head, hold for three seconds, flex toes inward stretching the back and hamstrings and then release, repeat three times.

THE BALANCE DIET & LIFESTYLE

Sarvanga Yoga Poses

Sarvanga are excellent poses to aid in weight loss but also are good for many purposes. In Ayurveda, "Sarva" means the whole, "Anga" means body. Hence, the "Sarvanga" is the whole body. The name means that the whole body benefits from these poses.

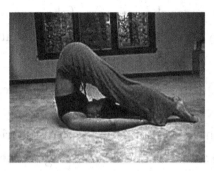

Regan's illustration gives you a visualization of the final pose.

Sarvangasan Yoga Pose for Improved Metabolism

Known as sarvangasan and pronounced simply, "Asana". The benefits of this pose are numerous. It helps with digestion, metabolism and weight loss, good posture, organ drainage, infections, hypertension, thyroid, sleeplessness, shortness of breath, constipation, urinary disorders, strength and balance.

Postural Instructions for the Asana Pose

Lay flat on your back
Keep your legs together
Raise up your legs, bend the knee push feet into air.
Balance weight onto your shoulders, head and elbows.
Use your arms to balance & support your body weight and hips.
Straighten your legs in the air feet pointing to the sky.
Tuck your chin into your chest
Rest the weight of your body on your shoulders and elbows

Hold Yoga poses for as long as 3 minutes. Relax and repeat up to 3 times

Always seek proper positioning from a certified yoga instructor to avoid injury. Not intended for people with neck problems or other weakness or injury. Not recommended for pregnant or menstruating women.

Downward Dog – Stand spread eagle, all arms and legs apart, bend knees slightly and lean forward inverting your upper body while touching your fingertips to the floor and come up on your tip toes raise your buttocks toward the sky as you straighten your knees, do not lock the knees in place. Drop your head forward between your arms and feel the reverse gravity in your internal organs as your spine lengthens releasing pressure. This helps purge the contents of the organs stimulates the nervous, digestive and visceral systems and speeds metabolic waste removal. Hold for a few minutes stand upright and release.

Ayurvedic Bow – On all fours, lean forward and keep your knees on the ground, press your elbows close to your ribs as you slightly bend them, supporting the weight of your upper body with the triceps. This is similar to a push up. The toes are straight then flexed gripping the ground and the buttocks are tight supporting the lower back as you arch your mid back toward the ground and tilt your head upward looking into the sky. Imagine a cat stretching forward and then reverse in a humping motion arching the upper back up toward the sky while dropping the head forward between the upper arms down toward the ground. The rhythmic pumping motion gets the organs and circulation flowing to stimulate metabolism.

The alternating intervals that yoga produces, allows the muscle to utilize the hold and relax technique that is beneficial in increasing muscle tone. A Yoga for Weight Loss video is a useful guided yoga exercise routine for home use.

Yoga and Meditation are exercises of the mind and body. Exercise is an important part of a healthy lifestyle. It is only natural that Mind Body Medicine will now play a powerful role in the future of weight loss and weight management with integrative medicine now coming to the forefront of healthcare. The Balance Diet & Mind Body Weight Loss Program fulfills the public interest in natural healthcare, when the demand for legitimate alternatives is at an all time high. Weight control has become our most pressing issue in healthcare, today. Both overweight and obesity lead to disease and they are both due to imbalance within the Mind and the Body that require adopting a healthier lifestyle which includes exercises of the Mind and Body.

CHAPTER 10

Therapies & New Medical Treatments For Weight Loss

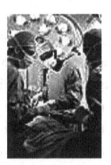

Medical Weight Loss, Bariatric & Plastic Surgery

IT IS AMAZING WHAT MODERN MEDICINE CAN DO. SOMETIMES, WE have problem areas that seem to stay fat no matter what we do, even after we lose weight. A few surgical procedures may be considered in treating these problem areas once your weight loss goal has been achieved. Lasers, Far Infra-Red, Intense Pulse Light, Pico, Micro & Nano-Currents, Ultra-Sound and Radio-Frequencies; It all sounds like a Star-Trek episode, but the face of Aesthetic medicine is changing at the speed of rocket-science and there are some wonderful new non-surgical procedures. However, Surgery is the only method to achieve dramatic and permanent results. There are always risks involved when it comes to surgery. Under properly qualified skilled care, the risk is greatly diminished. Check the surgeon's credentials, before and after photos and record of accomplishment and ask about aftercare programs to ensure your safety. The more invasive the procedure the greater the risk involved. However, these are a few of the most popular procedures.

Laser Skin Tightening – After weight loss skin may sag and there are new non-surgical medical laser procedures that may help improve the appearance of sagging skin. Laser is a frequency of light. Many new therapies are light based.

Liposuction & Body Sculpturing & Lifts – Are types of surgical and non-surgical procedures which allows the Physician or health professional to either, topically or invasivelyinsert a candela and break up stubborn fatty deposits to be sucked out by vacuum or to lift and tack up or cut away sagging skin and permanently remove it, after extreme weight loss. Sometimes ultra sound is used to melt fat and tighten the skin around the area of fat loss however; sometimes tissue removal may be necessary to achieve the desired results. Surgical lifts may be needed after a rapid or major loss of weight. There is some degree of risk Involved, such as swelling, blood clots or numbness in the treated area. Healing time and final results can take up to one year to be seen. However, most people who resort to these treatment are usually happy with the results. Regardless, healthy diet and exercise are always important part of a healthy lifestyle to maintain and to achieve the best final result.

Mesotherapy Injections – fat dissolving injections that contain homeopathic medicines, high amounts of B-6, artichoke extract, or phospysydilcholine in a fat dissolving solution. Since it is a cocktail ingredients may vary. This can be a painful procedure this varies according to the individual's pain tolerance. Sometimes there is a reaction immediately following the injection. It can be a painful procedure, the pain level peaks within ten minutes after the injection and subsides over time. However, many report satisfactory results after the swelling subsides and a decrease in measurement at the injection site. This process can take two weeks to a month and may require a series of weekly injections until the desired results are received. Itching or rash is a rare side effect.

Anti-Aging & HGH Injections – Human growth hormone and other some other anti-aging type injections have been shown to increase fat metabolism, weight loss and to renew youthful muscle tone and in some cases, reverse signs of aging. These are effective forms of anti-aging medicine and these injections are under anti-aging specialist or doctor's supervision only, within the United States. Caution and blood monitoring should be used to detect and decrease the risk of possible adverse side effects. It is a good idea to take an anti-antigenic and anti-angiogenic substance, which blocks apoptosis when using this approach to weight loss for additional precautionary care.

Stomach Banding, Stomach Implants, Stomach Bypass & Bariatric Surgery – for obese patients with a few other health risk such as heart attack or cardiovascular disease. This is for patients who are over 30% over their body mass index ratio. Some people just seem to be unable to lose their weight any other way. When there is a risk of death due to grossly, excessive weight and obesity there are safer surgical options available. Newer and updated versions of theses types of surgery are available at your doctors' discretion and usually the risk involved is less than the risk of remaining grossly obese. One must always make lifestyle changes and take nutritional supplements and vitamins after this procedure because it can affect nutrient absorption or cause nutritional deficiencies.

Bariatric Care – Many people need help from their doctor to lose weight. The medical weight loss experts are called bariatric doctors. If you are severely overweight or obese it is considered a disease and it is a good idea for your medical doctor and his nurse to supervise your weight loss program. Especially, while on medication for co-morbidities or obesity related diseases, which are the number one killers of Americans. Regular check-ups are important and necessary in the early detection of adverse reactions or complications. Your doctor may find it to be a medical necessity for laboratory testing to analyze your general state of health prior to beginning your diet or exercise regimen. Your doctor may find that it is important to order blood, urine and saliva test to diagnosis any underlying conditions and to determine your quality of health before suggesting that it is beneficial to your health to begin a weight loss program. Bariatric physicians specialize in obesity. If you are excessively overweight, you may be a candidate for bariatric surgery. It is recommended that you visit a bariatric specialist for an evaluation before beginning any new diet and exercise program if you are obese.

Medical Weight Loss Plans – The Balance Diet and Lifestyle, is the foundation of the Clinical Mind Body Weight Loss Program, which is a multiple disciplinary approach to weight loss involving health professionals such as medical doctors, nurses, psychologist, physical therapist, exercise physiologist and dieticians/nutritionist. It is patient care weight loss program that utilizes unique teaching tools and it is available in many international medical sites and doctors' offices as a foundational part of their medical weight loss treatment plan. It is used to help patients achieve healthy weight loss goals in a medical and support group setting. The Mind Body Weight Loss Program is only available in certified Mind Body Weight Loss Centers, ask your doctor if they are in the Mind Body network as these medical sites are the only sites who provide this weight loss program, it is a healthy lifestyle training program and it is considered to be medical when provided under a medical doctor's care.

The more invasive the surgical procedure, the higher the risk factor which range from minimal to moderate and sometimes serious risk may be involved. Some surgeries may not be successful, resulting in a second surgery. It is usually not the doctors' fault, it is usually because the patient changed the body without changing the mind and tried to continue the same eating habits as before, or from trying to eat solid foods, too quickly, not allowing the body to heal from the surgery which can cause a tear in the incision that caused a need for a second procedure. However, patients lose weight, but, some patients gain back the weight because of a lack of proper aftercare or due to needed behavior modification that wasn't available or provided. If the advantages outweigh the health risk, surgery may be a good option for chronic or morbidly obese individuals who are already at risk for sudden death but who are stable enough to undergo

THE BALANCE DIET & LIFESTYLE

surgery. Most people state that whenever possible they preferred to make every alternative option before resorting to Invasive procedures, in the same regards it is recognized that sometimes there are a need for these procedures and effective results can be quickly obtained when otherwise it would be impossible without surgery. For more information, contact a specialist in these fields for a consultation to find out if you are a candidate for surgical procedures. Most doctors in the field of medicine, now, recognize the importance of diet and lifestyle in helping to provide better patient outcomes and satisfaction along with medical care or surgical procedures and now offer aftercare programs such as Mind Body Health programs.

Body Balancing Techniques & Mind Balancing Therapies

Postural Awareness

Good posture is important to the organs and digestive processes of the body. When we have poor posture the organs are being crunched up inside. It is important to keep the shoulders straight, chin up and spine erect so that the pressure of our weight is not cutting off visceral circulation and nerve flow from the spine and the spinal nerves to the organ systems. The sympathetic, parasympathetic nervous systems and the immune system run parallel within the body. The cardiovascular system regulates circulation. The digestive system is affected by improper posture. When we maintain good posture all of theses systems function in an optimum capacity. When we maintain proper posture it opens up the diaphragm so that we can breathe air in more deeply and it reduces the pressure and stagnation that may accumulate in the organ systems. Yoga and postural exercise may plan an important role in weight loss due to these factors.

Massage

Massage has been proven to reduce the site of cellulite in three to six sessions. Vibration Massage is quick and effective in smoothing the appearance of unsightly cellulite. Massage has always been a part of health care systems and has been around since pre-historic man, probably since the cave man stomped his toe, as the old saying goes. Massage increases circulation and filters out old cellular debris and toxins. Cleansing medicinal herbal poultices compliment massage in the loosening, breaking down and speeds the removal of cellulite.

In Ayurvedic Medicine, Garshan is the invigorating massaged useful for weight loss. A very fast paced massage is applied briskly to create friction on the surface of the skin. In Vishesh, increasing the subcutaneous circulation to assist in the breakdown and elimination of fats and cellulite formations. Instead of lotion or oils, the therapist wears raw silk gloves that leave the skin aglow with blood flow and increased circulation. Another effective Ayrvedic Massage is Vishesh. A firm, pump-type squeeze technique is designed to remove tough fat formations and deep toxins. This is a rather rough type massage that is not suited for everyone. There are also, a couple of aesthetic massage therapy devices on the market that combat the appearance of cellulite. The concept is to stimulate the area enough that the body's circulatory systems excrete the excess fluid through the urine/kidneys thus reducing the bloated appearance and revealing a smoother skin texture within a few Treatments. These types of treatments are valuable in reducing the appearance of cellulite. It is recommended that you have a few treatments as close together as possible until the desired result is achieved and then, receive one treatment per month throughout the summer months to maintain the results.

Structural and Spinal Alignment

A balanced structural system is imperative to any health and fitness program. Good posture and proper alignment of the bone and joints are crucial in maintaining the pain free level of health required to adhere to any exercise and fitness program. Neurologist, Orthopedic Physicians, Bone and Joint Specialist, Physical Therapist, Osteopathic Physicians, Cranial Sacral Therapist, Chiropractors, Podiatrist, Fitness Trainers, Yoga Instructors, Nurses, Doctors, Body Workers and Massage Therapist are integral part of maintaining health and wellness. They are an important and vital part of a balanced healthcare regimen. If you are in pain and cannot perform exercise due to discomfort, seek the help of a practitioner in one of these fields. However, if you are unable to find the relief you need through one of these do not hesitate to try another professional who can give you relief from pain. The discomfort of misalignment can interfere with your weight loss and exercise routines. Any therapy that keeps you in proper alignment and balance is good. Supports and orthotics, which absorb impact shock and reduce joint stress while balancing the body are important to help with proper posture and is important in maintaining good health and a healthy nervous system and helps enable one to exercise with ease.

THE BALANCE DIET & LIFESTYLE

Physical Therapy and Theraputic Modalities

Treatments which increase the circulation and metabolism of waste are good to aid in weight loss. The European culture have been know to utilize galvanic current to speed up fatty waste removal and cellulite. Sometimes using injectables or topical agents to speed up the process of elimination or to drive herbal tonics into the skin, by adjusting the machine settings to penetrate into the fat tissue layer using ultra-sound, galvanic current or needles, this is called ionto-phoresis or phono-phoresis. Micro current, interferential, ultrasound, hot and cold contrast therapy, submersion tanks, vibration massage or any therapy that gets the energy flow back into stagnant tissues can be beneficial for the break up of fatty tissue and weight loss. These treatments can only be preformed safely by qualified practitioners.

Reflexology

Reflexology is an ancient technique that can bring balance to the whole body including the organ systems. The science and art of reflexology originated more than 5,000 years ago by the ancient Indian's. However, the Chinese were using a similar therapy. And yet, there is other evidence linking yet another form of the ancient art as far back as the Egyptians! Dr. Fitzgerald, an American physician, developed the western reflexology in 1902, when he noticed the value of pressure in relieving pain during surgical procedures, he named it ZONE therapy which was further perfected by Eunice's Ingram who tweaked the therapy into the zone therapy we know today commonly used on the feet known as foot re-flexology. Reflexology is applied pressure, performed on reflex points on the feet, hands and ears. When performed professionally and properly, it has a positive effect on a broad range of health problems.

Reflexology Tips

1. Reflexology is usually performed with out lubricant; however, adding oil makes for a really nice foot massage at the end of your reflexology session.
2. Make sure nails are clipped before palpating the site
3. Note positive stress cues (unusual roughness)
4. Apply the same degree of pressure to each reflex point when examining and treating an affected area.

The reflexology points are located at specific sites on the feet, hands and ears. For weight-loss and maximizing digestion, metabolism and eliminating toxins, and when aiding the body in the break down of fats, and for the removal of fatty deposits, the following reflex points should be worked as often as possible: Thyroid, Liver, Stomach, Small Intestine, Pancreas, Adrenal Glands, Kidney, the descending & sigmoid colon reflex points on the whole body. Should you notice a "positive stress que" or hardness in any of these areas? The area should be worked at least once daily. You can do this yourself, however, you should be certain that you have made the right contact point on the reflexology map correlating to your feet. Take special notice that some points can be wrongly manipulated. If you are not 100% confident with locating the proper point, it is better suggested to seek reflexology therapy from a trained professional, which you will be glad you did. You can learn from their skills and they will usually point of the exact location of positive stress cue areas, and offer some personal reflexology techniques you may use at home.

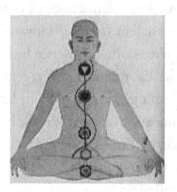

Marma Balancing
In Indian Ayurvedic Medicine, the Marma are the nerve root centers of life and good health. The Marma consist of one hundred and seven nerve conjunctions. It is important to prevent interference and imbalance from occurring in the Marmas. While in a weight loss or in any restorative health process because the Marmas provide the link between body and mind. According to ancient medical teachings, which are still practiced today in Ayurvedic medicine, if the Marmas become blocked or imbalanced, it may create emotional as well as physical illness. Deep pressure is applied to Marma points to purge them and injury to the Marmas, should be avoided completely, as adverse effects and illness, both emotionally and physically are sure to be set into motion. There are three major

THE BALANCE DIET & LIFESTYLE

Marma points, between the eyes similar to the third eye position on a Charkas chart. At the base of the sternum similar to the heart charka point and the third Marma is below the navel area in the abdomen which is similar to the there are also, important Marma points located on the soles of the feet, similar to reflexology or zone therapy. All Marma points are usually tender. Marma therapy can be quite uncomfortable due to this fact. The Marmas differ from acupuncture points in that they are connected directly with the nervous system are broad spectrum and very deep, unlike surface acupuncture points, Marmas cover larger areas.

Marma balancing can be achieved by practicing one of your weight loss exercises, such as, yoga, walking, stretching, swimming or alternatively by massage. Therapeutically, massage can be the performed at home or by an experienced therapist. A good daily self massage routine ensures constant rebalancing. Of course, you should use a good quality herbal detoxifying or cleansing oil such as sesame, clary sage, myrrh, or Mind Body Topical Weight Loss Gel/Oil. Remember to stimulate the points for at least three to five minutes.

Chinese Medicine & Acupuncture

For over 5,000 years, in China, herbal medicines, acupuncture and massage have been used to stimulate digestion and to maintain a healthy weight by restoring Qi. Qi is pronounced Chee. Unlike western or traditional medicine, in Chinese medicine the goal is to bring balance to the whole being. Qi is the perfect balance in the bodies energy flow to the bodily functions, the emotions and in sync with the energies of the earth. Qi is the energies between the five elements air, water, earth, wood and fire. The two opposite forces in the world, which are Yin & Yang.

Yin	Yang
Feminine	Masculine
Negative	Positive
Passive	Aggressive
Sedentary	Active
Cold	Hot
Dark	Light

It is recommended to balance the five elements in your environment. You should have all five present to avoid an imbalance of overpowering energy in your environment. Acupuncture is used to balance the bodies vital energy by placing burning herbal preparations called moxibustion to create heat in the needles that are inserted into the skin at the acupuncture sites along the meridians to channel energy and restore Qi flow and correct imbalance or disharmony within the body. According to Chinese numerology, it is possible to inherit an imbalance by being born where there is a missing element in your astrological chart. If this occurs then you must add the missing element to your environment. Say if you were missing a wood and water element, it can help to correct the imbalance with Feng Shui. You would create an area in your environment that you could spend time in to bring those energies into balance. An example to balance the missing wood element, you could bring a tree into your home or cover the walls and ceiling with wood paneling. You could have a fountain, hot tub, or aquarium to bring the water element energy into your life. A candle or fireplace can add fire energy. Wind chimes and fans can bring balance in the air element. To balance the earth element you can use crystals and minerals. This brings balanced energy to the environment to accommodate healing energies for the person dwelling in the environment. It is important to create a supportive healing environment that accommodates your weight management goals, internally and externally.

Detoxifying Therapies – Everyone should cleanse with some form of therapeutic detoxification therapy on a regular basis to keep the body invigorated and functioning at a maximum capacity. There are many environmental toxins and bad diet factors to justify utilizing therapeutic practices to achieve effective weight loss success. Sluggishness and Toxicity hinder weight loss. Eliminating stagnation in the organs, glands, cells and tissues are especially important, while on a weight loss program. Detoxifying treatments are required when maximizing the removal and elimination of metabolic waste from the body. When we are losing weight, we need to use some method of detoxify the body on a daily basis. There are many options for detoxifying therapeutic practices. Detoxifying the body can release toxins from the stored fat, where, metabolic waste and toxic residues are stored.

THE BALANCE DIET & LIFESTYLE

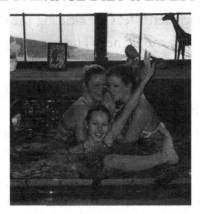

Invigorate Your Body & Mind With Cleansing & Balancing Therapies
Taking relaxing baths are a simple way of detoxifying the body of impurities. By adding herbs or essential nutrients to the bath, you can target specific toxins to detoxify them from your body. The Romans and Greeks perfected bathhouses and spas. They practiced skin brushing and beating with olive branches, this sounds harsher than it actually is. This practice increases circulation in areas of fatty deposits. The lack of circulation is culprit in having areas that are prone to fatty accumulations. Sluggish tissues lack energy and vitality these treatments help energize your system. Another option which makes a nice equivalent modern day practice, is to use a bundle of fresh rosemary branches tied to gather and lightly spank problem areas when the skin is softest while wet in the bath until reddening of the skin occurs and a nice, warm tingle is achieved. It is also, beneficial to add a few drops of essential oils of rosemary to the bath because it is one of the best essential oils for weight loss. Toxic conditions should be eliminated within the body detoxification is necessary in maintaining good health, optimum digestion and in achieving weight loss. Detoxification involves purging the body's excretory systems, or eliminative systems, which consist of the colon, the lungs, the liver, the kidneys and the skin. These extensive cleansing rituals are achieved by using, Natural or Medical detoxification therapies and treatments. These treatments are designed to purge the body of toxins and waste products that are affecting, interfering with or slowing down the metabolic rate of the body. Detoxification speeds up waste removal within the body. One of the best approaches to the detoxification process is of course, internal cleansing. Fat is solid waste. Solid waste has to be eliminated by the liver and come out through the bowel. A good liver and colon cleanse is usually necessary. There are several nice herbal hepatic cleanse treatments on the

market, there are several nice detox teas for clearing the liver as well. There are also organ clearing Homeopathic medicines. The main organ to filter out fat is the liver. It filters out the fat and regulates fat metabolism.

By soaking the body in substances such as Epsom salts can rid the body of lactic acid buildup which ease sore muscles after over exertion. You should not use the bleach in hot tubs or Jacuzzis, as the vapors can be toxic if inhaled. These are basic home remedies. However, in extreme cases a physician may be required to assist in treatments. Physicians usually assist in procedures such as, Intravenous Chelation Therapy, Bio Toxic Reduction Therapy or there are some new Homeovitic Medicine Flushes of Heavy Metals and some new oral Chelation options, now available through natural health practitioners that are much less invasive and that work wonderfully. The following are some of the most effective and simplest forms of therapeutic detoxification practices. Always rinse residues from the skin with a fresh shower after any detox soak. In addition, drink plenty of steam distilled water during and afterwards.

Medical Spas, Salons, Day Spas and Health Resorts

Check with these facilities to determine what is available. There are plethora of body treatments, skincare and therapeutic choices available depending on your needs and desires. Salons & Day Spas are quick, easy to book into and offer more of a pampering type setting and involve skin care and image consulting in some instances. Medical Spas offer much of the same but offer more invasive and comprehensive procedures such as facial fillers. The Medical spa setting is usually more clinical and based on health care treatment protocols; such as laser procedures some are even covered by insurances, if a licensed physician supervises them. Health Resorts and Retreats are very beneficial when you need an interruption from your lifestyle to make the necessary behavior modifications. In Health Resorts, all consumable meals and drinks are usually prepared for you and food intake is controlled. Individual and group therapy meetings are part of the program and wonderful relaxing therapies are part of the daily regimen. Resorts take you away from the environment that may be sabotaging your self–help plan. This can be a beneficial experience, as it demonstrates how you should be eating, thinking and feeling in a healthy living environment. Having this experience allows you to mimic the regimen after you return home as it gives you a healthy structured lifestyle example.

THE BALANCE DIET & LIFESTYLE

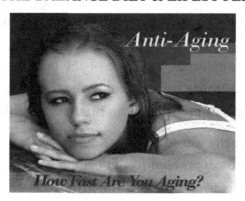

There are many different types of therapeutic treatments that are beneficial in weight loss and weight management. These treatments are good for children and adults that are battling weight loss. This section is dedicated to several of the most effective therapeutic treatment modalities that are easily available. There are too many to list them all. this is a general overview of some of the effective treatments available for use during weight loss and weight management.

THERAPEUTIC TREATMENTS FOR WEIGHT LOSS

Water – is of course the most cleansing, purifying substance on the planet. Pure Steam Distilled Water is by far the first and foremost of importance in any cleansing or detoxification process. Fasting and Juicing are a close second. Enemas and High Colonics are more invasive and should be used as well. Then of course, there are special diets and medicinal herbal cleansing supplements and teas, which should be consumed on a regular basis.

Heated Hydrotherapy – induces sweating. The skin is of course the largest excretory organ. A lot, of toxins can be eliminated through the skin. Hot Cleansing Baths with a variety of particular herbs suited for the individual's toxic condition and sea salts or Baking Soda baths are ideal, as well.

"Infra Red Saunas – boost the immune system and are detoxifying to the body. There are infrared versions on the market that only heat up the body core instead of the old coal method that heats the air in the sauna, making it difficult to breathe. The far infra-red sauna has been proven to speed up fat metabolism, helping to burn stored fat and break up stubborn fatty deposits and also to increase lymph and hemoglobin counts in the blood, inducing a controlled, fever response in the body's natural healing mechanisms. This type of "Hyperthermia Detoxification Therapy" has even proven to be useful in the treatment of cancer; yet, it is so safe that hospitals use it to warm premature babies.

<u>Sun-Bathing</u> – usually stimulates sweating, this is very naturally detoxifying. You should protect yourself from burning with an umbrella if necessary. The purpose is to induce sweating, not to burn the skin. You can sweat under an umbrella or tree. However, direct sunlight for a limited amount of time, is healthy for you. Providing vitamin D and other positive stellar influences on the natural bio-rhythms of the body. Sunbathing is not recommended for more than two hours if you have a base tan and as little as fifteen minutes when health reasons do not permit extended sunbathing. Therefore, exposure times vary by skin type and from person to person. Always be sensible in the sun and avoid over exposure. Never over expose yourself or allow your skin to burn in the sun.

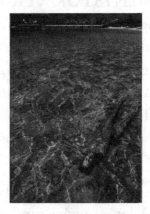

<u>Water Flotation</u> – Studies in the U.S. Navy show that floating in water increases the Mind Body Connection. This was discovered in submersion vessels during test on sub-marine studies.

<u>Body Wraps and Herbal Poultices</u> – Body wraps are a similar concept as the minerals detoxify waste products and toxins from the body. Seaweed body wraps are a commonly used beauty treatment helping people loose inches instantly. Instant inches lost are usually from sweating out toxins from bloated tissue which is carrying toxic water retention. However, it has been documented through the ARE in Virginia Beach that Edgar

Cayce a famous holistic healer, recommended people to apply castor oil packs mixed with herbs to draw toxins out of the body and break up dead cell debris and excess tissue formations inside the body. Many people have followed his instruction and had miraculous recovery of symptoms. Today, people still follow the holistic health plans that Cayce channeled in during hypnosis. The Cayce recommendations have proven to be quite effective.

<u>Aesthetic Cellulite Massage</u> – Uses a suction device that has been clinically tested and proven to reduce the appearance of cellulite and unsightly bulges. It helps to break up hardened areas of accumulated fat. It separates the adipose tissue from the epidermis to minimize the appearance of cellulite; it is especially beneficial to smooth the orange peel and dimpling effects of cellulite.

<u>Exercise is detoxifying to the body. Exercise creates sweating. Sweating is an effective form of detoxification. Exercise is crucial to detoxification and is necessary in any weight loss program. It is a wonderful way to push toxins out of the tissues and to speed up the removal of metabolic waste. The sweating response is the body cleansing in itself. Exercise is probably the best way to trigger this response and is one of the only ways to burn stored fat. Exercise is imperative, because you have to use more than you consume to loose weight, exercise uses stored fat and converts it into beautiful radiant energy.</u>

<u>Vibration Massage</u> – Is a therapy device, which creates a vibration that increases the circulation and removal of metabolic waste, including excess bloating and fat in the tissues. Is considered a form of massage therapy. It increases the blood flow and creates a red glow to the skin, bringing blood and nutrients into the tissue being stimulated. It is good for breaking up accumulated fatty deposits and helps tighten and tone the skin after weight loss.

<u>Compresses and Body Wraps</u> – In many cultures in European Spas and Sweden Seaweed solutions soaked in cloth and wrapped in fatty areas have shown to reduce water weight gain. Mineral Mud clay mask, coffee wraps and cayenne pepper are all noted to have benefits in cellulite

reduction. The clairvoyant, Edgar Cayce recommended castor oil packs and herbal medicinal to break up excess tissue formations and growths which proved to be effective on many occasions.

Aromatherapy – Aromatherapy is the essences of essential oils from botanical sources. These all-natural fragrances hold powerful properties, which are of a medicinal nature and can be useful in your weight loss program. The following are only a few that aid in digestion and fat metabolism. They can be used in the bath or in body preparations.

Essential Oils For Weight Loss

Peppermint – is a wonderful digestive tonic. It is stimulating to the skin to increase circulation and the removal of toxins as well that it is energizing. Sniff a few drops before a workout exercise to rejuvenate and energize! Make a cup of peppermint tea and sip while breathing the energizing vapors

Castor Oil – dissolves abnormal accumulations within the body.

Juniper – is a good cellulite tonic; they use the berries to make gin, which was once beloved to be a cure all in England.

Lemon – is closest to our own digestive enzymes and is good to shift cellulite.

Geranium – is good to stimulate the lymphatic system and rid the body of excess toxins and fats.

Rosemary – is excellent for the liver and lowering cholesterol levels and aids to metabolize fats. It is also good for the gallbladder and aids in digestion.

Oregano – aids in digestion breaks down and helps digest fats in Italian foods

Dill – Aids in digestion and can be blended with cucumbers applied to the body and wrapped with cellophane wrap as a detoxifying treatment.

Hot Stone Therapy – Stimulates the Immune System and Speeds Metabolic Waste Removal

Lymphatic Drainage – is a massage technique to stimulate the body's deep healing potential. It encourages the elimination of toxins and edema. It is a pumping technique, which promotes increased lymph flow and waste removal throughout the body. It is a wonderful therapy to help tighten and tone the skin as you loose weight especially on the face, chin and neck. Lymphatic Drainage is also good for stretch marks or from being overweight. Sagging skin can often can be improved or diminished in appearance with Lymphatic Drainage. It helps reduce the appearance of cellulite, usually the spongy orange peel look improves noticeably after one to two treatments.

Manual Lymphatic Drainage – Skin brushing, yoga, walking, swimming, jumping on a mini-trampoline, singing, deep breathing, dancing and other exercises all benefit the body as a sort of manual lymphatic drainage and is good for toning.

Colon Cleansing & Waste Removal

Colon cleansing is one of the most detoxifying therapies that one can do for their health and improves metabolism and weight management, as well. The average American adult, depending on their age and diet, may carry between fifteen and twenty pounds of dehydrated fecal matter in the colon. This matter can slow down the metabolic processes and the elimination processes of the body.

The sluggish or slowed elimination of fats and other solid waste toxins and may contribute to an increase in body weight. When we are dehydrated, we may be re-absorbing toxic fluid from the bowel, this is reason enough for colon hydrotherapy. Dehydration of the colon can lead to structural atrophy and dysfunction of the intestines. Colon hydrotherapy flushes out the colon to cleanse it. Other methods are laxatives, enemas, herbs or other cleansing products. Colon Hydrotherapy is beneficial to our health and is an effective therapy in weight loss and weight management plans. However, we cannot move all of the contents of the bowel with colon irrigation alone. Peristaltic action occurs with the consumption of foods containing fiber. Colon health relies on chlorophyll, calcium, magnesium and sodium bile salts. Keep in mind that people who are constipated usually are dehydrated or have a deficiency of silicon, magnesium or fluorine. If the large intestine is not functioning properly, waste backs up into the small intestine creating a layer of mucosa. This mucous restricts the absorption of essential nutrients leaving the body feeling hungry and unsatisfied, leading to overeating.

Regularity of the bowel is imperative to weight loss. If you eat three meals a day you should eliminate four times a day to lose weight. The purification of waste build-up in the colon is very toxic. The reabsorption of these toxins can cause lowered metabolism, lowered energy, water retention, abdominal sustention, water weigh gain, bloating and cellulite. Proper elimination of waste is imperative to maintaining a normal weight. A high fiber diet and lots of water is required to keep the colon healthy. The flushing and elimination of accumulated and toxic fecal matter through Colon hydrotherapy is one of the most hydrating treatments available Colon hydrotherapy helps hydrate the dehydrated matter so that it can be effectively eliminated or evacuated from the body. The water may help to neutralize acids that create bio-chemical imbalances. Colon hydrotherapy use to be considered a treatment of Hollywood film stars because so many rich and famous people in the movie and entertainment industries rave about the cleansing, detoxifying and anti-aging effects of Colonics, today, many people utilize cleansing Colonics or enemas as a basic part of their health care regimen and use it as a form of preventative health care. Most of the previously mentioned modalities are offered in combination at many Health Centers, Medical Spas, Salons, Day Spas & Health Resorts.

Heavy Metal Detox Soak

In cases of heavy metal toxicity, when excess metals are blocking the absorption of nutrients (which the body may use to maintain healthy metabolism) or when there is blocked liver function. You may use 1 cup of Clorox bleach in a basic tub of hot water sitting for 30 to 45 minutes until a sweat has broken and the water changes to gray, which is an indication that some of the metals have been released through the skin.

TRADITIONAL & RECONSTRUCTIVE OPTIONS IN WEIGHT LOSS
Traditionally, general guidelines for the treatment of obesity include:

THE BALANCE DIET & LIFESTYLE

Low fat diets
High fiber diets
High Protein diets
Low Carbohydrate diets
Low or Excessively Reduced calorie diets
Invasive Surgery/Stomach stapling
Appetite suppressants
Medications

New & Traditional Methods

Providing specific recommendations to the dieter
Mind Body Techniques
Setting goals for weight loss.
A slower rate of weight gain
Weight maintenance/Behavior Modification
Exercise & Diet prescription
Nutrient dense/more balanced diet
Stomach banding/Removable Implants/ Safer Bariatrics
Healthy Lifestyle programs
Cleansing & Metabolism Boosting

CHAPTER 11

Ancient Secrets For Balanced Weight, Health & Longevity

AYURVEDIC MEDICINE IS SAID TO BE THE MOTHER OF ALL medicine and it was the first form of Natural Medicine that is now, implemented in Mind Body Medicine a modern approach to health and longevity. The secret to this ancient approach to healthcare is about living a healthy and balanced Lifestyle. It is the root of Naturopathic practices and Naturopathy a health science which integrates almost every form of natural healthcare on the planet. Naturopathy has proven to be a very effective natural approach in losing excess weight and keeping it off for good. Just as Ayurveda, is the foundation for Mind Body Medicine. This ancient approach to healthy living is about achieving balance in Mind and Body to create a life that the primary focus is lifestyle awareness. It was part of the healthy living practice of peoples of ancient India but was almost abolished after the British invasion of India.

Ayurveda is now accepted as the most valid of all forms of natural medicine because it has stood the test of time for obtaining an optimum living experience on all levels of existence as it stresses the importance of achieving all-round health. Physical, psychological, emotional, spiritual and perhaps in other ways we are unconsciously aware of or may not be consciously aware of at our present state of conscious evolution. It addresses and corrects the causes of health problems and illness in additional consideration to the physical function of human body systems with respect to the traditional approaches to physical healthcare. Naturopathy utilizes traditional while integrating alternative approaches to psycho-social, psycho-emotional and stress related influences to created a program that brings balance to all of the bodily systems. Naturopathy also, mandates that the key to well being is balance in all realms of life and existence. Balance within the mind, body and spirit. Balance in all activities experienced in life, within the self, the inner self, the higher self, the spirit self and the god self.

The naturopathic approach to living ensures quick and permanent results in helping one to achieve and maintain their ideal weight. Any form of excess is viewed as an imbalance, being overweight is an imbalance. The ancient secret to life is balance. In order for one to understand the value of Integrative principles in weight control one must understand how to apply the basic principles of Traditional and Non-Traditional Medicine from around the world by knowledge of the history and usage of these modalities in order to achieve "balance". Ayurveda and Naturopathy are the two better-known forms of Holistic healthcare. Ayurveda and Naturopathy are both very old forms of Medicine originating from Europe and India and are the major basis of Mind Body Health Programs. In the fourth century Socrates was a Greek philosopher who stated "there is no illness of the body apart from the mind" it appears that there has been this observation throughout the history of mankind. Any imbalance in the body affects the mind and any imbalance in the mind affects the body. To correct an imbalance in the body you also, would seek to correct the imbalance in the mind, which may be hidden, and vice versa.

COMMON QUESTION AND ANSWER:

What are Ayurvedic, Naturopathic, Homeopathic, Botanical and Herbal Medicines? Forms Of Natural Medicines based on healthy living.

Natural Medicine has been used throughout all recorded history and time by humans and animal species on this planet and are all part of the Holistic approach to healthcare. Some animals seem to know instinctively which plants to eat when they feel sick. The focus of many ancient shamans was to restore health and prevent disease by using natural medicines that are derived from

222   •

DR. JOYCE PETERS

botanical or natural sources. Naturopathy & Homeopathy are "Holistic" blends of centuries old, natural, non-toxic therapies with consideration to current advances in the study of health. Behavior modification is an intricate part of the Naturopathic health care system for achieving a healthy state of mind for good overall health and longevity.

These two healing traditions are a holistic healthcare approach, in the respect that it is based on the care of the whole person; the basic principle is that,

One has to be in balance with their environment, be it the natural environment, biorhythms of the earth and planet, healthy social interactions and relationships, and spiritual and emotional balance as well. Covering all aspects of family health from pediatric to geriatric care. In weight loss, Naturopathy and Homeopathy prove to be a very effective program. One of the most important keys to successful weight management is lasting permanent lifestyle support to maintain the ideal weight of the individual. Each weight loss plan is usually specifically designed for the particular & unique individual.

Naturopathic Medicine is effective in treating most health problems, both acute and chronic, including weight loss counseling. There are three types in this field. A Naturopathic Physician is an expert that is bound by the same or similar oath as other doctors, "First of all, do no harm" and is one whom may or may not be licensed, a national board accredits some of the doctors who has received a diploma from a Naturopathic Doctorate Degree program, in most cases, most of the nations Traditional Naturopathic Doctors and Physicians are members and are accredited by the American Naturopathic Medical Association and Accreditations Board. However, there are other associations. The main thing to remember is that in general, all Naturopaths have one main purpose and mission, to naturally trigger the body's self healing potential by restoring balance to the system as a whole through supporting the body in a natural way.

Naturopathic Medicine has been a distinct American healthcare profession for over 100 years. Only a few states have licensing requirements, and the reason to be licensed as a Naturopathic Physician is if they are trained and practicing in minor surgery and pharmacy. Most Naturopathic or Homeopathic Doctors, are accredited, and are trained in nutrition, immunology, homeopathic endocrinology, anatomy, neurology, pathology, biochemistry, pediatrics, physiology, radiology, microbiology, botanical and herbal medicine, psychology, homeopathy, laboratory testing, physical therapeutics, natural childbirth and care, orien-

THE BALANCE DIET & LIFESTYLE

tal medicine, acupressure, reflexology, and other clinical sciences. Naturopaths are people who live as healthy and as naturally as possible to preserve health. Naturopaths promote green living, clean living and preserving the purity of the environment. Naturopathic Doctors, spend 4-5 years earning their degree depending on their specialties and are considered scientist and teachers of natural health to their patients.

HOMEOPATHIC WEIGHT LOSS MEDICATIONS
&
THEIR ACTION ON WEIGHT CONTROL

Abies Canadensis	Suppresses cravings
Ammonium Bromatum	Reduces appetite & headaches from sugar withdraw
Ammonium Carbonicum	Reduces appetite
Ammonium Muriaticum	Reduces sluggishness
Antimonium Crudum	Helps cleanse the body of fat
Argentum Metallicum	Silver supports immunity reduces detox catarah
Argentum Nitricum	Reduces cravings for sweets
Calcarea Carbonica	Reduces craving for indigestible things
Fucus Vesiculosus	Rejuvenates slow or sluggish Thyroid or Metabolism
Graphites	Reduces hunger pains/ stomach
Kali Bichromium	Enhances digestion
Kali Carbonicum	Suppresses strong desires for sweets
Kali Phosphoricum	Curbs the desire for sweets
Lycopodum Clavatum	Eliminates excessive hunger
Natrum Muriaticum	Curbs the appetite
Phosphorus	Decreases hunger soon after eating
Phytolocca Decandra Berry	Assists in killing fungi and related sugar cravings
Pulsatilla	Decreases desire for fatty foods and warm food
Sabadilla	Helps suppress appetite for sweets
Silicea	Tendency to bring balance in the body
Spongia Tosta	Decreases excessive hunger
Staphysagria	Helps you to feel stronger and less weak

HOMEOPATHIC WEIGHT LOSS MEDICATIONS
&
THEIR ACTION ON WEIGHT CONTROL

Sulphur	Helps to supress excessive appetite
Veratrum Album	Suppresses voracious appetite.
Thyroidinum	Creates thirst for water. Improves thyroid function

All of the previously listed homeopathic medicines are listed in the Homeopathic Materia Medica and are tried, proven and tested to have these reactions and side effects in a healthy individual. If you administer too strong a dose or too much of a dose, you can actually create the symptom you are treating. In the smaller dose, it stimulates the body's innate or natural ability to detect and initialize whatever means available to rebalance normal function. Better results are achieved by using smaller specific doses. It is recommended that these only be used under supervision of a health care provider as these are homeopathic medicines and improper dosage can be toxic, harmful or even fatal. Do not let that alarm you too much, because they are powerful. They are just as effective as prescription weight loss medications when administered properly and are natural and non-addicting; therefore the body can utilize them more efficaciously to achieve the desired result but, the main goal is to develop a healthier lifestyle.

Ayurveda The Basis Of Mind-Body Medicine

Ayurveda is said to be the mother of medicine. As the face of medicine evolves it seems that what goes around comes back around. Ayurveda originated in India as a way of life. Ayurveda is Mind Body Medicine Ayurveda is much more than a way of life. Ayurveda is a holistic medicinal approach to health and longevity. Ayurveda implements, healthy diet, healthy lifestyle, yoga, and meditation practices to prevent disease and maintain good health in mind and body. Ayurveda focuses on balance in mind and body by daily practice of meditative healing states of consciousness while utilizing natural foods, spices and herbs as medicine. Ayurveda is the oldest system of medicine on earth. It is the "Mother of Medicine" and it is the most recognized of all of the great heal-

THE BALANCE DIET & LIFESTYLE

ing systems of the world. In Ayurveda, food is medicine. If you eat the right foods, keep your dosha balanced, then your body will automatically heal itself. If you eat the proper food in the right proportion, you will not be overweight. The British invasion of India, had replaced Ayurvedic Medicine with Western Medicine in India. Traditional medicine had almost wiped out all other forms of medicine until Mahatma Gandhi took the first step to salvage Ayurveda by opening the first new college of Ayurveda in 1921. Gandhi saved Ayurveda and it is the foundation of Mind Body Medicine, today. Mahatma Gandhi practiced Ayurvedic practices in his daily life and lived to be very old. He was slender and healthy and led an example of balance and harmony in all levels of his existence. He worked on a spinning wheel every day of his life. He once stated that he felt that he had to work for his food or it was as if he was eating stolen food when he ate. Spinning is repetitive and methodical. Spinning may have actually helped to induce a form of hypnotic trance.

Ayurveda For Weight Loss

Ayurveda can help you to lose weight. By applying Ayurvedic principles and following these simple steps to weight loss, you will have success. Day by day, you will see your dream becoming your reality, as you loose the weight. Continually, abiding by these principles will help you achieve your desired destiny of maintaining a healthy weight for a lifetime through personal self-discovery and self-realization.

INDICATORS OF WEIGHT GAIN DUE TO A LIFESTYLE IMBALANCE
Group 3 "Dieter's Dosha Type Test"

A) Kappa Dosha Type

Are you of strong build? Do you have a tendency to eat big meals? Do you tend to avoid change? Do you tend to feel sleepy, tire easily, feel lethargic or unmotivated? Do you tend to like large or heavy meals? Are you generally slow to lose weight? Are you slow to start but once you get going do you tend to outlast the crowd in your endeavors? Are you reluctant to alter from your set routine? Does change make you feel outside of your comfort zone? Do you have slow digestion? Do you have irregular or bulky stool? You are Kappa.

B) Pitta Dosha Type

Do you have a fast metabolism which leaves you hungry all the time? Are you often hungry and thirsty? Do you have stomach or digestive irritations or problems? Do you get grumpy, anxious or disoriented when you are not eating? Do you feel euphoric just after eating and then tired a little later? Do you eat to avoid nausea, dizziness or irritability? Do you crave cold food and drinks? Do you tend to over do everything? Do you like a variety of foods and flavors during a meal? Do you tend to eat anything and everything? Do you feel overheated? Do you fluctuate between watery diarrhea to loose stools. You are Pitta

C) Vata Dosha Type

Do you need four or more small regular meals a day to feel well? Do you prefer warm as oppose to cold foods? Do you tend to stick to certain foods instead of a variety? Do you prefer quiche' casserole, soups and stews to get a mixture of foods instead of cold mixed salads? Do you tend to have gas or to get constipated stools? Do you tend to need more in between meal snacks than others? You are Vata.

The first step to weight loss success is to start with self-realization. Understand your own thoughts and feelings. The ultimate love is self love. Love and accept yourself unconditionally. Create a vision in your mind of your new self image. Devise a plan, utilizing the information in this book. Plan your weight loss success. Believe in your self, become self reliant that you will lose your excess weight. Picture yourself already there and project yourself forward to your goal. See your slimmer healthier physique. Know that losing the weight can be simple when you change your thoughts about food. Make your daily food choices healthier ones which help your body to lose weight. Develop healthier actions in your eating habits and watch your thoughts carefully, because…"your thoughts become your reality". Mahatma Gandhi, one of the world's greatest philosophers, inspired people with his philosophy on how important it is to stay in a positive state of mental consciousness. He recognized the power of positive thinking. These words, written by Gandhi, encourage people to utilize the power of their own positive thoughts. The words continue to inspire self-discovery and self-realization by encouraging positive thinking. This statement by Gandhi makes it clear that how we think actually creates our reality. We create our own reality, because our thoughts will manifest in physical form and project us into the future we create.

THE BALANCE DIET & LIFESTYLE

Gandhi was an inspiring example of teaching others how to achieve self-realization through meditation and Ayurvedic principles which are the basis of Mind Body Medicine. The spinning wheel was used to spin cloth by Indian peoples in India. Gandhi worked on his spinning wheel up until the time of his death. Many common things can be used as a meditative tool. The spinning wheel resembles the hypnosis wheel which is used to induce a deep hypnotic state of consciousness to allow the hypnotherapist or counselor the ability to gain access to the subconscious mind.

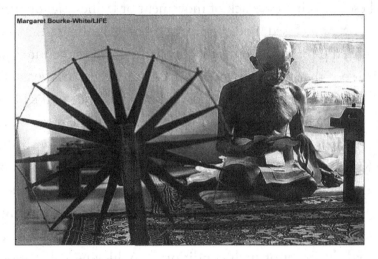

Keep your beliefs positive

Because...
Your beliefs become your thoughts
Your thoughts become your words
Your words become your actions
Your actions become your habits
Your habits become your values
Your values become your destiny

Mahatma Gandhi

In Ayurveda, food has three distinct basic qualities light, passionate and sluggish. Which of these three food types do you think will help you loose weight? It is simple. The more complicated aspect is that Ayurvedic foods are categorized by six "taste" which are: astringent, sweet, sour, salty, pungent, and bitter. Characteristics are Heavy or light. Oily or dry, and lastly, hot or cold. You should maintain all six tastes in your diet at the same time avoiding the foods, which negatively affect your dominating Dosha.

The word in India for Light is **Satvic**, which brings the mind into a harmonious state. Salads, Veggies, Fruits, Nuts, Herbs, and healthy herb teas and tonics all have a light quality. The word for Passionate in India is **Rajastic**, which stimulates a person's sensuality trait. Passionate foods are all highly spicy, salty, hot and dry. Some of the Passionate foods and drinks are wine, coffee, dairy, rice, wheat and tea. These are only acceptable in moderation. The word for Sluggish in India is known as **Tamasic**. These foods increase lack of movement or laziness, ignorance and greed. Over cooked, over processed foods, meats, and heavy liquor are Tamasic foods and should be avoided if possible. Foods that are natural and that create balance in the body are the foods that will help you achieve your weight loss goals. Because it is easier for the body to digest natural foods and bring balance to the body.

Ayurveda is a science of life. A philosophy based on the interaction of Mind-Body & Spirit. It is to enhance the relationship of the self with the universal energies or Kundalini. These energies manifest in each individual and every person has all three energies. Being overly dominant by one energy may indicate what disease states a particular individual may be prone to developing, therefore Ayurveda is preventative medicine as balancing the Dosha may be an effective means to avoid the onset of such conditions. . Achieving balance of energies is a primary priority in Ayurveda. In the hands of an experienced practitioner, the use of Ayurveda can achieve sometimes-miraculous results.

Ayurvedic care teaches one how to maintain a healthy lifestyle. Determining and balancing your Dosha type. Focusing on diet and eating habits or eating patterns, rest & sleep, attaining work schedules which are more in tune with your Dosha type, exercise, yoga, meditation and controlled breathing regimens.

Your Dieter's Ayurveda Dosha Type

The first step to Weight-Loss is to begin with balancing your Dosha. Our dominating Dosha type is called our Prakruti (Our Body-Mind type) will influence the kind of foods we should eat, what type of exercise we need and even the things in life that we enjoy as hobbies or past times.

The ultimate goal of Ayurveda is to maintain perfect health in Body and Mind. In Ayurveda, each molecule in the body is comprised of the five elements. Ether, Earth, Water, Fire and Air. In Ayurveda, an imbalance in any of the five elements can lead to disease. Therefore, the major focus is to correct or prevent any imbalance in any of the

THE BALANCE DIET & LIFESTYLE

five elements to prevent disease and maximize physical and mental health.

Kundalini Energies
EARTH, WATER, FIRE, ETHER & AIR

The Three Types of Dosha's

There are three Dosha types. Vata, Pitta and Kapha. Our Dominating Dosha type determines our Prakruti.

<u>Vata</u> – Air and Space-The moving force of body & mind-circulation & neuromuscular functions

<u>Pitta</u> – Fire & Water-Biological fire-digestions and metabolic application of nutrients-hormones, mental intelligence

<u>Kapha</u> – Earth & Water-Stability, patience, support and strength to mind and body-promotes healing & immunity

Vata People– tend to eat smaller portions. Vata's prefer sweet, sour and salty foods. Vata's are active and energetic. Vata's have better short-term attention spans and forget long-term because they are prone and adapt well, to change. In mind, they are scattered instead of centered but the autonomic responses are superior.

Pitta People – tend to get hot easily. Have hyper-coloration of the skin. They have a big appetite. They are quick to anger. In addition, tend to be over emotional.

Kapha-tend to be large framed. Slow learners. They are affectionate and emotionally secure. They are very virile, strong and muscular.

Meditation

Meditation is an Ayurvedic practice. It takes you to a place in your mind that you are your purest self and to your deepest level or understanding, which can help you realize what created your weight imbalance, in the first place. Meditation provides a means to do this. People have received a myriad of health and personal benefits from their meditative practices. Being in a State of Meditation is a state of mesmeric consciousness. Meditation is excellent for weight loss as it allows the organ systems to take a break and recalibrate their functions into greater more efficient functioning in synchronicity with the rest of the body and the mind. Through meditation, we are able to release the clutter, and negative energy of our cares, worries and concerns and work toward our goals. It is through meditation that we may bring ourselves into an altered state of conscious awareness that brings us more in tune with all that we are connected to in the universe. In this altered state of consciousness we tap into the collective consciousness of the universe. In this realm of existence, we become connected with the all knowing. This state of consciousness is in tune with our higher self. Our higher-self knows what is best for us and when we can get in touch with this part of our psyche, it is there that we can reach our full potential growth and deeper healing states. We can resolve our problems and channel in our best creative energies. Meditation brings us closer to our personal purpose and meaning in life. Through meditation, you are sending out an energetic thought projection of what you are meditating about, into the universe of what you want sent back to you through karmic energy.

Dieter's Lifestyle Dosha Type Test

What is your favorite hobby?

- a. Sitting on the on the lawn reading a good book or having a picnic by the water
- b. Being with someone special or family and friends anything we can do together
- c. Sky dive, bungee jump, scuba dive, skiing, jet boat/ fast cars & racing

What is your favorite TV show?

- a. Documentaries/Soap operas/Series/Frazier
- b. Talk shows/Reality Shows/Oprah/Dr. Phil
- c. Sports/Cops/Game Shows/Friends/Seinfield

What is your favorite food?

- a. Meat and potatoes
- b. Casserole/ Soup/ Dressings/Cheese
- c. Salad/Spicy/Rogan Josh/ Mexican

Dieter's Lifestyle Dosha Type Test

Describe your Body?

    a.   I am BIG and Beautiful but I want to be thinner

    b.   I am slim in certain areas & a little overweight in others – because I don't exercise consistently and over indulge occasionally.

    c.   I am fairly normal, but have some fat prone areas I want to loose.

How do you gain weight?

    a.   Just looking at food/can't loose – keep gaining

    b.   Just in spots/ mostly slim

    c.   I can gain or loose easily

Describe your activity level?

    a.   Mildly active

    b.   Active

    c.   Hyper-active

What is your favorite exercise?

    a.   Lifting the remote/walking

    b.   Brisk walking/swimming/jogging

    c.   Running/aerobics

How would you describe your personality?

    a.   Stable/dependable/secure

    b.   Talkative/caring/dedicated

    c.   Assertive/enthusiastic/outgoing/reliable

What type of work do you prefer?

    a.   Sedentary/desk/paper work/ relaxed

    b.   High work load/deadlines/goal oriented/physical

    c.   Active/thinker/problem solver/mental

How does stress affect you?

    a.   I could care less…. I let the rest of the world do all the worry (Calm)

    b.   I am going to lose it if I don't get out of here… (Avoid)

    c.   Watch Out! I am not putting up with this! (Angry)

> ### Dieter's Lifestyle Dosha Type Test
>
> How are you in a romantic relationships?
>   a.   Like The Rock Of Gibraltar-Steadfast and True
>   b.   Close and Emotional-"Like Two Love Birds in a tree k-I-s-s-I-n-g"
>   c.   Passionate and Exciting/Hot & Cold/Fire & Ice
>
> ---
>
> What is your idea of a vacation?
>   a.   NATURE-Camping out in the Wilderness by the Water/Trip to the Beach/Sand-dunes & Salty Air-Cool Fruity Drink
>   b.   TRAVEL-Hiking through ancient ruins in Peru, Egypt, Mexico, Italy Spain-Quaint Little Villages Here and There & Wineries….
>   c.   CITY-Viva' Las Vegas/The SUPER BOWL/ Party Animal
>
> Which of the following three describes your lifestyle?
>   a.   Same-ole' Same-ole' What ever Will Be—Will Be,
>   b.   Follow the Yellow Brick Road-Lions and Tiger and Bears, Oh-My – "We're off to see the wizard the wonderful wizard of OZ"
>   c.   Born to Be Wild! Looking for Adventure, always on my way going somewhere.
>
> ### Dosha Type Score Evaluation
>
> Add the number of each a, b, & c answer. Total each of the a, b & c answers individually. Add up the number of a, b, or c answers that you had.
>   a.   Kapha _____
>   b.   Vata _____
>   c.   Pitta _____
>
> The highest total score of indicates your Dosha Type.
> My Dosha Dieter Type is _____

Your weight loss diet is important to maintain balance within, as well. Follow the diet that is right for your Dosha type. Pure organically grown whole foods on a daily basis are important. When you are fasting, it is important to include the veggies and fruits that are right for your individual Dosha type in your juicing recipes. (See juicing section in this book)

THE BALANCE DIET & LIFESTYLE

BALANCING DOSHA WITH DIET

You can determine your Dosha type and bring balance to your Dosha by the determining your true characteristics.

Balancing VATA

Follow a calming diet to comfort and soothe Vata, Vata people shout eat at regular times in a relaxed atmosphere. A diet that is warming and nourishing. with salty, sour and sweet tastes.

Vata Diet Foods Recommendations

Eggs, Milk, Yogurt, Cheese, Rice, Wheat, Barley, Oats, Fruits Bananas, Melons, Berries, Veggies, Carrots, Garlic/Onion, Potatoes, Herbs, Sage, Oregano, Thyme, Basil, Ginger, Nutmeg, Cloves, Cinnamon, Spices, Black pepper, Mustard, Cumin, Coriander

Balancing PITTA

Pitta people need to cool their chemistry. Pitta needs to quietly relax at meal times and set aside the daily stresses at meal times. Do not skip meals or eat fast food or junk foods such as Mexican or other hot and spicy foods.

Pitta Diet Foods Recommendations

Beans, Legumes, Barley, Rice, Wheat, Oats, Egg Whites, Fresh Water Fish, Chicken, Pheasant, Veggies, Cabbage, Brussels sprouts, Bean Sprouts, Alfalfa Sprouts, Zucchini, Asparagus, Mushrooms, Cucumber, Lettuce

Balancing KAPHA

Kapha People should consume high fiber, low fat meals that are as raw as possible but with spices. Avoid anything high in fat or heavy foods in general.

Kapha Diet Foods Recommendations

Skim milk, Buttermilk, Butter (Real), Snow Peas, Carrots, Pumpkin, Seeds, Sunflower Seeds, Barley, Buck Wheat, Corn, Apples, Millet Rye, Rice, Zucchini, Dates, Plums, Pears, Herbs (All), Spices (All)

The following are Ayurvedic food supplements. Ayurvedic herbs and teas are useful to balance dosha for appetite control and weight loss. These supplements can be found in combination in herbal tea and spice formulas. They are excellent in helping to balance Dosha and have wonderful medicinal qualities to bring balance within the body and to improve quality of health.

Dosha balancing teas that aid in balancing the dosha's contain spices:

Vata – cinnamon, ginger, nutmeg, and licorice.

Pitta – chamomile, spearmint, coriander, fennel and hibiscus.

Kapha Tea – cinnamon, ginger, peppermint, cardamom, black pepper, orange peel.

Chai Tea – usually contain spices for balancing all dosha types, cardamom, clove, ginger, star anise, cinnamon, nutmeg and black peppercorn, fennel.

Adding spices to your food can help balance your dosha.

Examples of Ayurvedic Spices:

Vata – cardamom, cumin, ginger, cinnamon, nutmeg, asafetida and salt which are warming and soothing spices

Pitta – cumin, coriander, fennel, turmeric, sugar and salt which are cooling and calming spices.

Kapha – coriander, ginger, mustard, turmeric, cinnamon, and cayenne which are warming and energizing spices.

Ayurvedic weight management involves improving digestion and metabolism with blends of enzymes and ancient Ayurvedic herbs that stimulate metabolism, balance excess and at the same time, will ease and soothe digestion. Usually, Ayurvedic Weight Loss Supplements contain herbs such as:

Ayurvedic Weight Loss Herbs

Amla – helps decrease body fat and increase lean muscle.

Banaba – a medicinal plant that grows in India. Banaba can reduce elevated blood sugar levels and can aid in belly fat weight loss within 1-2 months according to double-blind studies in the U.S. and Japan.

<u>Guggul</u> – is the most important cleansing herb in Ayurveda, normalizes blood fats, cholesterol and triglycerides levels. It enhances thyroid function and can aid in weight loss & fatigue.

<u>Triphala</u> – an adaptagenic herb that assists in the body's removal of fat and waste, while increasing immunity, energy and good health by supporting the endocrine system and its organs, tissues and glands.

<u>Gymnema Sylvestre Leaf</u> – aids in weight loss as it stimulates and energizes the metabolism.

<u>Neem</u> – cleansing herb that flushes out excesses and helps to block fatty tissue from forming while it helps to prevent over-indulgence.

<u>Mangosteen</u> – known as "the fruit of the gods" scientific studies in several countries have shown that it aids metabolism on all levels. It has proven to decrease obesity, cancer, blood sugar, blood cholesterol and blood pressure while it increases fat and carbohydrate metabolism, immunity, health, energy and weight loss. The fresh fruit contains anti-fungal, anti-parasitic, anti-bacterial, anti-viral compounds as well as xanthones an anti-oxidant which increases oxgen in the blood thirty times more effectively than most other fruits or vegetables. It is a most effective anti-aging food and is at it's enzymatic best, in its preferred natural fruit state, however, the juice makes a healthy tonic for over all health.

The Use Tea's, Supplements, Natural Hormone Replacement

Indeed many natural substances can aid the body in increasing metabolism and to aid in weight loss and maintenance. Too many to be listed individually. Vitamins, Minerals, Enzymes, Amino Acids, etcetera. What is important to know is that every known essential nutrient, as established by the FDA, has a specific roll in body functions. When you are dieting, you need supplementation. The daily-recommended allowance is the minimum required by the body to maintain proper functioning. Weight Loss researchers show that the daily use of these substances can help you lose two to three pounds per month when used with proper diet and exercise. These substances can be bought in supplement formulas like the Mind-Body Weight Loss Formula. Always tell your physicians of all supplements and natural medicines that you are taking to avoid interactions with other medications. If someone tells you not to take, any of these substances carefully consider what his or her motives are. Positive and Negative Reports have been put out on most of these substances, however, in moderation most of these are perfectly safe for daily use while on a weight loss program to aid in losing weight. Any substance in excess can be harmful, even water taken in the wrong manner can kill you. It is advisable to take a normal dose as directed on the label and no adverse affects should occur, if you notice any, discontinue use and consult your physician. Always make sure that you select substances from a pure and organic source.

The following are examples of the most effective, natural weight loss substances known. Locate a doctor that is familiar with these natural substances. You should always check with your doctor first before using any of these. It is important to remember that a specific dose of these botanical substances is imperative. The way Homeopathic Medicine works is "like treats like". In other words, a homeopathic dose or small dose of a plant substance in a larger dose would actually create the symptom that you are treating.

Basic List of Natural Medicines and Weight Loss Food Substances

"Let your medicine be your food and your food be your medicine"
Hypocrates

Hoodia – Used by African peoples for appetite control & energy for centuries.

Lemon – is one of the miracle weight loss foods and perhaps the most potent weight loss food on the planet when used properly. Lemon is similar to our own hydrochloric acid, it is high in enzymes which help break down food particles for digestion. Lemon thins bile within the gallbladder and makes it more effective for use by the liver to break down and metabolize fats. They are in a food class of their own. Grapefruit & Lime produce similar properties and are good diet foods.

Collostrum – helps the body produce insulin-like growth factor (IGF) growth hormone which has a specific effect on fat metabolism as they stimulate fat-burning by shifting fuel metabolism to fat stores and away from carbs which is believed to help burn more stored fat during exercise.

Pyruvate – stops fat from forming, protects lean muscle tissue, and lowers cholesterol. It is safe, available without prescription and has been studied through 27 years of research.

Enzymes – full spectrum enzymes are needed by everyone. Digestive enzymes are needed to properly digest food, everyone needs enzymes for digestion and many other metabolic functions. Some produce growers irradiate of fields of orchards as pest control, this kills many of the enzymes in produce. Enzymes that act on protein is a proteolytic enzyme. As we age enzymes decrease. As enzymes decrease, toxins increase in the body resulting in metabolic putrification and poisoning of the body, an imbalanced body chemistry and decline or loss of homeostasis, the body's self healing ability.

Garcinia Cambogia – is an herbal extract called HCA that is good in reducing appetite, burns fat and aids weight loss.

Ginkgo Biloba – increases circulation and removal of toxic waste including excess fatty deposits and contains enzymes which enhance metabolism.

Black Walnut – high in organic iodine stimulates thyroid function helps expel parasites that may be feeding off the nutrients in the body

St. John's Wort – Has Seratonin boosting ability. Which is great for regulating the appetite and reducing hunger. It also reduces cravings for sweets because of the effect on the compensatory functioning hormone system and seems to aid the pancreas in regulating balance and function reducing cravings for sugar. It reduces stress and depression, which drain our energy and fatigue us. St John's Wort reduces fatigue, as well, so you will have more energy to exercise.

Alfalfa Sprouts – contains cholesterol & fat lowering saphonoins and estrine extract & enzymes that aid in fat metabolism & lowering serum cholesterol levels.

238   •

DR. JOYCE PETERS

Green Tea – loaded in anti-oxidants which break down fatty deposits in the body and contains EGCG (epigallocatechin gallate-a plant chemical that triggers your production of noradrenalin, an appetite suppressing hormone)

Amino Acids – found in protein, amino acids play many roles in the body and some help the liver metabolize fats. Amino acids are excellent supplements for weight loss. Amino acids that enhances weight loss, suppress appetite and help increase lean muscle are: L Carntine, Arginine, Methionine L Orinthine and Tryptophan (banned in the U.S. occurs naturally in turkey and milk) should not be taken individually as it can create an imbalance of other amino acids. Examples are taking L-Arginine without L-lycine can trigger dormant viruses. There are twenty amino acids, nine of them must be obtained from food, eleven of them biologically transmutate or are manufactured in the body as needed.

Chromium – regulates the pancreases metabolism of sugars and increases the effectiveness of the hormone insulin. Excess insulin turns to fat, Chromium helps the body to turn sugar calories into muscle instead of fat. The more muscle you have the more calories your body burns. If you a take plant based chromium supplements, you can expect less fat and more muscle. If you exercise 45 minutes every other day, along with taking chromium, you can expect to loose three pounds per month.

Vandyle Sulfate-Vanadium – regulates pancreatic function and the metabolism of sugars. Helps balance and stabilize blood sugar levels.

Protein Supplements – give high energy that is low in fat. The body is 20% Protein, it is the most abundant substance in the body next to water. Protein will help you keep muscle while you loose weight especially with exercise. Protein is required by the liver to produce enzymes and bile. Protein increases the breakdown of toxins However, all proteins like all carbs are not created equal. Some forms of protein can create too much acid, it is important to get enough protein but not from bad sources. Nor should we over consume protein so much that it generates an acidic body chemistry.

Conjugated Linoleic Acid – supplemental forms are available however, a natural source is livestock that is grass fed contain conjugated linoleic acid. CLA's help the body to produce lean muscle and decreases fat storage. Two pounds of muscle burns ten pounds of fat per year.

Bladderwrack/Irish Moss – good in building up and fighting against thyroid disorders. It is high in Iodine to speed metabolism and increase optimum thyroid function. It comes from the sea and is loaded with Iodine, which affects the thyroid and one of the best weight loss substances known. It helps with the appearance of cellulite and aids with the female hormonal aspects of cellulite formation.

Energy Herbs – that give a gentle lift in energy levels are – guarana, ginseng, gotu-kola which also increases carbohydrate metabolism and reduces stress while decreasing appetite. MaHuang – increases circulation and the metabolism of fat. It is a thermogenic herb but should be used with caution under the supervision of your healthcare provider.

Bitter Orange – contains synephrine which resembles ephedrine. It suppresses the appetite and burns fat. Ephedra works because the ephedrine alkaloids simulate your body to release noradrenalin, an appetite suppressant. Care should be used as it can affect your temperament and moods and may also increase other hormones associated with agitation and anger if you experience a change in moods or have mood disorders these should not be used ad well as caution to heart and hypertension patients are not recommended to use herbs without always checking with your physician before using these herbs.

Fiber – cleanse fats from the digestive track and speeds the removal of waste Fiber in supplement form and in food, makes you feel full longer resulting in the consumption of fewer calories. Fiber blocks cholesterol buildup in the liver. If you increase your fiber intake to 25 grams a day you can expect to loose an extra pound per month.

.DIM – Balances and stabilizes the endocrine system including the thyroid, stomach, duodenum, jejunum, and pancreas. Therefore, aiding the metabolism of the digestive system to balance the proper functioning of these organs and glands. DIM helps to restore optimum functioning of these organs and glands.

DHEA – safe when taken in small doses. DHEA is a hormone that blocks the enzyme that produces fat tissue.

SAMe – derived from an amino acid, helps brain manufacture neurotransmitters, helps with addiction withdrawl, promotes healthy liver, healthy brain function, decreases stress and mental fatigue, increases phosphatidyl choline which aids in fat metabolism.

Androstenedione – hormonal support for production of lean muscle.

Parsley, Dill or Oregano – All aid in digestion, add flavor to foods and can be added to food as easily as salt or pepper.

Thermogenic herbs – increase thermogenic and boost fat metabolism. Include cayenne, ginger, cinnamon, fennel, clove, coriander cilantro, parsley, dandelion, garlic, cranberry and mustard.

Evening Primrose Oil – is a good fat it contains Gamma-linolenic acids which aid weight loss. Gamma linolenic acids block the formation of cellulite, fatty adipose tissue around the organs, and decreases bloating and water weight gain by eliminating excess sodium levels and fluid retention. Gamma-linolenic acids create prostaglandins that stimulate calorie usage and increases metabolism.

Coconut oil – offers much promise today to sufferers of hypothyroidism and slow metabolism. It is a known fact that the fatty acid chains in coconut oil offer wonderful health benefits. Medium chain fatty acids produce energy and speeds up sluggish metabolism to promote weight loss. There are many side affects of a sluggish thyroid gland and the resulting slower metabolism. First, it affects your energy level greatly, and with a slower metabolism and subsequent reduction in activity there is often unwanted weight gain.

Letcithin – helps the liver generate bile and the gallbladder to manufacture and release high quality bile which helps the liver to break down and eliminate excess fat. Eggs are high in Lecithin which is essential for healthy liver function. Eggs contain sulfurs and sulfur type amino-acids which are required by the liver to manufacture enzymes. Studies show

THE BALANCE DIET & LIFESTYLE

that eggs are not responsible for heart disease it is the way that they are prepared that defines the risk. Boiled eggs are healthy for you and the average person can safely eat 1 or 2 eggs per day. Egg does not apply to food combining rules, they are in a food class of their own.

Soy – Studies also show soy helps you lose weight by blocking storage of fat. Soy is great for increased energy and stamina! Soy can supercharge your energy levels, increase stamina and improve your workouts!

Fenugreek – dissolves fat in the liver

Artichoke Extract – may help to dissolve the appearance of cellulite.

Fennel – removes fat from the intestinal tract and may suppress the appetite.

Cranberry concentrate – may flush fat and excess fluid retention.

You may find that all of these natural remedies are helpful. However, keep in mind that pills & supplements alone are not the solution to weight management.

CHAPTER 12

The Mind Body Lifestyle for Weight Management

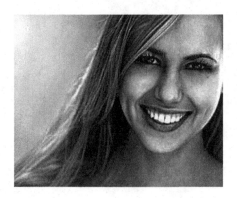

You Can Do It!

LIFESTYLE IS THE SINGLE MOST IMPORTANT DETERMINING FACTOR IN PREVENTING MOST CONDITIONS. THE MOST basic cause of most conditions, including obesity is an imbalance in lifestyle. There are many other factors involved,but all are related to imbalance. Balance is affected by hormones, genes, DNA, biochemical toxicity, inflamation triggers, emotions, hunger signals, stress, portion size, habits, poor food combining and even your thoughts. All of which can be improved with knowledge, good nutrition, healthier lifestyle, wellness therapies and simply knowing how to make better choices at each meal on a daily basis. Therefore, Balance is the solution in maintaining a healthy weight throughout a lifetime and in preventing many other diseases.

Your lifestyle transformation requires change. The changes that you will be making will accommodate a lifetime of successful weight control. To achieve this it will take behavior modification. As your lifestyle transformation occurs you will be learning to eat properly as well as developing the skills to stick to a daily exercise regimen. Making healthy lifestyle changes can help you to achieve your fitness goals and maintain them for life. Effective weight management is a lifelong process which begins with learning to see yourself as a winner at the end of the race in your mind. Make a mental picture yourself of how you will look and where you will be once you have achieved your goal. Change involves recognizing where you have been, what is needed to make a positive change, setting lifelong goals and then taking action to get the desired outcome, and lastly implementing a strategy not to repeat the same health mistakes that have jeopardized your health in the past, making a commitment to stick to the healthy lifestyle principles that worked for weight loss and making them work for you for a lifetime by adopting a caring lifestyle that accommodates proper self care.

> *"When we have self love our self confidence is high and we believe in our own abilities to achieve our goals; this is a sure recipe for success. Loving yourself unconditionally is the only true source of emotional independence and stability. When we love ourselves it is a true source of joy, peace and happiness. Psychologist say that an overestimated sense of self worth is actually healthy because it accommodates psychological growth".*

Lifestyle Awareness

It is time to face reality! The rate of sedentary lifestyles is alarming. The lack of physical activity is very high in the U.S. According to a report by the National Center for Health Statistics, 40% of American adults engage in no physical activity during leisure time. The report showed that women are more sedentary than men are. I propose that many of our main health concerns stem from a "lifestyle imbalance". The Balance Diet and Lifestyle is an educational tool to learn of the sometimes hidden imbalances that occur from living a life that is indeed "out of sync with nature" and "out of touch with our true inner selves". When our Mind is out of Sync with our body, we are out of synchronization with our full health potential. Imbalances with our environment or when we are not in our natural element, it may create a disruption in our body's ability to maintain balance and homeostasis which greatly affects our inner healing abilities. Imbalances may create health problems, because as humans, we were designed to live in harmony with the earth and nature.

Another study on the quality of the health of the participants in the study, it showed that one in 10 Americans age 45-54, one in five of those 55-64, one in four of those 65-74, and one in three of those 75 and older, reported being in fair or poor health. Another government study by the National Center for Health Statistics that indicated Americans spent 1.3 trillion on health care in 2000. This equates to 13.2 percent of the gross national product, far more spent on illness than any other nation on the planet. This equates to one third of the health care dollar was spent on hospital care, one-fifth on physicians, and one-tenth on prescription drugs. Prescription drugs used to treat disease and illness associated with obesity and related conditions. The report also states that the cost of prescription drugs consistently increased 15 percent a year from 1995 until present, faster than any other category of health care spending some of which were for prescription drugs. A large portion of this was spent on weight loss medications. Some of which caused even more illnesses, mostly in the form of heart damage. More than 60% of the adult population is overweight or obese and the medication we use to treat it is making us ill and sometimes even causing death. Being overweight makes us ill and the other illnesses that it causes are what is killing us! Which equates to this, if the disease doesn't kill us, then the treatment likely will. The equation is simple. Healthier alternatives and behavior modifications must be made. We are what we eat. We create our own state of health. It is time for an effective change.

Lifestyle Balance Is the Key to PSW
Balance allows you to tap into your (PSW) "Powers Stored Within" & "Psycho-Somatic- Wellness" (PSW) you must observe the basics of a healthy lifestyle. Living a balanced lifestyle is key to good Mind and Body health and wellness.

THE BALANCE DIET & LIFESTYLE

Going through life out of balance is stressful on the Mind and Body and leads to illness. Living in an imbalanced state of existence throws your whole being off kilter with the natural laws of nature. For example, picture a four legged table, in many ways, we can be compared to a table, a table can support a lot of things as long as it's support structure is in place, but, if you over- load a table on one end, with heavy objects, it can topple over, or if you take one leg off it will fall down. To stay balanced, we need to maintain a strong support system in life. It is important to replenishing the mind with positive and encouraging information to continue handling the mental struggles in a positive mental state and replenishing the body with proper nutrition will help you handle the physical load. If either, the Mind or the Body lacks receiving the nourishment that it needs an imbalance occurs. To tap into your (PSW) "Powers Stored Within" & "Psycho-Somatic- Wellness" (PSW) you must restore balance to your Mind-Body Connection, mentally and physically. There are many health counselors and coaches that offer supportive health programs for both and mind body exercise sessions can help you learn how to restore and maintain your inner balance. Just remember when we fill ourselves or our lives with too many things that drain us and not enough things to replenish us, our life becomes robbed of Joy. Without Joy, faith and hope is destroyed and illness or misery sets in. Persistent discord and imbalance in our life signals our mind to escape and if we ignore the warning signals the body can manifest into a symptom or an illness. When we become ill, we are forced to stop what we are doing, slow down and rest, this takes us off the imbalanced life-path that we were on and makes us start back into living again more slowly, when you are laying in bed sick, you do a lot of thinking. Why wait to become sick to inter-rupt our life. The moral is, take time to allow your body rest, restoration and self-healing or your body will shut down and take it in a not so pleasant way. If you make sure you are living a balanced healthy life and lifestyle, you should become ill less often. Take time to meditate on wellness, visualize your ideal health, ideal self and ideal lifestyle. Allow the "Powers- Stored- Within" your mind and body to process your visualizations and manifest them into "Psycho-Somatic-Wellness"(PSW). Use the following chart to show you how.

DR. JOYCE PETERS

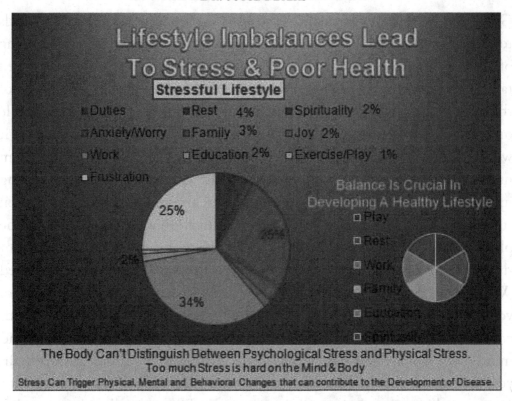

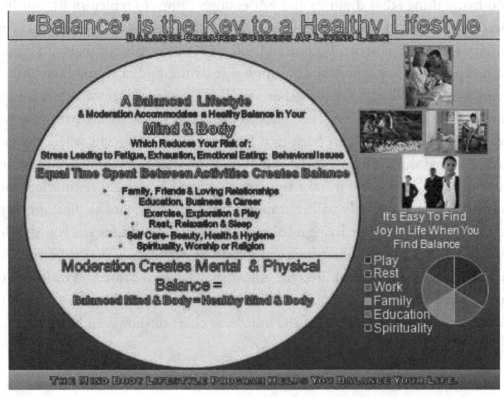

THE BALANCE DIET & LIFESTYLE

In Home Lifestyle Additions

You spend more time in your home than anywhere else, we are exposed to more toxins in the home than you can imagine. The hidden toxins are in simple everyday household items such as cleaning products, food products and packaging, bedding, furniture, personal care products and the list goes on. I recommend that everyone invest in these healthy home products to detox the body from toxic exposures and help restore healthy balance:

Juicer - start juicing! Juicing is preferred for cleansing the body and nourishing it at the same time as you get a concentration of nutrients and anti-oxidants that are safer and more effective than taking a supplement, however, if you do not like vegetable juice, you can add a slice of apple to sweeten the taste. Eating vegetables is an important lifestyle change that can improve your health, eat the vegetables that are recommended in the juice recipes, too. Juicing alkaline veggies is an easy way to help balance body chemistry, especially if you regularly eat or drink acid foods such as meat, coffee or wine. The most alkaline juices are from alkaline vegetables such as; cucumber, wheat grass, cabbage, celery, parsley, cilantro, sage. These are is good for your health and improve internal balance. Experiment with the recipes, until you find the taste that you like, you can always add a little apple or pineapple to improve the taste. Keep your portion size to 6 ounces 2 x weekly for three months.

Water Dispenser- Every home needs a hot and cold water dispenser as it makes drinking clean, fresh, pure water and hot tea an easy part of your healthy lifestyle. Drinking water is important, but drinking hot herbal spice teas offer rejuvenating benefits. Many cultures around the world drink teas on a daily basis. Herb teas and spice teas such as Chai or Mullen spice offer many health benefits, Pau'd arco,, yerba'matte, and green tea are rejuvenating and some offer parasite prevention, too.

Far Infra Red Sauna - (FIR home sauna) because every household needs one. I recommend this therapy as it offers many health improving benefits. A FIR session increases deep breathing therefore each time you exhale you excrete carbonic acid which helps maintain homeostasis and internal balance. It is excellent as a weight loss aid because it's burns calories, increases fat metabolism, and great for skin tightening . In addition, it's mimics' a fever and mimic's a cardio-work-out and improves cardio-health, it's great for detoxification, and helps to boost immunity, improves skin ailments, it's good for the anti-aging benefits, it helps increase metabolism of stored fat, cholesterol and helps normalize blood pressure.

> FIR delivers these three things that will help improve your health.
> #1 deep heat,
> #2 increase oxygen (breathing increases)
> #3 Alkalinity in the chemistry to help restore balance.

Why are these three thing important helpers in restoring health? It can be a part of a prevention lifestyle and healthy addition to regular medical care. It's not the answer to health care but it can be a useful preventative tool. Many diseases, including cancer cells hate these three things; oxygen, heat and alkalinity. Most opportunistic infections, and microbes such as bacteria, viruses and other parasites, usually can't proliferate under these three conditions. The best saunas have FIR heat, and some have oxygen. There are precautions to use, always ask your doctor if this therapy is right for you. After each FIR session, it is important to replenish the body by drinking an electrolyte replenishing drink. Chemistry balancers such as coral calcium with trace minerals can help replenish your body from trace-mineral loss from sweating and help alkalize. If you think about it when people get sick they often have a fever and often the urine will become alkaline, the body will pull buffers from bone and perhaps stem-cells with it to repair and heal the body from imbalance and illnesses, then the fever subsides and the chemistry becomes balanced again as people get well. First ask your doctor if it is safe for you to take extra calcium. I think when you start on far infra red sauna therapy you should do it daily for the first week then 3 times weekly for two months drinking lots of water during the sessions. The goal is to sweat, sweat and sweat to get the toxins out of your body through the skin. There is a home sauna that is compact, more affordable than wood units and just as good plus; it can be stored under your bed after each use so it's great for college student or those living in small spaces. I use this type of FIR sauna, personally, and I think you may like it, too. To view more healthy home products visit http://www.shop.mindbodyhealthprograms.com

Example Cleansing Regimen
Far Infra Red Sauna- 30 minutes 3-5 times a week working your tolerance up to an hour in the FIR sauna, be cautious not to overheat. You should drink ad-

equate amounts of water and mist the body with water to prevent overheating while in the sauna.

Drink 60 ounces of water every day & use distilled water to make your cleansing herb teas and green tea. Take trace minerals and amino acids and drink well prepared Kombucha Tea daily to help replenish your electrolytes and pro-biotics after sweating and doing colon cleansing. Also, kefir cultures, is a good replenisher of friendly intestinal flora during cleansing.

Hydro-therapy or Enemas- Another option for cleansing the body, is colon cleansing.1 - 2 x week in three quarts of distilled water taken 1 quart anally at time by holding 15 minutes while massaging your abdomen before releasing. Always take pro-biotics if you opt to do this type of cleansing. Some people swear by the benefits of cleansing your colon, some drink colon cleansing herbal teas or juices such a cabbage juice, others oppose using laxative and prefer the use of colon hydrotherapy other health professionals oppose using hydrother-apy for colon cleansing. If you are comfortable with this concept find a good colon-hydro-therapist or to test yourself first try conditioning yourself by taking enemas. Coffee enemas increases Glutathione levels in the liver which helps in removing built up colon and liver waste. Start using a tiny douche bag sold at most pharmacies and work up to a volume according to your own individual comfort level. Some conditions will not allow certain individuals to use these cleansing methods; ask your doctor what is right for you before starting any type of colon cleansing.

The Mind Body Medical Weight Loss Program offers doctor supervised life-style program with customized diets delivered daily by e-mail or text, variable daily exercise reminders, behavior modification counseling sessions and weekly therapeutic treatment modalities such as non-surgical Beautiful Image body sculpting and toning. Visit the site locator at http://www.mindbodymedical-weightlosscenters.com to join.

Controlling and Curbing Your Cravings For Sweets or Deserts

The sweet-tooth, is always the hardest food craving to control. This is another lifelong battle in weight management. Falling off the sugar "ban-wagon", like an alcoholic, you need to give the sugar up and take it one day at a time to sugar so-briety and ironically, enough, it is the substance you see most in alcoholic anony-mous meetings. Craving sweets can be a craving for the sweetest things in life or the sweet and simple pleasures in life or things in life associated with childhood. When it is hard to find friendships or loving relationships we may find ourselves craving the carefree, youthful relationships we had as a child. Candy is often thought of as a treat for kids. Craving sweets can be that you miss child hood and the carefree, worry-free emotions of childhood. Like walking through the morning dew, bare-footed as you go out to play with your neighborhood childhood friend on a Saturday morning without a concern in the world other than playing and having a fun day. It may be that you are missing the days when the only thing you had to do was to take a break from playing to have lemonade or a Popsicle. Get in touch with the carefree feelings and emotions of your inner child in other ways than eating sweets. Alternatively, craving sweets may indicate that you are "sweet on someone" that you are attracted to and are having difficulties expressing or showing these emotions and feelings to that person. Or maybe you are lacking a sweet and loving relationship. Another reason could be that your own personality is lacking sweetness. Do not use sweets to compensate for a lack of sweetness in your life. If emotions are weighing you down too much to interact effectively seek professional help.

Positive Thinking Leaving Negativity Behind
One must take the necessary actions to bring about positive change to overcome negative learned behaviors and eliminate sabotaging influences. It is your life, live it. Sometimes it is not what we are eating it is what is eating us on the inside, emotionally, so to speak. The final step to ensure life long success in Mind-Body Weight Management is to develop a healthier lifestyle. Find your inner peace and tranquility. Now is the time for a happier, healthier future.

"Mind Body Lifestyle Temple"
Smile
Feel & Express
Get in Touch with
Yourself &Your
Feelings & Emotions
Relax/Meditate/Pray
Deep Breathing/Panchakarma
Practice Healthy Daily Activities
Be open to change and accept it gracefully
Learn to Defuse Stress and Negative Emotions

THE BALANCE DIET & LIFESTYLE

Use the Power of Positive Thoughts & Self Talk
Eat Right, Exercise, Get Adequate Rest and Sleep
Listen to soothing music & enjoy a soothing Bath
Daydream of Pleasurable Environments and Joys
Create a spiritual sanctuary to practice your Faith
Share in Laughter – Watch a comedy or funny movie
Give and receive hugs – & Reflect on Happy Memories
Visualize yourself already having achieved your goal
Connect with the Bio-Rhythms & Energies of Nature
Ground, Focus and Center your mind body and spirit
Look to the future with Positively, Hope, Love and Faith
Surround yourself with positive people you enjoy being with
Take care of yourself so you may continue to help others.
Spend time in peaceful, natural, and comforting atmospheres
Love yourself and experience the loving feelings of others
Spend Positive Quality Time with family, friends, and Pets
Make peace with negative feelings of the past, practice forgiveness
Seek fulfillment in your work and do the activities that you enjoy.
Major Lifestyle Tips
Stay socially & physically active in your life and active pursuing your dreams.
Set Goals & Practice daily-self reflection of your success in your weight management progress.

The Importance Setting Personal Goals in Weight Loss

Fad diets do not work for very long. The goal has to be in goal setting and behavior modification. It is important to set your goal and design a personal action plan in order to achieve permanent weight loss. The diet is a very important aspect in weight loss. There have been many diets designed for this purpose. There are over 300 diets at any given time on the market. Most all have good intentions behind them.

Appetite suppressants only work while you are taking them. Diets and diet aids are all right to jump start your weight loss but it is your healthier new lifestyle and positive outlook on achieving your goal that works the most effectively. The food you choose to eat and the healthy choices you make is the only "magic pill" that is going to keep the weight off permanently. However, the diet is only the tip of the iceberg. By now, you have realized how imperative it is to modify beliefs and lifestyle to be successful in your weight loss and weight management. It is crucial to set your goal to adopt a holistic lifestyle based on healthy living in order to achieve lifelong success and lasting results. It is important to set a goal and make a commitment to yourself to loose your excess weight. Use the Mind Body Weight Loss Goal Form in this book to monitor your progress and to keep a record of your success. Keep it as a momentum to your success once you have achieved your weight loss goals.

Reasons Why We Put Off Losing Excess Weight

Fatigue –	Too tired or not enough energy.
Denial –	Still looking for that "magic" pill. Denying that beauty comes from within. Do not want to acknowledge the fact that your behavior is affecting your health.
Fear of Change –	I am comfortable with my self.
Hypochondria –	I have aches and pains. Therefore, I CANNOT exercise.
Procrastination –	I am going to loose weight but I have to take care of some other things, first.
Stress –	I am too busy to have a healthy lifestyle & diet.
Self-Sabotage – Self Defeating Beliefs –	have accepted struggling with your weight is just a part of life.

They are all lame excuses…Set your goals and devise a plan to stick to them.

If our attitude is too negative, it is time to make a positive change. It is important to read the chapter on learned behaviors to gain a more complete understanding of behavior modification for weight loss.

The Main Reason That People Are Overweight Is Bad Habits

1) Overeating – consuming calories in excess of physical exercise. Overeating is learned by watching caregivers who excessively overeat or by parents forcing their children to eat and "clean their plates." Children forced to eat out of frustration.

2) Bad food choices-overeaters tend to snack on fattening food items instead of healthy ones. Overweight people usually consume high fat and sugar snacks. Overweight people tend to eat junk food instead of healthy snacks.

3) "Emotional eating" – eating for other reasons than true hunger – the more overweight tend to become satisfaction eaters. Eating when they are not truly hungry. Reasons include eating because of emotional stress. Eating for approval of parents. Satisfaction replacement or as a substitute for other emotional needs. Lack of satisfaction in other areas of life and other rea-

THE BALANCE DIET & LIFESTYLE

sons such as relationship dissatisfaction.

4) Excessive Food Intake Rate – behavioral scientist have discovered, that the overweight tend to eat too much and to eat faster while chewing less before swallowing than slender people swallow. The satiation or full signal takes 20 minutes to reach from the stomach to the hypothalamus in the brain. During this time the overweight, tend to continue to consume calories that add on the pounds.

5) Eating Times – eating too late in the evening and laying down full. The calories turn to stored fat and interfere with rest cycles creating fatigue the next day that is then creating overeating for energy lost from lack of restful sleep.

6) Having a glass of wine, a beer or cocktail, each night to relax before bed.

7) Having a cup of coffee late' cappuccino every morning that is full of sugar.

8) Pretzels are thought of as low fat, but they are made of refined white flour. Air-popped, Popcorn is a better choice.

9) Low-carb energy bars, are made from flour, sweeteners and additives.

10) Drinking calorie, sugar, caffeine & sodium loaded sodas or other drinks.

While developing a healthy lifestyle for weight management, supportive relationships are crucial. Creating an environment and surrounding yourself with like-minded individuals with similar health goals can contribute to your success. For example, a recovering alcoholic is not going to hang out at the bar and be successful for very long. Therefore, keeping company with overindulgent personalities can be a constant source for bad influence and may sabotage your weight management plan.

Mind Body Weight Loss Goal Form
Your Name: _____ Date: _____
List Your Top 3 Health Goals–
1) _____
2) _____
3) _____

Mind Body Weight Loss Goal Form

List Obstacles That May Interfere–

_____

_____

List Goals to Eliminate Obstacles–

_____

_____

List Past Attempts to Loose Weight–

_____

_____

List past Failures Avoidance Goal–

_____

_____

List Food Elimination Goals:

_____

_____

List Food Consumption Goals:

_____

_____

List Exercise Goals

_____

_____

                                              Recheck

Signature: _____ **Date:** _____

---

12 things you should know to achieve weight loss success
Know that you can and will achieve your weight loss goals.

THE BALANCE DIET & LIFESTYLE

Know and avoid or eliminate the root cause of your weight gain.

Know and believe that you will not starve to death, while dieting to loose excess weight.

Know that once you are at a healthy weight, you will resume eating again to maintain your healthy weight balance to sustain health, energy and life.

Know thy self and to thy own self be true, get in touch with your self, your true hungers and desires.

Know that it takes 20 minutes after you are full, to receive the satiation signal from the stomach to the brain.

Know that it is not necessary to eat until you feel full. Know that if you eat a normal healthy portion you will feel full and satisfied within 20 minutes.

Know and believe that by eating smaller healthier portions you will loose your excess weight and look and feel great.

Know that you have control over your weight and what you put in your mouth.

Know that your thoughts are powerful and help to create the image of yourself that you reflect.

Know and believe that you are strong enough to stick to your diet and achieve and maintain the healthy body weight that you desire.

Know and accept that exercise is a mandatory part of weight management and that improves the body and mind physically and psychologically.

KEEPING A DAILY FOOD JOURNAL

Since we are what we eat, it is important to keep track of the foods that are being consumed on a daily basis. This is a simple way of monitoring caloric intake and assessing the quality of your diet.

Date/Time	Food Item	Calories	Liquid Drink/ Juicing	Calories
Breakfast:				

Date/Time	Food Item	Calories	Liquid Drink/ Juicing	Calories
Mid Morning Snack:				
Lunch:				
Mid Afternoon Snack:				
Dinner:				
Evening Snack:				

Developing Conscious Awareness

Many times people that have a weight condition go though their lives ignoring the fact that their lifestyle is the reason that they have a weight issue. They seem to block out the need for being responsible for their weight and health status or some seem to be unconscious of their weight issue. Focus your attention, in an analytical way, about your body. What do you observe about your body, what does an outsider observe about your body. What do you believe has caused the weight issues in your life. For each reason you think of, carefully, think of ways to correct this situation in order to resolve the habit, influence or behavior to correct your weight condition. Meditate on the answer and write the solution down on paper. Write it down, three times.

Daily Totals

Number of Carbohydrates Consumed:	_____	Total Calories from Carbohydrates:	_____
Number of Proteins Consumed:	_____	Total Calories from Protein:	_____
Number of Fats Consumed:	_____	Total Calories from Fat:	_____
Total Calories From Food:			
	_____		
Ounces of Liquids Consumed:	_____		

THE BALANCE DIET & LIFESTYLE

Ounces of Water Consumed: _____	
Total Calories from Liquids: _____	
Daily Grand Total Caloric Intake: _____	
Areas of Over Indulgence:	
Areas of Under Indulgence:	
Problem Areas:	
Diet Correction Plan:	

Recognize Self-Sabotaging Behavior

Eating healthy as an individual but when going out with others, giving in and eating junk, because everyone else is doing it.

Losing a few pounds and treating yourself with junk food as a reward for weight loss. Eating healthy all through the week and blowing your diet on the week-end.

Coming off the diet before your original goal is achieved.

Fasting and binging, gaining and loosing.

Yo-Yo dieting addict.

Eating healthy foods, but eating a portion large enough for three people.

Skipping meals and doubling up at the next meal. Consuming calories at a rate faster than the body can tolerate the sugar rise creating fat storage.

Neglecting your exercise regimen, skipping all or part of the routine.

Before you think of more reasons to procrastinate your weight loss program remember these:

Tips For Ending Procrastination

1) There is no time like the present.
2) Now Is The Time For A Happier Healthier Future.

3)   Carp Pei Deim – "Seize the Day"
4)   "Gather ye rose-buds while ye may, for old father time is a flying"
     Walt Whitman

How to Create a "Mind Body Weight Loss Journal"
Purchase a journal and label your journal "Mind Body Weight Loss Journal".
In this self assessment journal. Write about your weight control journey. Have
progress sections in your journal. Keep a progress record what others are saying
and what you notice about how other people change perception of you as you
transform your physical image.
    Measure yourself.
    Weigh yourself.
    Record your clothes and shoe size.
    Write how you feel about your size
    How does your body feel in this size.
    Write what you have been eating that caused weight gain.

I noticed that people seemed to stare or look at me more than before, when I
began looking deeply at myself. After I lost 25 pounds, I noticed that younger
people naturally were more attracted to me as I became more physically fit.
People with common interest attract each other.

How to Form A Weight Loss Journal
    List ten things that you think will change in your life, when you loose
    weight.
    List ten things that you know you should do to loose weight.
    List ten things that you could do to speed up your weight loss.
    List ten things to describe how your new, slender, healthy, body will look.
    List ten ways that you can make your weight loss goal a reality.
    List places and events you wish to go when you loose weight.

Date your journal each time you write your weekly update story. Once a week
insert a picture of yourself to track your weight loss accomplishments and fitness
achievements. Reinforce your determination by feeling your success. Bask in your
success, this empowers you and builds up your self-esteem and confidence.

THE BALANCE DIET & LIFESTYLE

How To Start a Progress Photo-Album

Start a progress photo album. Reinforce your determination by visualizing your success. Taking pictures is one way of positive visual reinforcement and makes a wonderful before and after example of your own personal transformation process. It is a reminder of how things were and how things can be.

Take pictures of yourself eating healthy meals.

Take pictures of yourself exercising.

Take pictures of you in smaller sized clothes and take a picture of you in your old clothes that are too big, holding out your old waist line.

Be the leader, form a group hike, beach walk, neighborhood walk with current friends, neighbors and relatives. Take pictures. If no one you currently know is interested, it is time to make new connections it is important to have supportive others around you in your daily environment.

Join an active group such as a scuba club, exercise class, hiking club, travel club the people in these groups are active by nature. Take pictures of your new activities

Take pictures of yourself out while having fun at a group event with these active new found friends.

Take a vacation and take pictures. Wear colorful bright clothing, enjoy your new self and new life, you deserve to really let yourself go and live life to the fullest.

Review your weight loss journal, do all the things you listed that you wanted to do after you lost your weight and always, always, always take pictures.

It is important not to judge your total self worth by your appearance or your weight. These journals make a good reminder of what you have been through in the past and what you do not want to go through again in the future. Whenever you may be tempted to gain the weight back or revert to old habits and patterns, look at the photo album and read the journal. It is a great deterrent for yo-yo dieters.

CHAPTER 13

Balancing The Mysterious Powers of Your Mind

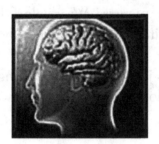

IN ORDER TO INCREASE THE POWER OF YOUR MIND OVER your body, you must understand how the mechanisms work. The brain is a physical body part. The mind is your conscious awareness. When someone says, "I changed my mind" what does that mean? It doesn't literally mean that the brain made a physical change. It was a thought that changed, and thoughts are not thought of as being physical, but, we believe that thoughts can change the physical body, and that thoughts can manifest into reality. Life is like a painting that we create. Life doesn't just happen we have to get out there and live it to make it happen.

Distinguishing the mind from the brain is one of the most complex scientific mysteries. There are mysterious mechanisms in understanding brain function and why, what, when and where a separation between the brain and the mind is still a mystery to us on many levels. The Body is a reflection of the Mind.

Mind Facts:
>   Human beings are creatures of habit. We form habits, easily.
>   If you do something for 30 days it becomes a habit.
>   The mind desires to be comfortable, we are pleasure seekers.
>   The mind seeks things that create a pleasurable or rewarding feeling.
>   Will power is in the conscious mind.
>   Learned Behaviors are in the subconscious mind.
>   The conscious mind is the ten percent of the mind that we use.
>   The subconscious mind is over eighty percent of the mind.
>   The subconscious mind will easily over power the conscious mind.
>   To make an effective change it has to come from the subconscious level.
>   The subconscious sees changes in habits as unpleasant.
>   We tend to make habits of things we enjoy.
>   The mind gives very strong signals to avoid unpleasant experiences.
>   When a weight loss plan is too difficult to follow it increases the failure rate and increases the risk of yo-yo dieting.
>   To stay successful, it is important to develop a healthy lifestyle.
>   Choose a lifelong weight control plan that you enjoy and that is reasonably satisfying to you on every level of your existence in Mind, Body & Spirit.

How the Physical Brain Works – The choices we make are usually made in order to maintain our physical comfort zone, to survive and exist in life, to attain comfort and satisfaction of the senses. The more repetitive our experiences are the more prone we are to become stuck in a pattern of doing things in a certain way and then it becomes a habit, and it becomes harder to make change from the way that we have become accustomed to doing things. It is hard to teach an old dog new tricks, but, we are not dogs. Human beings are the slowest to develop independence but we are the most advanced mental form that exist on the planet and we are of the highest in intelligence. Therefore, as a human being, you have the level of intelligence to understand the consequences of your actions and to make a decision to change.

It is said that even before birth and beyond the time that we exit our human existence on earth, that everything that we experienced in this lifetime, has been recorded in incredible detail in the memory banks of our mind, which is housed somewhere in our brain. We are born with the ability to learn to make decisions and choices, we use our memory, to recall experiences and we begin to use information, this is a god given ability that starts at conception and continues through out our entire life and perhaps beyond? You may ask how consciousness can transcend beyond the physical life of our brain. Think about this for a moment. The brain is only alive as long as our heart is pumping and the blood is flowing through our veins. The brain is the control center as it sends signals and bio-electrical impulses to regulate all bodily functions and mental actions. The brain can do this even when in a coma, therefore, there must be innate intelligence working with the brain that is so powerful, yet, we can't see it. It is a power that just as the wind can't be seen but felt and this energy may be magnified and concentrated to great intensity with certain practices of intention.

When our mind body connection is in balance and synchronized it is a powerful state of consciousness. When we want something with our entire mind and body there is really nothing that you can't change your mind about and improve about your health when it comes to managing your weight. However, the physical mind, the brain's decision making abilities are subjective to brain chemistry. An imbalance in brain chemistry can affect our decisions; for example, when the blood sugar drops it affects our mood, rationalization, reasoning skills and logic. It is common for a hypoglycemic person to have an inability to concentrate, experience mood swings, food cravings and irritability due to drops in blood sugar due to the imbalance in the brain chemistry which are due to the imbalances in blood sugar fluctuations. Any imbalance in brain chemistry affects behavior that is why there are so many medications for the treatment of imbalances in brain chemistry.

Leonardo DaVinci once said that ultimately everything connects with everything else. This is true, because according to many scientific studies, we are all connected to everything at a deep and spiritual level through what Sigmund Freud called the collective consciousness which is like the air, you cannot see it, but you know it is there. Tapping into the collective conscious is tapping into the knowledge and the energy that has all of the answerers to all of our problems. There is an answer to every problem, deep in the sub-conscious mind. Believe in the powers that are deep in your mind. Believe in the powers in your mind and put your faith in your ability to tap into this power, while remembering that we generally only use about a tenth of the brains capacity, unless we tap into our own unused resources, which can be done successfully, though meditation, prayer and hypnosis. The physical brain functions normally when it's neural chemically balanced. Even if we were born in a completely balanced state, the environment, environmental factors, stress, emotional trauma, drugs, synthetic substances, processed substances, refined substances, food, chemicals and other things do affect our brain function and may alter behavior. Brain chemistry is constantly changing by the process of life and these changes affect our physiological existence, too. The mind/brain affects the body/physiology in an endless loop. The mind affects the body and the body affects the mind. This occurs according to the events that happen to take place in our life and it is how we respond to the daily change that makes the difference. This is why a healthy lifestyle is important.

Life is about change. It is important to seek a lifestyle that is nurturing to us and that can accommodate a positive state of mind otherwise the cycle continues and wears the mind and body in an unhealthy or negative way which results in imbalance, disease and even weight gain by forming a protective layer of fat. The formative years of life up to age 12 are imperative in subconscious programming, the programming that occurs during the various stage of development from birth up until puberty will affect us through out the rest of our life. We are born with two basic emotional instincts, fear and love. All other emotions are derivatives of these two basic emotions added with perception formed with the use of our other senses triggers the release of the neuro-chemistry to fire other emotions. Our brain is a computer that we use as a memory storehouse of information to reference back to as we go through each day and make decisions and choices based on past experience and the sensory perception that we are experiencing at the moment we are making the choice. The only thing we have in the present to make new choices is reprogramming and creating new patterns of change with reinforcements from our five senses. Our sensory perception is formed with touch, site, smell, sound and taste. This is one of the main reasons that it is important, in initial programming, that children learn to develop a taste for healthy food early on in life. The brain receives thousands of forms of information experiences continual processing in life.

In a perfect world, life would be free of fear, chemicals and contamination;

our brain chemistry would remain in a balanced state of love and total bliss. The Ayurvedic word for this state is Moksha. Living in a modern society is far from Moksha as there is an imbalance balance of the two primary emotions, fear and love. We can create a new set of rules by changing our lifestyle to include practices that give us balance. Balance is the most important thing to blissful existence. We developing our sense of self in early years and mind body programs for children are ideal to bring about change in the society. Any perception that triggers fear instead of love adds to feelings of being threatened or attacked, negative perceptions, sets off the stress signals, triggers our survival mechanisms which release a chemical response that forms our beliefs about the world in which we live. Our response to this trauma is stored in our memory logs for future defense until a similar experience triggers a recall of the memory at a later date. The problem is that we become conditioned to act automatically if something accidentally mis-fires the stored mechanisms, and our response come out as an over reaction to new situations because our perception becomes clouded and we can no longer see the newness in new situations because we are associating everything to something that has already happened in the past. This association causes behavioral patterns in society that are fear based. This is why a new mind set is important to stop perceiving future events with the opinions that were formed by experiencing entirely different situations from the past. Once a threat has passed it is in the past but the brain has difficulty in trying to perceive that a new situation is entirely different and not related to anything else that you have experienced in the past.

Every time you do something different or visit a new place do you try to relate it to some other place you have been to in the past. The brain tries to relate everything to something else, the brain often does this with everything new that it experiences. With every new experience new chemicals are released, the more times they are released the more we perceive things to be the way that we think they are, when they may not be the way we think they are because the continuous reinforcement of a belief makes it harder to change the belief because our mind is keeping a record of every time that we have ever experienced anything similar or anything that remotely resembles the belief and reinforces it deeply into our mind. The brain forms a new baseline with every similar experience and the senses have been elevated in anticipation of the next potentially threatening similar situation. Over years and even decades of constant fear we become conditioned and the automatic mechanisms of perception in the mind affects the physiological responses of the body. The continual release of stress hormone and the cortisol effect is commonly associated with imbalance, disease neurological dysfunction and weight gain.

The ever-present stress thousands of chemicals, food additives and toxins in our environment affect brain function, as well. Repetitive exposure to these toxins, over time, accumulate in the body slowly but eventually may erode receptors, decreasing cognitive abilities, and adversely affecting the body's ability to cope and slowing neurological responses and reflexes. Toxic heavy metals are block the normal conductivity of the natural bio-electrical mechanisms in the body. As the brain naturally strives for balance or homeostasis, heavy metal toxicity can cause damage to the body but it can also be the hidden cause of the triggering of false cravings, over stimulated signals to the eating centers in the brain, including the amygdale areas that are associated with binge eating and may be related to other eating disorders, alcoholism, drug addiction and dependency.

Proper medical evaluation is necessary in the treatment of brain chemistry imbalances but there may be alternative treatments with Mind Body Medicine combined with a balanced diet and lifestyle that can provide effective results with or without the use of prescription drugs that generally mask symptoms of the imbalance rather than correcting the underlying bio-chemical imbalance in the brain. It is understandable, that drugs are generally designed to neutralize or block receptor sensitivities but without eliminating the original cause, the condition tends to worsens over time or relapse if medication is discontinued. Instead of using stronger drugs or to mask symptoms, it is a more ideal approach to change behavior, detoxify the body and correct the imbalance to attempt to prevent the physical manifestation of disease. As research is probing the hidden depths of neural chemistry and it's effects on the behavior of humans, we begin to look for more natural and effective means of balancing brain chemistry. By adopting healthy lifestyle practices, dietary changes, cleansing and detoxification along with specific herbs and dietary supplements are a great place to start rebalancing of your brain chemistry. As we take the steps to cultivate good health and bring balance to our body and brain chemistry, we develop a strong healthy mind and body with a renewed perception about life and an invigorated approach to life that allows us to experiencing Moksha in a world that we perceive as a positive place and we begin to enjoy the beauty and splendor in life.

Behavior Modification

Behavior Modification is the answer to struggles with weight control and is clearly related to developing a healthier lifestyle and eating behaviors. Most of the time we are totally unaware of the hidden blocks that stand in the way and keep us from attaining our deepest desires and dreams. Behavior modification is important and "awareness" of the consequences of bad dieting habits and the importance of a proper diet. Most importantly, "awareness" of the significance of the balanced diet and lifestyle in achieving total health, in Mind Body & Spirit. It is imperative in the treatment of weight related conditions that we develop healthier more positive lifestyles, to achieve and maintain permanent successful results and increased health, energy and endurance from our weight management care plans. Due to the epidemic of obesity, weight related health care cost continue to rise.

Recognizing Denial

If we do not realize the hidden obstacles that are blocking us from our goals, we can never reach the goal and we hit a wall which we cannot penetrate or break through. Put your weight situation under the microscope. In other words, pick it apart and analyze your weight situation with a fine tooted comb until you understand yourself and why you became overweight. This will help you understand yourself and your eating habits. Investigate all clues that will help you to decipher where the over eating issue is coming from. Face the emotions head on. Seek counsel if need be. Get to know yourself inside and out this is the only way to achieve self acceptance.

Usually when we are overweight, there is something, imbalanced, lacking or missing in our life or our body that we are trying to compensate for. Do not compensate this need, what ever it may be, with food. Honor this need, but, not with food. Put your eating habits under a magnifying glass and shed light to expose all of the real issues with your weight. Seek help from others who are more experienced than yourself, but ultimately, let your intuition be your guide. Listen to yourself for the answers and look at all of the answers with your intellect, heart, and gut instincts or mind, body and spirit. From a holistic perspective we can then determine what the true answers are and muster up the courage to follow through to resolve the issue. By doing this, you are defusing negative effects and reclaiming control of your health.

Learned Behaviors

Learned behaviors and thought patterns may cause weight gain or obesity as well as other psychosomatic illness and other health related conditions illustrate the power and control "Learned Behaviors" have in our lives and how important Behavior Modification is in overcoming the Root Cause of our problems of excess and imbalance. These may help you gain greater understanding about learned behaviors as the possible cause of excess weight and obesity. The names of these patients are held in strict confidentiality and consent was obtained to share their story anonymously, in their desire to help others who may have experienced similar situations that contributed to an excess weight problem. It is very important that we are careful not to blame ourselves or other persons who may have contributed to our weight problems. We are all human, and most of us are doing our best to make it though this life and carry our responsibilities in the best manner that we are capable of due to our beliefs and learned behaviors. Unfortunately, as it turns out, the majority of the time, weight issues or the problem that we struggle with has some emotional aspects that may be linked to past hurts from other people. Usually, someone who is very close to us, who would never intentionally, create dysfunction in our lives. It is important to realize we cannot stuff down unresolved emotions with food.

Covering our body with layers of fat does not protect us; it only hurts us and isolates us more, from our feelings. We cannot work out unresolved emotional issues through other means. If we have unresolved issues we have to dig through the old emotions until we can release them and let them go. The one's that we tend to hold onto usually stem from childhood, when we felt that we didn't have the right to get mad or angry with people who caused the unresolved emotional issues, with our parents. These old emotions must be released because they are damaging and cause a built up in negative emotions. Many times learned behaviors are passed down from generation to generation. It takes an intelligent and strong individual to break the chain or the cycle. These chains are sometimes what keep us together as families. Such is the case in Co-dependant behaviors. This is not to insinuate to break up family ties or abandon certain individuals; this is merely a recommendation to form healthier relationships and to gain awareness to the deepest root of the problem or issue affecting your health and your weight.

An Example Cause and Effect of Learned Behaviors

A Female patient that I was working with had been overweight since she was five years old, after our third counseling session, she realized and shared with me and incident when she believed the over eating started in her life. The incident definitely created a "Learned Behavior". She shared with me that she remembered a particular holiday dinner when she was 4 or 5 years old, where they had an abundance of food and deserts and she stuffed herself like everyone else had, and remembered her aunt made the hurtful comment to another aunt that the little girl was getting fat! , And they gawked at the amount of deserts she had eaten. When the grandmother saw how it embarrassed the little girl, she went over in a comforting manner and patted her on the knee and told her," now, don't you let that worry you one bit, you cant help it, you are just like your mother and me, you are just going to be fat because you are built big like us." The little girl was comforted, continued eating and grew up to be fat just as her grandmother predicted. She believed all those years that she was destined to be fat, and she was. However, as it turns out, she is not built like her mother's side at all and mostly resembles her father's side much more. She had a false belief imprinted into her subconscious mind; it was a false learned belief about her body. We had to reprogram the false belief and restore it with a truth, that she has ultimate control of her body and the destiny of her health, as we all do. Within three months of beginning her program, she had lost 30 pounds.

Mind-Body Weight Loss Yogic Mantra's

"I forgive myself and all others who may have contributed to my excess weight"

"I release the deepest cause of my weight problem, from my Mind Body and Spirit"

"My mind, body and spirit, now work together to achieve & maintain my healthy normal weight."

"I will achieve my weight loss goals, I alone control the appearance of my body."

"Smaller healthier portions satisfy me, completely."

THE BALANCE DIET & LIFESTYLE

Understanding the Subconscious Mind

The hidden or false belief that was formed is still implanted in the sub-conscious mind at the exact age and level of understanding as when we originally formed it, the false belief has the same logic and reason that we had when we began to believe it. Your three year old inner child may be telling you to eat all your food or you'll get sick or die! It may sound silly, but these are the types of unconscious behaviors that drive us to do the things we do. Sometimes, we can't change our behavior until we work to bring out the hidden issues and beliefs and make a change in belief. Sometimes this requires professional counseling.

How The Subconscious Mind Works

Example: You are standing in front of a window directing your attention to the person in the room with you and involved in conversation, the conscious mind is focusing on the information you are exchanging in conversation with the other person. However, your unconscious mind is calculating every car that is passing outside of the window, everything that is going on in the surrounding environment that you may be unconsciously seeing or hearing out of the corner of your eye or hearing from other rooms in the building. At the same time the subconscious mind is communicating with the nevous system as well as the organ systems regulating and controlling homeostasis, your breathing, respiratory, digestive and heart rate and elimination systems. The subconscious mind does many involuntary functions that we are consciously not aware of unless we deliberately direct our attention to them consciously through meditation. The unconscious mind has the ability to take in information while you are sleeping and even if you are unconscious or comatose. Your subconscious mind absorbs everything and for cxample, knows exactly how many cars that has passed by your house even though you are not consciously aware of this information it is programmed deep within your mind. The unconscious mind gathers this information through the five senses and the other senses which have not been recognized as of yet by medical science. Even though we are not consciously aware of these senses, they are collecting information and this information influences and affects our behaviors. It is even more influential on the subconscious mind, if the information is repetitive. The more times that the subconscious mind is receiving the message the deeper, it goes until it is recognized on a conscious level. That is one of the reasons that positive music lyrics are so important

DR. JOYCE PETERS

for the youth in our society. We need more positive lyricists that do not teach or encourage dangerous or self-sabotaging, negative and unhealthy behaviors. Thoughts are powerful and program the subconscious mind to create all that we have in our reality. Notice fast food and junk food advertisements. The music is catching and sticks deep in the mind. This triggers a response to go out and get junk food.

The Left-brain assimilates emotion, creativity, vision, and mission in life, leadership, long-term goals, group thinking, and teamwork. The right brain assimilates, logic, reason, words, short-term memory, and tension, order and control and individual perspectives. And right in the center top of the cranium, lies the corpus callosum, this is where all new information is accepted in synchronicity. Below the conscious mind is the subconscious mind it is also the subliminal mind. This is a state of awareness of which our conscious mind is unaware of. It is said that we only utilize less than ten percent of our total mind potential. In reality, the subconscious mind is very powerful and is possibly 90 percent of your mind. Therefore, it makes sense that there are things unknown to us that are driving our actions and to be able to tap into the incredible power of your unconscious mind and command it to assist you in achieving your weight loss and weight management goals that you will have weight loss success.

MIND BODY WEIGHT LOSS BEHAVIOR MODIFICATION CD

Reinforcement exercises are recommended, as reinforcement to the subliminal subconscious reprogramming that you keep a copy of you individual mantra's by your bed at night to read before sleep. It is recommended repeated use for a period of six to eight weeks to boost implantation the new behavior into the subconscious Mind. The Mind Body Weight Loss CD is good for behavior modification. It is helpful when repetitively used on a daily basis for at least a month. The Mind Body Weight Loss CD delivers positive and powerful subliminal messages to the subconscious mind. Since is subliminal, it is programmed into the subconscious mind. The individual mantras should be repeated as necessary, repetitiously 3 sets of 10 on a daily basis for four weeks. Behavior modification occurs at the subconscious level. To effectively help the overweight individual, they have to recognize and release any and all obstacles that are blocking their will power from successful achievement of the goal. Our conscious effort to lose excess weight or our willpower is not as powerful as the self-sabotaging behaviors that were programmed into our subconscious mind while our eating habits were being developed. Any subconscious blocks in the mind body and spirit must be released if they are creating an interference or hindrance in achieving weight loss goals.

Subliminal Behavior Modification

Subliminal Behavior Modification is a powerful method of changing Learned behaviors are deeply imbedded in our subconscious mind and are very hard to break the mental bond with what we believe to be true. Subliminal behavior modification and hypnosis techniques have been used successfully, many times. Examples of military and governments for using these tactics to conform soldiers into fighting life and limb for their collective cause. Brainwashing and convincing soldiers to commit kamikaze missions with the believe of rewards in the afterlife. Therefore, we can use similar techniques for our personal good and gain, because we can see the results in our present physical life when used properly, this is a very beneficial and necessary thought process that creates positive transformations. Subliminal behavior modification stimulates the learning centers of the brain by creating images in the brain through visualization techniques. As the images emerge from the imagination the thought forms are connected to the mind and body. If the mind is in a suggestive state of awareness, the mind and body can accept the new image into memory and override old self sabotaging learned behaviors with the new more pleasurable ones. Repetitively, the thought forms are transported to very cell in the body through neuro-transmitters and recall memory. The more times one listens to the subliminal messages and memorize the information the deeper into the subconscious mind it goes until it becomes part of the long term and subconscious mcmory which instructs the cells how to act to hormone or peptide messages. The Mind Body Weight Loss CD – is filled with positive thought affirmations on both a conscious and subconscious level. Repeated use of the Mind Body Weight Loss CD can help reprogram the subconscious mind and help you develop an action plan to ensure permanent lasting results in weight management.

Subliminal Self-Help Recordings

The "Mind Body Weight Loss" CD's from "Mind-Body Health Programs" can be an effective form of behavior modification. The recordings combine relaxing sounds with very positive messages to use as a reinforcement to any behavior modification program. The Mind Body Health program recordings are an effective tool in reprogramming the subconscious mind from negative habits and learned behaviors. The Mind Body Weight Loss CD is excellent in helping you to develop healthier eating habits and to help you avoid self-sabotaging behaviors. It helps reduce cravings for junk foods and contains messages that aid in weight loss. Changing bad habits is a powerful way to permanently achieve and maintain a normal healthy weight for life. The Mind Body Health Program series offers other self-help recordings that are available for various life issues. Mind Body Health Programs offers versions for Men, Women and Children that contain imprinted messages designed to reprogram the subconscious mind so that immediate results may be obtained.

Hypnotherapy and Self-Hypnosis
There is nothing to fear, hypnosis cannot make you do crazy things that you would not ordinarily do or things that would be dangerous to your health. There is no doubt about it, hypnosis is a positive and effective, drug-free, natural appetite suppressant and is highly considered a healthy alternative to diet pills. There is no question that hypnosis works. The reason why our will power fails us is that we only use a small portion of our brain's potential. Hypnosis is a quick and effective treatment to aid in unlocking the power in the subconscious mind to overcome obstacles and self sabotaging behaviors that may ruin your diet. The conscious mind is approximately 15-20% consisting of will power, logic, reason. The subconscious mind is approximately 80-85% consisting of learned behaviors and beliefs. Filtering out sabotaging fears and behaviors through hypnosis may be a major key to long lasting and permanent weight loss results. To unlock the power of your subconscious mind and utilize powers that are deep within you, hypnosis and self-hypnosis may be the answer. Many have reported results by utilizing the power of hypnosis.

Hypnotherapy has become quite an accomplished profession. There are over 127 known states of hypnosis. Professional hypnotherapist are worth the expense of their sessions because learning all of the states, the suggestibility types and induction techniques takes time. Just one session with a professionally certified hypno therapist can be very powerful. Most people report successful weight loss and habit-control with hypnosis. Hypnosis dates back to France in 1779. Although it was not referred by hypnosis back then. Franz Antonmezimer is credited as the being the first hypnotist, Therefore the term "mesmerized" was developed. It was in 1849 that a Scottish physician, John Braid coined the term hypnosis from hypnos, which was the greek god of sleep. Hypnotherapy has gone through much great opposition, Benjamin Franklin was head of a church orchestrated forum which came to the conclusion that hypnosis was hocus-pocus, this assessment of the validity of hypnosis was the key factor which drove Franz Antonmezimer out of France before the French Revolution. The church was the reason that so many stigmas were placed around hypnosis that we are still overcoming, today. The church's views stemmed from the false believe and assumption that hypnosis was possibly a form of sorcery because they did not understand how or why it created these miraculous results and therefore the practice was banished. Hypnosis is an overload of message units that disrupt the critical area of the mind, triggering the fight or flight mechanisms which creates a state of hyper suggestibility allowing access to the subconscious mind to make post hypnotic suggestions which create a more positive behavioral changes for the purpose of self-improvement and motivation.

I feel that this approach is one of the most effective ways to implant healthier new thought patterns and behaviors to achieve quicker results in overcoming self-sabotaging and false learned behaviors about food. Hypnotherapy has become more accepted in the medical community since Freud and Jung endorsed hypnotherapy as an effective treatment. Hypnosis had little validity until in 1950 when the AMA determined and made a statement that hypnosis works. Now, many doctors and major hospitals use trance hypnosis for pain reduction and speedy recovery.

During my research in hypnosis, I discovered many credible and incredible examples of the efficacy of hypnosis. For example, a medical doctor in Los Angeles shared her story with me about her experience with hypnosis, a medical doctor at a hospital in Beverly Hills stated that she had a cardiac arrest patient, which she intervened with a shock induction technique and stopped attack by utilizing a specific shock induction hypnosis technique. She reported that within seconds the patient's heart monitor resumed normal heart rhythms and the patient made an immediate pain free, recovery without damage to the heart. This story is an inspiration to the efficacy that can be achieved when we take an integrative approach to healthcare. This is only one example of the incredible results that can be obtained when we utilize traditional and alternative healthcare approaches in combination. Many people are effectively using hypnosis to under

DR. JOYCE PETERS

go dental work and surgeries which can be included baratric programs as well.

Hypnosis is a powerful tool in behavior modification, as well. Hypnosis is proven in research studies to ease the discomfort of acute and chronic pain with a very high success rate. Therefore, hypnosis can ease hunger pain and take the focus away from the feeling of hunger. The state of Hypnosis is created by an overload of message units, disorganizing critical thinking patterns, this over stimulation triggers the fight or flight responses within the body triggering a state of hyper-suggestibility, this provides access to the subconscious mind. When a person reaches hyper-suggestibility, new information can be introduced into the subconscious mind and can be a powerful tool in weight loss and weight management.

A simple self-hypnosis technique:

Find yourself in a quite comfortable room. Stare into the flame of a candle and allow yourself to become very tranquil. Breathe fully and deeply relaxing every part of your body. Feel your eye-lids relax and your eyes beginning to blink. Think of your weight loss goal, and allow yourself to drift into a relaxed conscious state where you can vividly visualize your self at your goal weight. As you become more and more sleepy. Feel the weight of your body become heavier and heavier as you become more and more sleepy. As you body relaxes completely feel the burden of the heaviness being lifted away from your body, feel your body becoming lighter and lighter until you have lost all of your excess weight. As the burden of the extra weight is lifted, Imagine how good you look and feel having achieved your goal. Before you bring yourself up from a hypnotic state, make a post hypnotic suggestion that you allow your subconscious mind to go to work for you in daily life to bring about a reality of weight loss. As you bring yourself back into full waking conscious reality each and every time you do this practice, enjoy the feeling of knowing that the burden of excess weight has been lifted. As you smile with the feeling of accomplishment of having finally achieved your goal, repeat in your mind and whisper to yourself:

"I have lifted the burden of carrying excess weight."
"I am now, achieving my weight loss goals".

Repeat these thoughts over repetitively as you drift into a hypnotic state
I see myself slender, healthy and beautiful. I am permanently slender.

THE BALANCE DIET & LIFESTYLE

I am satisfied and content with low calorie, healthy foods.
I am the magician of my own life and successful weight control
program.
My old habit of hungering for junk-foods and sweets is gone forever.
I am strong, powerful and I create my life and the image that I reflect

Results from self-hypnosis will gradually occur in time. Regular practice is required for a behavior modification to take place in the subconscious mind.

Caution: observe caution to avoid fire and never leave a burning candle unattended or in a dangerous container or area where fire may occur.

Metaphysical Psychology

According to the concept of metaphysical psychology. Hidden thoughts in the subconscious will begin to present physical signs in our environment. As our thoughts create our reality. This believe system states, there are no accidents, every thing is cause and effect. If a bug is flying around your head, ask yourself, what's bugging you? If your losing your sun-glasses, what is it that you don't want to see? Take the blinders off and see things more clearly. If you are over weight, what do you really want to gain? What do you want to gain excessively? What do you really want protection from? What do you want to hide behind? Why do you want to hide the real you underneath the weight? The outer self is a reflection of the inner-self.

Mind Body Weight Loss Kinesiology

There is an energy that is exchanged between a patient and a healer. It is important, believing that you are going to achieve your health goals to regain wellness. Learned behaviors and thought patterns may cause psychosomatic illness and other health related conditions including weight gain or obesity. Dr Peters designed Mind Body Weight Loss Kinesiology as a tool to reprogram the false beliefs of the subconscious mind using a technique that is designed to distract the conscious mind to get the message deep into the subconscious mind. To set the new positive thought into the subconscious mind the words are repeated while a series of tapping contacts are made on trigger points along the meridians of the body. This procedure is performed while the patient is in a state of deep meditation to implant the new message into the subconscious mind. This is usually achieved after helping the patient achieve a deep relaxing state of consciousness. Relaxing therapeutic touch therapy & guided imagery techniques are useful. A session of Mind-Body Kinesiology takes the patient into a relaxation exercise that brings the mind deeply into a meditative state. Once the power of suggestion is established at a deep mental level of concentration, mantras are repeated after the therapist states the words to be repeated by the client. As the client repeats the mantra, the therapist taps along meridian points in the body to energetically charge the new thought pattern. Negative phrases are never used. All phrases and mantras must be positive and project a positive outcome as the technique is applied the positive mantra is repeated as the therapist creates a psychological distraction by tapping the meridian point.

A positive thought mantra concerning the correction of the negative cause, is repetitively repeated by the patient and the practitioner while the points are stimulated with repetitive acupoint tapping on the specific meridian points associated with emotional Kinesiology. You may use fingers for tapping or a quartz crystal piezo instrument on the points. Each point is associated with an emotion. Such as, humiliation, shame, pride, stress, ect… the therapist carefully observes the speech of the client to find clues as to what area of existence is out of balance. Warning signs are positive stress clues. stuttering, inaccurate repeat of the mantra or forgetting the mantra during the session. When the point indicates a positive stress cue, this can be an indication of the emotion that is suppressed and that is contributing to the weight issue. The patient is encouraged to practice self-reflection to achieve self-discovery and self-realization. The patient may then eliminate self-sabotaging behaviors. The behavior may reflect back to unresolved emotional traumas and falsely imprinted beliefs about eating behaviors. Awareness allows us to recognize and eliminate the cause and replace negative thought patterns with a more positive truth that will better serve them in helping them to achieve their weight loss goals. Most every patient enjoys this method and reports improvement from this therapy.

Psychological Balancing Techniques

There are many balancing techniques in use by counselors, therapist and psychologist to help people balance their mind and make healthy psychological changes. Learned behaviors and thought patterns can be hard to break away from just because you want to change, doesn't mean you can easily change, unless you are able to tap into the source of your real power, furthermore, these hidden subconscious super powers may cause psychosomatic illness and other health related conditions including weight gain or obesity. I developed two techniques to help people tap into the power of the subconscious mind, one is for hemispheric balancing and behavior modification and is called "Hypno-Hemispheric Balancing Technique and is designed to help stop binge eating and the other is called Mind Body Weight Loss Kinesiology as a tool to reprogram the false beliefs of the subconscious mind using a technique that is designed to distract the conscious mind to get the message deep into the subconscious mind and to set the new positive thought into the subconscious mind. These techniques are designed to stimulate the learning centers in the brain so that you can make change.

The therapy stimulates visual, auditory and kinesthetic learning centers. Words are repeated while a series of tapping contacts are made on trigger points along the meridians of the body. This procedure is performed while the patient is in a state of deep relaxation to implant the new message into the subconscious mind. This is usually achieved after helping the patient achieve a deep relaxing state of consciousness. Relaxing therapeutic touch therapy & guided imagery techniques are useful. A session of Mind-Body Kinesiology takes the patient into a relaxation exercise that brings the mind deeply into a meditative state. Once the power of suggestion is established at a deep mental level of concentration, mantras are repeated after the therapist states the words to be repeated by the client. As the client repeats the mantra, the therapist taps along meridian points in the body to energetically charge the new thought pattern. Negative phrases are never used. All phrases and mantras must be positive and project a positive outcome as the technique is applied the positive mantra is repeated as the therapist creates a psychological distraction by tapping the meridian point.

A positive thought mantra concerning the correction of the negative cause, is repetitively repeated by the patient and the practitioner while the points are stimulated with repetitive acupoint tapping on the specific meridian points associated with emotional Kinesiology. You may use fingers for tapping or a quartz crystal piezo instrument on the points. Each point is associated with an emotion. Such as, humiliation, shame, pride, stress, ect... the therapist carefully observes the speech of the client to find clues as to what area of existence is out of balance. Warning signs are positive stress clues. stuttering, inaccurate repeat of the mantra or forgetting the mantra during the session. When the point indicates a positive stress cue, this can be an indication of the emotion that is suppressed and that is contributing to the weight issue. The patient is encouraged to practice self-reflection to achieve self-discovery and self-realization. The patient may then eliminate self-sabotaging behaviors. The behavior may reflect back to unresolved emotional traumas and falsely imprinted beliefs about eating behaviors. Awareness allows us to recognize and eliminate the cause and replace negative thought patterns with a more positive truth that will better serve you in helping you to achieve their weight loss goals. Most every patient enjoys this method and reports improvement from these therapies.

Another technique is psychological kinesiology. Psych-K techniques are beneficial in weight loss. Dr. Rob Williams developed Psyck-K therapy. Psych-K is used for balancing the right and left hemispheres of the brain to achieve holistic global balance between the mind and body. Psych-K therapy enables the conscious mind to make new connections to the subconscious and accept healthier thought patterns through a new direction, resolution or VAK balance. This involves imprinting a Visual, Auditory and Kinesthetic cue into memory, to help overcome the negative behavior. The practitioners ask the patient specific questions and test the answer with Kinesiology to identify true or false beliefs. A new direction balance and statement is then introduced and meditated upon to allow the brain to accept the new thought pattern. After completing the technique the patient is tested with Kinesiology to ensure that the new statement was accepted by the subconscious mind. If the message was imprinted into the subconscious mind the subject will test strong, if they test weak, there are specific techniques to help imprint the new message into the subconscious and a specific technique to overcome or release blocks which may pose as an obstacle or interference in absorbing the healthier new thought pattern into the subconscious mind. Psych-K is a beneficial therapy for weight loss as it aids the mind in accepting healthier thought patterns about food and compulsive behavior. It is important to recognize which part of the brain helps with weight loss goals.

THE BALANCE DIET & LIFESTYLE

Left Brain	Right Brain
Emotional Thinking	Physical Thinking
Goals/Dreams/Visual Picture	Logical/Reasonable Thinking
Team work and Leadership	Details/Action/Words
Rest and Relaxing	Management/Maintenance
Freedom/ Adventure	Tension/Stress
Creative and Spontaneous	Control/Order/Structure

The Corpus Callosum is the brain center where right and left brain information is integrated to be utilized.

Quantum Medicine

On the quantum level the brain is separate from the mind and the mind manifest as the body. Due to research that has been conducted in the study of Quantum mechanics and Quantum Physics it is now believed that when we act on our desires those thoughts become messengers of change in the universal consciousness to perpetuate a physical change. Quantum mechanics relates to the early work of several German scientists. Albert Einstein and his work in the Theory of Relativity which inspired scientist Heisenberg among many others to delve into the realms of quantum physics. Through massive scientific research testing, proving and disproving, it is now widely believed that you can achieve instant success in attaining your desires by tapping into the layers of your quantum mechanical body through quantum mechanics. Thought patterns have a frequency and harmonic oscillation. Studies indicate that what we think, we send out into the universe to signal the universe to send it back to us and confirm the power of our existence. The downside is that we may have the ability to draw what we don't want or what we fear.

Long ago light was thought to be in wave form. However, Planck discovered the energy of light to be discontinuous through the "blackbody radiation experiment". The blackbody radiation experiment proved that the energy of light is discontinuous and not continuous as the energy of a wave should be able to have any value along a continuum of values. Quantum mechanics is the science of examining the relationship between people observing the behavior of an electron and the response of the electron being observed. It has been more than sixty years since the development of the "uncertainty principle" of Heisenberg and Bohr, and there have been no theories to indicate that the uncertainty principle is invalid. The uncertainty principle is this, if an electron is not being observed it is like wave, when it is being observed it is like a particle, implying that thought affects the action of an electron. Every cell in our body has an electron. Dr. Bruce Lipton, PhD, an American Cell Biologist used these principles to discover that human cells actually do a similar thing, according to the cell owner's thoughts about the perceived environment and found that our perceptions can affect the behavior of cells and change our health and this is called the biology of human consciousness.

Quantum Projection Exercise

To make your thoughts work for your weight loss goals, focus your thoughts deeply into each and every excess fat cell. Focus mental energy on blasting the fat cell to bits. Visualize the fat cells leaving your body every day and your body shrinking down to your healthy ideal weight.

A very basic explanation of the quantum mechanical body is the synchronizing of the Mind-Body connection with the universal consciousness to achieve the belief, but more favorably, the desired goal. Instructing your body through its innate intelligence to go into a slimmer form by projecting yourself forward to a healthier slimmer future through your own thought processes may be effective. In weight loss, the use of Quantum Mechanics, may be beneficial in the energetic emission of thought being energy and matter being the physical manifestation that occurs at a rate faster than light on a subatomic and muti-dimensional level. By pondering something in thought imagination, you are propelling thought energy from the MIND by physical brain waves to affect the BODY as electron-particle of matter at a faster rate than the speed of light as indicated by the most brilliant minds in history and the scientist who discovered quantum mechanics, with the possibility of upwards of nine dimensions, electrons have the ability to jump through space and time according to scientist, Born and Schrodinger's "visual model equation" in Quantum Physics. On a quantum level we are "endless possibilities" meaning that what ever we can think we can be as we are the creator of our own reality. The face of medicine is changing, today. As we realize our individual ability to create the health we seek by utilizing our own healing powers and tap into the innate power of Mind Body Medicine that comes from within to materialize our goals including weight management. We know that illness can be caused by thinking we are sick, it is called psychosomatic illness and we may be able to produce psychosomatic wellness, but the possibility has to become real to us, we have to believe and we have to live the life in our mind that we want to create, long before we see it begin to manifest in the physical world.

Potentially terminally ill patients have been noted to have gone into spontaneous remission and many patients have experienced a miraculous recovery while utilizing meditation and these types of Mind Body techniques, because when we stop seeking an outside answer and look within ourselves, we become a mind with a body, we release from our consciousness the belief of being powerless as we are conditioned to believe. The health that we display is the product of conditioned reflexes. This goes to show that what we believe with our entire mind becomes reality within our body. We have to do our mental work then the dream becomes a reality and our thoughts manifest to become part of our existence. It all starts within us. We still have to take the steps in the physical world to make it happen, because life doesn't just happen the way we want it to, we still have to do the physical work, too, but we can accomplish much more than we ever dreamed with our thoughts just as Mahatma Gandhi had expressed in his insights, our thoughts do become our reality.

Guided Imagery

Guided Imagery is visualizing in the mind, the health goal of the body. Egyptian hieroglyphics suggest that they were using powers of the mind to manifest great accomplishments. Making a mental picture in the mind of already having achieved or accomplishing your goal. Seeing ourselves the way we really want to be, gives us a goal to work toward. A person, who is on a weight loss program, should regularly visualize themselves already at their ideal weight. This gives them a goal to work toward and a measurement to measure their success by.

To achieve it you have to see it…Visualize Yourself having already achieved your Weight Loss Goal. Imagine how relieved you feel having the burden of excess weight lifted. Visualization and Guided Imagery are powerful Mind Body techniques. Studies show that just imagining that you are exercising can improve your muscle tone by 14% in six months. So imagine you are exercising on a daily basis and imagine the results you can achieve in your weight loss plan.

Studies show that Imagery can improve physical performance. Many great athletes have used visualization techniques. One of the greatest examples is Michael Jordan. Jordan often said that he would visualize the ball successfully going through the hoop. No one can dispute the success Jordan had by doing this mental exercise to perfect his mental game. If you can see yourself making things happen, you can make things happen. The mind sets the goal with intent and the energy of the intent manifest in physical form if the intent is focused on the goal. This is a form of a visualization technique and Jordan has been documented saying that he visualized making the shot, many times. This means that in combination with his phenomenal talent he visualized it happing in his mind first. Another example is an Olympic runner who injured her knee six months prior to the Olympics and could not practice until the competitions began. She states that each day she practiced in her mind and come time for the games she competed and won the gold metal.

The Benefits of Guided Imagery

Guided Imagery helps us imagine becoming your new self-image
Meditation helps concentration on achieving the "new you" goal.
Guided Imagery allows you to project a thought into the universe to manifest in the physical world.
Guided Imagery is visualizing in the mind, the health goal of the body.
Make a mental picture in the mind of already achieving or accomplishing the goal
Seeing ourselves the way we really want to be, gives us a goal to work toward.
A person, who is on a weight loss program, needs to visualize themselves already at their ideal weight. This gives them a goal to work toward and a measurement to measure their success by.
Meditate on the Goal – Keep your Minds Eye on the Outcome.
Imagine the feeling of accomplishment repetitively.

Do a daily visualization having already achieved your goals until you actually achieve your weight loss goal. The Mind Body Weight Loss CD takes you through a detailed meditation this should be used every day for at least a month during your initial reprogramming phase. The messages will work for you and help you achieve hypnotic and meditative states of consciousness where great levels of positive change can occur. The more you use it the better it will work

THE BALANCE DIET & LIFESTYLE

for you. Some say that the term "Mind Body Medicine" means the power of the mind over the body. "Mind Over Matter".

The Mind Body Weight Loss Meditation with Guided Imagery Session

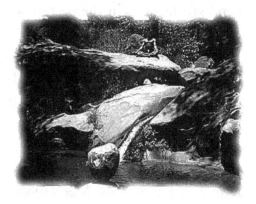

Take five slow breaths and as you breathe in, breathe in all of the energy that you need to help you achieve your weight loss goals. As you exhale, release everything that may be between your successfully achieving your weight loss goals. Close your eyes and begin visualizing yourself having already achieved your weight loss goal. As you lock this image into your mind step onto an imaginary scale and state the exact number of your ideal weight. Imagine yourself as having already achieved your goal. As you see yourself at your ideal weight, imagine how great you now feel at your ideal weight. Imagine how great it feels knowing that the burden has already been lifted.

Bring yourself to a state of conscious awareness where every thought and feeling is released and you are in touch with the collective consciousness.

Relax every part of your body individually until you come into deep meditative consciousness. As you visualize the steps you are taking to achieve you weight loss goals, allow the mind and body to go to work for you as you clear your mind of all obstacles. See yourself having already achieved your weight loss goal. Feel it with emotion. Want your new image with your entire mental mite. Your thoughts become your reality. Stay in this meditatative state of consciousness as long as needed and practice this meditatation on a daily basis.

Dr. Joyce Peters

Using Meditation To Achieve Your Weight Loss Goals

Scientific studies that were conducted at top medical schools show that meditation is beneficial to our health. Meditation has been proven to lower body weight, decrease acid, decrease blood pressure, decrease stress, and decrease appetite, and inner peace and satisfaction. In the past, it was thought that there are only three levels of consciousness, Waking Sleeping & Dreaming. There are upwards of six levels of consciousness and it is in the higher states where we are able to heal ourselves and solve our problems in life. The best way to enter into the higher states of consciousness is through meditation. In this state, we break through normal consciousness and expand our awareness because in this state of acceptance thoughts and feelings are not acted upon. Meditation helps us to get in touch with our higher self and our thoughts and emotions so that we can make decisions that are more conscious. Meditation is to become in tune and synchronize with all aspects of our lives, not to get away from it all. When we are meditating, we do not want to focus on the weight problem. When we meditate, it re calibrates our natural healing systems within to function and help to heal imbalances in the body. Meditation is not just relaxation, it is about becoming present in mind and body or some refer to meditation as a state of super alertness. Meditation is not so that we may escape from it life, it is so that we may get in touch with life.

Meditation is a state of "peaceful connection with everything that exists, it is a way of getting in touch with it all. Carl Jung, PhD was a German psychologist named the "ALL" as the collective conscious and universal intelligence. It is by consciousness that we are "All" connected. It is being in a grounded state of consciousness at the deepest state of reality where everything in life is inseparably connected and where we "ALL" exist in unison in the same quantum field, simultaneously. In meditation we are "ALL" connected to each other and with everything that exist. Once we achieve the ability to meditate we understand this awareness, and can utilize the ability to manifest our fullest potential and to gain power and control over our lives and our health. Our destiny can be abundantly enhanced through meditation. This is the reason that meditation is an important part of weight loss and healthy weight maintenance. It enables us to be aware and to get in touch with the cause of being overweight.

While meditating the goal is to push all fleeting thoughts out of your mind, every time an issue comes up, discard it until you get to the innermost thoughts and true inner self, when you get to your deepest hearts core, you can feel the euphoric energy that connects us all to one another and to the higher power. We become more focused and grounded with Meditation. One becomes more centered and aware through meditation.

To achieve a state of meditation, it is important to find an environment, in which you are blissfully comfortable. Some people make an area of their home as a sanctuary or refuge, some go to spas, churches, synagogues or Ashram houses and all of these are fine, all that matters is if it works for you, individually. Also, when out in nature exposure to the environment helps bring us into a state of meditation, as well, try using a nature sounds CD. The soothing sounds of nature can be quite hypnotic. Being in contact with the earth and the heavens above with all of the earths' natural energies and to bask in the beauty of nature attunes us more perfectly than any other meditative environment be it night or day. Ultimately, it is up to the individual to determine which environment is more meditative and gives the best results from the time spent meditating.

Sometimes, we may not realize it but we are meditating. Some people eat mindlessly while in deep thought and use food as an escape. Usually, they are trying to get to the required level of consciousness to resolve their problems. If you have a problem with eating food when mulling over your problems, put the food away and try meditation. Discard all thoughts of food and allow your mind to slip into utopia. You will know you have had a successful meditation when your consciousness level of awareness comes to a level of consciousness of missing time. In other words, you will feel that it has only been 15 minutes and an hour may have actually passed with out your recollection. This state of consciousness is believed to stop the false hunger, stress and survival instincts and hormones from being released and gives your immunity and resistance a chance to catch up. Meditation on a regular basis has shown to decrease blood pressure and increase immunity. The psychological and mental benefits are immeasurable.

In weight loss, we need to set our goal and practice a daily meditation toward achieving the goal. In daily life, we can become distracted from our goals. Daily meditation on our goal can bring us closer to achieving our goals. We need meditation because we are bombarded with distracting energies that create a cluttering effect on our senesces and state of consciousness.

This is a form of quantum medicine that is connected to quantum physics. What we first create in our mind we can manifest in physical form.

Easy Method Meditate

At first, use a candle as a focal point for meditation. Focus on the flame to relax and center your mind; stay focused on the fire, the dancing flame, and discard all unpleasant, negative or worrisome thoughts. Try using a word mantra such as "Ohm". Push all thoughts out of your mind. Release all feelings from your body. Breathe in deeply and slowly. Free your Mind and Body into a state of Moksha or bliss. After you have mastered this technique, you may no longer need a focal point and may easily transcend into a meditative state of consciousness. Alternatively, if you feel that you are unable to reach this state of consciousness, seek out a meditation class in your area, classes are very beneficial when you are first learning how to meditate.

An excess of weight is of course, an imbalance. In meditation, we achieve silence, which is a disruption of conditioned reflexes, which interrupts the pattern of disease or believed disease. What we believe on a deep level of metaphysical awareness within our deepest levels of consciousness becomes reality. This was also similar to Gandhi's philosophy that our thoughts become our reality. Through meditation, we are developing the ability to stand back and become a silent witness of what is happening in the brain or in our mind and body. When we become still and quite we experience silence of the body and mind, the innate and infinite energies spontaneously wake up and miracles may occur on our behalf, this allows the healing processes of the body to work, and we can only do this through meditation.

Comatose patients are quite often in deep healing states after trauma. In the mere non-judgmental silent awareness of a negative thought pattern, as the state of consciousness while in meditatation, it is a disruption and dissipation of the negative thought pattern or false belief. This can rationalize and overcome as a limitation. When we do meditation, this triggers the natural, infinite energies (Kundalini energy/ the interconnected power of the universe) and the innate or natural inborn healing knowledge, which synchronize the energies of the mind and body. The body can utilize the innate healing powers of the mind. In deep meditative states, the pharmacy within our body is activated to create the perfect medicine to heal itself. Transcendental Meditation is where one takes a mantra and uses the mantra to experience abstract levels of thinking, and ultimately experience deeper levels of thinking until experience the silence of consciousness and experience a state of pure awakeness, of pure silence with out thought consciousness. In meditation, we are connected with everything else that exists.

Mind Body Mantras

Repeating a mantra can help bring mental focus and clarity to your weight loss goals and aspirations. Chant the following mantra out loud three times each, on a daily basis for a month and once a week there after until you achieve the desired result. Remember your thoughts become your reality.

> I give my body full permission to lose the excess weight.
> I am achieving personal success because I depend on my self
> Two pounds of muscle burns ten pound of fat per year
> Exercise the closest thing to a magic weight loss pill.
> Exercise makes me stronger and physically fit.
> Exercise helps prevent disease.
> I forgive myself and all others who have contributed to my weight gain
> I realize that I alone create my own realty and control my weight
> I control what I swallow.
> I only eat fresh foods that aid my metabolism.

Conscious Thinking as Vibrational Medicine

If there is psycho somatic illness, then there must be psychosomatic wellness. Through senses that are yet to be fully understood, possibly the placebo effect, the body can pick up on the vibration of our thoughts and manifest them in our body where they may become a physical reality. Practice thinking yourself well. If you can think yourself sick you can think yourself well. If you can think yourself fat you can think yourself thin. How we perceived our body we may be able to create the though manifestation in a physical form. This is a form of quantum physics. It has also, been proven in microscopic laboratory experiments that a cell responds differently than when the cell is being observed and that the cells respond to different thoughts that the observer projects onto the cell. This proves that thought affects the behavior of cells, therefore, if we are constantly looking in the mirror calling ourselves fat and ugly we are going to become fat and ugly. Look into the mirror and tell your self you are slim and beautiful everyday. I had a patient to write "flat" on her stomach so that when she looked at her stomach, it reminded her to think "flat" not "fat". The human body is comprised mostly of water. Studies have also been performed on water by imprinting the water with emotion. The molecular structure of water can be altered by subjecting the water molecule to an emotional thought. According to some scientist, therefore, since the human body is mostly water thoughts and emotions can change the molecular structure of the fluid and chemistry within the body as well. Many over eaters have the same mental state of most obsessive-compulsive people and addictive type personalities, expressed in the form of food consumption. Over indulgence of anything, is not good for you. Meditation helps you to work through imbalances and to see the person you really are while it gives you a chance to project yourself into the future as the image of yourself that you want to be by concentrating on your new image in your daily meditation sessions.

Cellular and Molecular Biology

The face of medicine is changing, today. Cellular and Molecular Biology Is the science of observing the influence of negative and positive thought patterns and the effects of thought projections on an individual cell. It is the study of how thoughts during observation can affect the function and the proponents of the cell and counter wise the response of the cell creating effects in health. There is an innate intelligence aspect to human health. Our thoughts dictate to our cells respond by our emotions. Neuropeptides carry information throughout the chemistry and cellular fluid this can provide some insight as to how emotions can be felt in the body. Studies have shown that thoughts evoke emotion and send an energetic imprint into the body's water content and may change the molecular structure of the molecule. Love appears to have positive effects on health and appears to strengthen and purify while the emotional energy of hate appears to disrupt and destroy the molecular structure of the water molecules. Our body is over 70% water. It only makes sense that our thoughts can affect the health of our body, as well.

Research provides insight to the power of the Mind-Body dominion as opposed to genetic factors in imbalance and disease within the body at the molecular level. We know from studies that the more fully ingrained that the perception is, the more real it is perceived by the brain and the stronger the information signal becomes on a cellular level to trigger a cascade of changes on a cellular level. Dr. Parker founder of Parker Chiropractic College, promoted "The Infinite Oneness" theory and the Innate Intelligence of the Universe" both of these are phenomenal discoveries in how we evolve, exist, and survive in the world of natural science and respond to stimulus created by the outside world on a deep cellular and conscious level. Both theories relate to quantum physics and contain empowering information on how to maximize our own human potential in controlling our own destiny and potential for boundless health. Both show how negative thoughts from others as well as affect health that may lead to disease and how positive thoughts from others and ourselves create good health and wellness. There has been many scientific studies conducted that have documented these findings beyond typical cell biology studies. Keep your thoughts, beliefs and attitudes about your self and your body positive. It is important to think yourself thin just as it is important to have a healthy diet and lifestyle.

Science & Spirituality-Faith & Belief

Plato a great philosopher of scientific background, said that we each have a purpose and that we make sacred contracts to create scenarios that will ensure that our purpose is fulfilled in this lifetime. He believed that we make contracts before coming to live this life on earth, it is said that we chose our parents, siblings, children, lovers, spouse and co-workers and that they too, made contracts, prior to coming to earth. These contracts are to ensure that learn something from each other that makes us better souls in the end. Being able to make choices is empowering. There is a difference between spirituality and religion. Religion doesn't believe in metaphysical thinking, such as this. Religion has often been distorted and caused many conflicts. These conflicting thoughts may affect our thoughts about self, however, we are each entitled to our own beliefs. It is important to believe in a way that provides you with a healthy self-esteem. I believe that a healthy belief system allows you to have self confidence and to nurture personal growth and power. Science and spirituality are heading on a path to merge, again. Achieving your personal best can be a very moving and spiritual experience.

Having faith in yourself and believing in your self and your natural abilities to achieve your goals will ensure your weight loss success. Truly wanting to lose your excess weight and being willing to do what is necessary to lose your excess weight is the first step to ensure permanent success. It is also very important to allow the body-mind to experience deep levels of inner intelligence, known as the innate intelligence or the collective consciousness of the universe that is only tapped into through meditative states of consciousness. The Native American Indians believe that spirit forms of grandfather sun and grandmother earth unite their energies yearly to spring forth all of creation. There is a time of death and rebirth. The sun is the source of light that allows photo-synthesis that triggers the plants of the earth to grow and to produce the air that we breathe to sustain life. As father medicine uses the plants provided by Mother Nature's garden we are seeing the creation miracle cures, everyday. Accepting that all is interconnected creates a deep spiritual awakening and a positive loving connection for everything and everyone on the planet. Compared to the interaction that occurs between a patient and a healer. Amazing results can occur energetically between two energies when they are focused with intent to achieve a goal. When we make a choice to consciously blend our energies with the combined energies of the universe, we can pull all the power and determination that we need to give us the strength and power to achieve our weight loss goals. The conscious meditative effort to get in touch with the all knowing universe enables us to become more in touch the healing energies of the natural universe and to harness this power for the purpose of weight loss and weight maintenance by utilizing those energies to achieve our weight loss goals.

Reclaim Your Power & Energy
Frequently, recall the slender image you have created in your mind in your waking consciousness through out the day everyday until you achieve your weight loss goal. And always think of yourself in a state of good health. Your thoughts are powerful and manifest in physical reality. A clue of how you have neglected your health to the point of becoming overweight is by utilizing this technique. Find the sources which are draining your energy and eliminate them by doing the following exercise. Afterwards, work to remove energy vampires from your life. Claim and demand ownership of your power.

THE BALANCE DIET & LIFESTYLE

Energy Renewal Exercise

Dim the lights and Relax as you breathe deeply for 5 minutes laying flat of your back with your eyes closed. Imagine yourself as a plasma ball, imagine your energy becoming brighter and brighter as you imagine energetic sparks exuding from your skin and begin to fly off of your body in search of other energies lost or left behind. Find lost energy and draw it back inward.

Think about your current life situation, Where do you visualize that your energy and power is going? Where is most of your energy focused, or to whom is your energy going to?If it is going to people you want to keep your attachments to, do not withdraw your energy, simply pretend as if you draw your sword and slice away the energy connection. The most important thing is to stop your energy from being robbed and to draw all of your wasted energies back to yourself to recycle and reuse as needed to achieve your weight loss goal and to exercise.

Collect all of the energies that you are being robbed of or that have been robbed from you. Ground yourself. Find all of your energies, hook your energies and reel them back into yourself. Take what is only yours, do not rob others. Reclaim your full energies and then seal them inside of yourself. You have just renewed your power in life. Feel yourself powerful, whole and complete. Now, utilize this power every day until you reach your ideal weight and then to create the life that you desire and deserve for the rest of your life.

By cutting off energy losses, you are reclaiming your full energy, use this energy to do what you must do to lose your excess weight call on this energy when exercising to keep you fired up energetically to exercise off all of your fatty bulges. Realize that you are powerful; you are a mental, spiritual and physical power house.

Draining Sources Of My Energy & Energy Losses Are From:

_____

Picture your new slender self in this peaceful and most content setting. Imagine the clothes your slender self is wearing, visualize the size of your clothes and lock the number in to your cell memory, imagine your mood of joy and happiness as you are enveloped in happiness, see yourself smiling, imagine all the things you intend to do, imagine all the places you intend to go and visualize yourself already doing all of these things. Once you visualize yourself having already achieved your weight loss goal and experience the feeling and the image in your mind, then you are already creating that image in your physical reality. Use this guided relaxation exercise to begin projecting a new image upon yourself and is useful tool for stress reduction, too.

Guided Relaxation Exercise

Beginning Breathing, focus all your attentions on your breathing until you feel you have relaxed. Breath through your whole relaxation technique.

Start focusing on the toes, relaxing every little toe and up into your feet.

Feel your relaxation spreading like a pulsating wave, slowly moving up through the inside of your entire body.

Feel your relaxation moving up the legs, relaxing the calves, the knees, and the thighs.

Feel as you mentally move your sense of relaxation into your hips and abdomen.

Feel your insides and relax all of your internal organs.

Relax your buttocks and feel the tension slowly releasing from each part of your back. Allow the floor to hold you up and, as your body relaxes, feel as though you are grounding yourself.

Feel the relaxation coming into your chest, breathing very slowly and gently.

Bring your attention to your hands and fingers, relaxing each one in turn.

Then relax your hands.

Feel the relaxation moving up your arms, relaxing your wrists, fore-arms, and then your upper arms.

Allow your shoulders to relax. Feel the wave of relaxation moving up the back of your neck into the head and scalp.

Relax your face. Begin with your jaw and let your mouth hang open slightly. Relax your tongue and the muscles in the back of your throat.

THE BALANCE DIET & LIFESTYLE

Relax the chin and the cheeks, then the eyes and eyebrows, the forehead, and the scalp.
Relax the brain. Clear the mind of all cares and worries.
Allow the Body, Mind and Spirit to remain in this state of relaxation
until you experience bliss and utopia.

An excess of weight is of course, an imbalance. In meditation, we achieve silence, which is a disruption of conditioned reflexes, which interrupts the pattern
of disease or believed disease. What we believe on a deep level of metaphysical awareness within our deepest levels of consciousness becomes reality. This
was also similar to Gandhi's philosophy that our thoughts become our reality.
Through meditation, we are developing the ability to stand back and become a
silent witness of what is happening in the brain or in our mind and body. When
we become still and quite we experience silence of the body and mind, the innate and infinite energies spontaneously wake up and miracles may occur on our
behalf, this allows the healing processes of the body to work, and we can only
do this through meditation. Comatose patients are quite often in deep healing
states after trauma. In the mere non-judgmental silent awareness of a negative
thought pattern, as the state of consciousness while in meditation, it is a disruption and dissipation of the negative thought pattern or false belief. This can
rationalize and overcome as a limitation. When we do meditation, this triggers
the natural, infinite energies (Kundalini energy/ the interconnected power of the
universe) and the innate or natural inborn healing knowledge, which synchronize the energies of the mind and body. The body can utilize the innate healing
powers of the mind. In deep meditative states, the pharmacy within our body is
activated to create the perfect medicine to heal itself. Transcendental Meditation
is where one takes a mantra and uses the mantra to experience abstract levels of
thinking, and ultimately experience deeper levels of thinking until experience
the silence of consciousness and experience a state of pure awareness, of pure
silence with out thought consciousness. In meditation, we are connected with
everything else that exists.

Pro-Active Thinking – Repeat as many of these thoughts as possible.
Remember them and recite them as though they were bible verses. You can
loose weight and achieve a more positive mental outlook by reciting the following positive thoughts on a daily basis:

Daily Pro-Active Thinking Practice

I do want to lose my excess weight and I am losing my excess weight.

I am serious about losing my excess weight.

I am motivated to lose all of my excess weight.

I am increasing my activities I am loosing all of my excess weight.

I am passionate about losing my excess weight.

I exercise to burn all stored fat tom my body.

Exercise makes me strong fit and healthy.

I utilize the full power of my mind and body to achieve my weight loss goals.

I Have Learned To Think Pro-Actively In These Ways:

_____

Prayer Miracles can be achieved through prayer! Prayer has been proven to produce healing reactions in the body and miraculous healing has actually occurred with prayer, in hospital studies. Pray for your successful weight loss and weight management. In prayer you can ask God or whomever you consider a higher being for assistance in achieving what you want to happen in your life. Prayer is about connecting and speaking to what you consider the creator or God it is a state where out loud or silently we speak to spirit, what one cannot say they can literally see with the eye, can be felt with the soul. We must believe with all our being that our prayers will be answered. Numerous accounts throughout history and since the beginning of time, people have accounted that miraculous things have happened in their lives that they had prayed for. Through the power of prayer, waters have been parted and mountains crumbled to the sea. Say your prayer all throughout the day everyday. Believe your prayers will be answered. Have others to pray with you and for you, as well. It does not cost a thing in the world and it works. Praying is a very good practice for weight loss, the more you pray over it the more you send out Karmic energy that will come back to you to make it so. Most Prayers are finalized with a statement of belief, that what you have just said is true and complete and therefore the prayer, mantra or confirmation is ended with a statement such as "Amen", "It is so", I have spoken, or in the name of the Savior, Amen. The Hindu's chant "Ohm" or Aum" in respect to worship and praise the Omnipotent one. This started the belief that, "Ohm" it is the basis of all sounds in the universe. It became the sacred word "Hum" to Tibetans and the word "Amen" to the Egyptians, Greeks, Romans, Jews and Christians.

THE BALANCE DIET & LIFESTYLE

Examples :

1) "Dear God, I call upon you and your omnipotent power which you used to create the Universe to help me lose my excess weight, Amen"

2) "Oh Great Creator, Father of the Universe, Grandfather Sun, Grandmother Earth, I call the spirit guides of my ancestors I summons you, to help me overcome this spirit of gluttony and excess that has made me over weight and obese. I ask you to lead me and to help me shed my excess weight and regain my health - – I have spoken"

3) "Your Holiness, I call upon your energies that are within my Mind, Body and Spirit, to guide me that I will lose my weight and maintain a healthy weight through life. Satanama."

Incredible results can be achieved, when effective integrative practices or prayer is utilized. According to research performed in clinical and laboratory studies at New York University. The experimental groups showed increased hemoglobin counts and hematocrit ratios were measured and shown to increase, in the experimental groups when using therapeutic-healing touch. Statistically, the findings could have happened by chance less than 1 in 1,000. Which means we can learn how to help each other in ways that are too subtle than we currently understand. We are connected beyond the physical and conscious levels. In another controlled study conducted by Justas Smith, PhD researcher at the Human Dimensions Institute. A spectro-petometer was used to show the rate at which an active-enzyme will break down a protein compared to the rate of an active-enzyme would break down a protein, after it had been energized in the hands of a healer. The study showed that paranormal healing could be tested, monitored and demonstrated in a scientific laboratory.

CHAPTER 14

Rest, Relaxation and Sleep

REST, RELAXATION AND SLEEP ARE AN IMPORTANT PART OF A healthy Lifestyle. In fact, they are necessary to maintain good health and they are of equal importance as is a proper diet and exercise for a healthy Mind and Body. Include plenty of rest, relaxation and sleep in your life because they are necessary for you maintain balance in your life. Typically, simply ceasing activity is the way that most people rest; some sit down in their favorite chair and watch T.V. or read a book as a restful practice others prefer take a outdoor stroll, finding a grassy spot of earth and laying on a blanket outside surrounded by the sounds of nature. When weather doesn't permit basking in nature; sitting in a comfortable chair or laying down on a sofa, floor, yoga mat and doing basically nothing will suffice. The objective is, enjoying some peace and quiet time. These are a few of the ways that people rest or relax. Too much rest is not good for you, being sedentary is one of the worst lifestyle mistakes you can make. A balance between work and rest is key. Relaxing is shifting into a more rested or alpha state of consciousness. Sleeping is shifting into deeper states. Breathing alone can be totally relaxing by establishing a rhythmic pattern, rhythmic sounds induce a trance-like state of relaxation and this is a practice often used in meditation. Certain frequencies of sound and light can be used for relaxation and to even repair our DNA, according to some experts. Regardless, relaxation can help normalize cell function and bio-rhythyms. Low wattage soft- colored lights, night-lights, accent lamps or candles can be relaxing. Soft sounds such as lullaby or soft flute or harp music can be very relaxing, too. Chanting is a form of trance relaxation techniques, and some prefer total silence while others may use an Indian drum for drumming sounds from nature and even crystal bowls to produce a frequency of delta sound waves to induce a state of relaxation. If relaxing is difficult for you, a few bio-feedback sessions may help you learn the technique of relaxation. Try these simple relaxation techniques.

Body Relaxation/Physical Relaxation-
Start out with a few deep breaths. So many times we forget to breathe deeply. You should inhale for 3-4 seconds and exhale for 6-9 seconds. Then do yoga or basic stretches for various parts of your body, relax your arms, legs, fingers and toes. Lay down on the floor or yoga mat and relax your back and breathe in, inhale and exhale, several times with your eyes closed, relaxing the eyelids and the face and jaw. Relax the hidden parts inside your body and your hips, behind your knees and under your arms. Continue to breathe and relax until you feel a floating feeling in your physical body.

Mind Relaxation/Mental Relaxation-
Now that your body is relaxed, note the feeling in your mind and continue on to do a mental relaxation. Feel the experience of being totally relaxed, allow your scalp to get looser and more relaxed, let your forehead melt as you relax your eyebrows and temples. Relax your eyes more and close your eyes. Allow your jaw to drop open as you relax the muscles in your neck and throat and ears. Now move the mental relaxation inside your mind, pushing all thoughts out of your mind until all you think about is nothing.

Finding and Balancing Your Center -
Imagine being enveloped in a soft and soothing, oscillating flow of radiating energy all around your body, similar to warm sunshine circling around you body and through you, cleansing away anything that is unhealthy. Then, when you are physically and mentally relaxed you can begin to bring the cleansing energy inward to the deeper parts of your inner self, to your core and that is where you

will find your center. Once you feel this space inside, lay on your side and curl up into the fetal position under a soothing, relaxing, colorful silk veil or sheer breathable cloth. Solid Jewel-toned colors work best. Start out laying flat on a comfortable floor mat, on cotton, hemp or other natural fiber quilt or blanket and allow your body to stretch into poses and positions that feel good and release tension. Once tension is released, lay on your side and pull the blanket over your head, leaving room for air but close the light out. Breathe several, slow deep breaths. Position yourself on back with knees to chest or on side in fetal position to feel total comfort and inner stillness. Next, slowly, sit up in yoga pose, Indian style, keeping the drape over your head, again feel inner stillness. Allow every part of your body mind and spirit to align in one oscillating stream of universal love for self and all of mankind. Allow this love to flow from your heart out to everything and everyone in the world until you reach a feeling of peace, harmony and tranquility. Allow yourself to feel grateful for life and kindness, love and forgiveness toward others. Allow yourself to feel gratitude for all your blessings and gifts. Sit in this state of loving consciousness until you feel at one with all, or until you can imagine what it would feel like to be as one with everyone and everything. Bring the thought of being your best self within every cell, and then bring that feeling inside yourself until you feel it centered deep in to your heart and soul. Then say, I am centered and whole.

People who are trying to lose weight need to improve their sleeping habits as well as their eating habits. The pineal gland is part of the endocrine system. The pineal gland produces the hormone Melatonin, which regulates the body's wake/sleep cycles and therefore if we are low on sleep energy, we may have tendencies to eat to compensate for lost sleep resulting in lowered energy. Therefore, better sleep habits may be instrumental to the success of any weight management plan. Sleep deprivation can create a bio-hormonal imbalance, as the pineal gland is the gland, which regulates our wake/sleep cycles and affects our tissue & organ repair processes and slows metabolic waste removal as the body repairs and renews itself during sleep. The endocrine system is a compensatory system. The glands and organs work synergistically to produce, regulate and maintain a healthy hormonal balance in the body. The thyroid, and key regulator of metabolism, is of course part of the endocrine system. If the pineal gland is affected by sleep deprivation, it could possibly affect the thyroid and metabolism.

Lack of Sleep can increase appetite and hunger, to compensate energy lost from lack of sleep. Sleep deprivation can affect the body's metabolism, which may make it more difficult to maintain or lose weight. Rest is important to your health, be sure to get your "beauty sleep". The lack of Sleep creates a form of stress and has been shown to affect the secretion of cortisol, an acidifying hormone that regulates appetite. As a result, individuals who lose sleep may continue to feel hungry despite adequate food intake. If you are eating to make up for lost sleep at night the lack of sleep is contributing to your weight problem. You may help regulate your hunger by taking a fifteen-minute power nap at lunch before eating. This also, re-boots your metabolic processes and increases fat metabolism. Loss of normal Sleep may interfere with the body's ability to metabolize carbohydrates and cause high blood levels of glucose, a basic sugar. Excess glucose in the body, promotes the overproduction of insulin. An over production of insulin promotes the storage of body fat. This is similar to syndrome x and creates an imbalance of the metabolism of carbohydrates.

Long-term sleep disturbances lead to imbalance and may lead to insulin resistance and adult-onset diabetes. Sleep deprivation is associated with alterations in hormone levels that help regulate the appetite and contributes to the development of obesity. In addition to changes in sleep quantity, reductions in sleep quality can also affect weight. Decreased amounts of restorative deep or slow-wave sleep have been associated with significantly reduced levels of growth hormone and a protein that helps regulate the body's proportions of fat and muscle during adulthood. The lack of Sleep disrupts metabolic & hormonal processes, which can be a contributing, factor in weight gain and obesity. If sleep problems persist you may gain weight due to an increase in your appetite due to lack of energy. Sleep deprivation can interfere with daily functioning, causing you to use food as a substitute for adequate rest. Try the following helpful tips, but, if the problem persists, visit your doctor.

Helpful Tips That Improve Sleep Aid Weight Loss

1) Do not work on computers or watch television for an hour before bed. Avoid artificial florescent lighting, it blocks the production of Melatonin hormone and contributes to pineal dysfunction. Under candle or low light read for a few minutes, make sure it is non-work related reading.

2) Do not go to bed feeling hungry, but do not eat a big meal right before bedtime.

3) Make love, receive a massage or do light exercise such as sit-ups or

stretching are helpful to relax and sleep more restfully. However, do not do aerobic exercises in the evening before bedtime.

4) Use natural sleep aids such as valerian root or Passiflora herbals instead of medications. You will feel more refreshed the next day, not hung over. Avoid consuming caffeine, nicotine, stimulating supplements, drugs and alcohol in the evening and keep water by the bed.

5) Follow a sleep schedule, set a time for sleeping and awakening that is in tune with your natural biological clock. Adjust bedtime so that you awake naturally for work time or in starting your day. Listen to your body, not your alarm clock. If needed, start taking short, daily power naps.

6) If you have trouble sleeping at night, try a Melatonin hormone supplement before bed instead of medication it is a natural hormone that your body produces to trigger sleep response, it is also a powerful antioxidant and aids in cell renewal and tissue regeneration.

7) Practice relaxing pre-sleep rituals, such as controlled deep slow breathing such as panache karma and meditation.

8) Take a warm bath with by candlelight. Add chamomile and Epsom salts to your bath to aid relaxation.

9) Create a pleasant sleep environment, light natural music or sounds of nature. Cozy, comforting supportive pillows and plush clean, fresh bed linens. Make it as comfortable as possible temperature wise.

10) Make sure your bedroom is dark and quiet. Noise and light will affect sleep quality. Change your environment. If you cannot sleep, switch to another room.

11) It is recommended to sleep with the head of the bed to the north, never the south and facing east to wake up naturally as the birds, do, with the rising sun. The gravitational pull of the planet will aid proper digestion and circulation.

Studies show that people of developing countries have less sleep disturbances and weight related problems than Americans. The diet may be the culprit to sleep disorders. The diets of Americans are filled with junk when people stay up late watching television and eating snacks before bedtime. Snacking before bedtime is not a healthy behavior, this can be a form of excessive behavior. There are also fewer incidences of sleep disorders and other diseases of excess in other countries where bedtime snacking is not an acceptable behavior. Generally, what this means is that the poorer peoples of the world are generally richest in health, they have fewer sleep anxieties and tend to rest more soundly. This is partially from their habits of avoiding bed time snack and not excessively consuming fatty, rich foods on a daily basis, three times a day as is common in the typical American diet. In comparison to the diets of Americans and ratio of related diseases of excess, in the poorer peoples of the world there are less sleep disturbances, heart disease, diabetes, heart attacks, high blood pressure, and cancer.

Dream Therapy

Physician and psychological analyst, Carl Jung, often referred to the collective unconscious as the universal source of knowledge and information. Each night as we sleep we access this source as we enter into the dream state. When properly interpreted this source, it can give us a strong intuition and awareness of what is going on around us that we may not consciously be aware of. When we dream we are creating a movie that embeds the messages that our subconscious is bringing to the surface of our conscious mind. If we are able to decipher the messages that our subconscious is brining to our attention, we receive a preparatory alert through our dreams to prepare us for a change in consciousness that are outside of our known knowledge. According to Dr. John Kappas, the inventor of Kappasanian theory psychology and founder of the Hypnosis Motivation Institute, our "known's" are the positive or negative experiences that make it through the filters of the critical mind and become part of the information stored in the subconscious mind. Information in the subconscious mind are our "known's". This information is what drives us to do the things that we do and may form our individual beliefs and behaviors.

The more we delve into dream interpretation; we realize that the answers that we are seeking in our awakening consciousness are deep within the collective unconscious that we tap into as we sleep. We access the answers we need to grow and change by dreaming. Research studies show that we keep our sense of reality and sanity by venting out the things we cannot accept and deal with or the things that are impossible for us to understand, as we dream. Therefore, dream therapy can help us get in touch with our most inner emotions and can decrease emotional eating. As we evolve human psychology evolves to adapt to times. Survival methods are ever-changing we adapt to this change through dreaming as we grow and evolve and cultures adapt and change. Each night, ask your subconscious mind to give you a dream to help you understand the areas of your life that needs attention. Ask you subconscious to give you a clue as to why you are experiencing your weight issues so that you have better conscious awareness to approach your weight issues effectively to ensure quick and permanent results. Write down the dream and decipher the meaning to find the solution. When people start eating the standard American highly refined and high fat diet, this is when disease ratios increase. The roots of our problems are not in deficiencies, they are mostly caused by excessive eating behaviors. Remember that until we establish moderation for ourselves individually and get away from excessive behaviors, our problems cannot be permanently resolved. Alternatively, we sleep to escape the stresses of the day. We sleep so that the body can heal and repair itself and so that the mind can process the message units that it has received throughout the day and process the new information for psychological growth. Our dreams are a sign of the new "knowns". As new information filters through the critical mind into the subconscious mind and back up to the surface to the conscious mind through dreams. This creates our current sense of reality.

If you are on a weight loss plan and you start asking for answers about how to increase your weight loss. Dreams about physical inactivity or exercise and physical activity can be an indication that we are not getting enough exercise for weight loss, health or even mental reasons. Just as not enough physical exercise causes muscles to atrophy and fat to accumulate, not enough mental exercise stuns psychological and mental growth. Sleep is very important to your weight loss program and in maintaining good health physically and mentally.

Keep A Dream Journal
Keep a dream journal beside your bed every night with a pen-light. Write down your dreams when you first wake up before you forget them. To understand how you feel about waking life decipher the hidden message to resolve all of your weight problems and other areas that you are growing in.

Imbalances Are Revealed In Dreams
Imbalances in our waking life and other things that our subconscious mind is trying to alert us about are often revealed to us in dreams. Things that may be hidden from our conscious view or awareness often come up in dreams. Our mind begins to reveal these hidden things to us in our dreams.

THE BALANCE DIET & LIFESTYLE

Example dream journal writings are as follows:

I dreamed I had a tumor on my neck and head and that it had doubled in size. the next day. In the dream, my brother and sister confirmed that it had grown overnight. In the dream I realized I had cancer, that it was malignant melanoma, and that I did not have much time to live. My boyfriend and I were sleeping on a pedestal, tree house, when we woke up we were very hungry and wanted food. I looked down off the pedestal, I realized we were really high from the ground and if we fell, we would die. He was going to climb down the pole, like Jack and the Beanstalk and I was afraid he would fall and die and I would lose him, forever. He said don't worry about me, you are the one who is dying.

Example Dream Analysis :

The dreamer awoke feeling hungry and went on a food binge. The dream symbolizes a hunger and need for love, nurturance, support and understanding. The next day, the girl expressed how her love had grown and expressed her growing disappointment that he did not feel the same desire for marriage. The boyfriend suggested that they should slow down their relationship even further, confirming an actual relationship imbalance and interpersonal loss. There was an "interpersonal imbalance" between the couple. One was focused on family and matters of the heart. One was focused on career and financial success. In reality, the dreamer was afraid of letting go of the relationship; in waking life the couple was in the process of a break-up, due to "relationship imbalances" in the couple's goals and companionship needs. The couple had been apart for a week and then back together for a day on the night of the dream. The dream symbolism was a secret warning of what her subconscious already knew. The subconscious was gently alerting the dreamer that the relationship was far from being grounded and in fact, it was over.

Through this dream, the dreamer's higher self was reminding her that equality is important in a relationship and that mutual feelings must be reciprocated for the relationship to work in a healthy manner. What she was "hungering" for, could not be found in the relationship that was failing in her waking life. The current relationship that she was involved in was in fact, creating stress and it was time to stop sticking her neck out, cut her losses, and move on, to a healthier more stable lifestyle. This was the subconscious alerting her that the relationship wasn't healthy and that the growth she is experiencing in her relationship is detrimental and that it is time to cut the stalk down to heights and remove negative growth. There is no nourishment in the air food is from the earth and relationships must be solidly grounded to take them to the next level, the food she was hungering for is unattainable from the boyfriend, he is a long way from satisfying her hunger for love, which was displayed as food in the dream. In other words, the dream was the minds way of preparing her and alerting to her that it was time to cut the cancer that is feeding on her, out of her life.

This is only one interpretation as dreams are open to other interpretations. The point is that your mind will reveal secrets of your subconscious through your dreams, to help you solve all the problems you face in life, including your weight control struggles and emotional eating cues.

Healthy Living will always be important. Please, support groups like the "The Environmental Children's Organization" (ECO) Sustainable Living and preserving the natural environment and the future of humanity and the planet with truth, love and light.

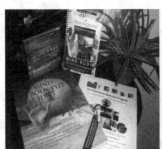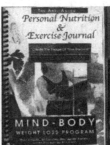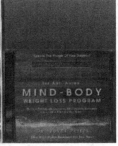

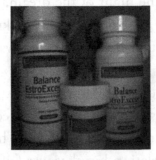

For other resources and health products such as these: visit http://www.shop. mindbodyhealthprograms.com

CHAPTER 15

Staying Motivated & Fit For A Lifetime

To MAINTAIN YOUR RESULTS FOR LIFE, YOU MUST DEVISE A maintenance plan. There are a few basic steps for staying motivated to live a healthy lifestyle in order to stay fit for lifetime. Realizing the importance of the diet and adopting the attitude that you eat to sustain the good health of your body. This means avoiding a diet that is lacking in foods that contain a natural balance of essential nutrients because when you jeopardize your diet with foods that have a low nutritional value, those foods will always leave you feeling hungry, unsatisfied and wanting for more. The diet solution can be as simple as eating quality fresh whole foods in comparison to eating processed foods that carry very little of the essential nutrients that your body needs to function, properly.

Eliminating Denial and Changing for Good

We are human beings, creatures of habit. Being in denial of overindulgences that are not as obvious as drug or alcohol abuse, can still kill us. Just as shooting up heroine or having, non-protected non-monogamous sex can. They are all forms of self-sabotaging behaviors that are detrimental to our health, just as a bullet is to the brain will kill you, over eating and being over weight will kill you, but only slower. In this day and time we have to make a choice to protect our health, just as we have to have self-control with our sexual prowess to avoid serious disease, we must develop self-control with our eating habits as well. What we accept at a deep level of awareness becomes our reality. Most people do not alter their set patterns very often. Yet, we each have a unique and individual pattern that we follow in our daily lives that is unique to anyone else's pattern, just like a finger print. Once we learn a pattern it becomes a known. To change a pattern is to step out side of our "knowns". Learned behaviors are "knowns". What we already know is comfortable, we are accustomed to doing things that way and doing things that way is easy. Few people alternate this pattern because to do so creates discomfort and effort. The first step to change is to eliminate denial that we have bad habits. We dictate our lives by what is known, comfortable and pleasant to us at the time. It takes 21 days to change a habit. If we change a habit for 21 days we can overcome it, for good, because the new pattern replaces the old habit and the new pattern becomes the habit. Addicts are at the greatest risk in the first 21 days. 21 is your lucky number when it comes to overcoming bad habits.

Human Beings are "Creatures of Habit"
Anything you do for 21 days can become a habit.
Change your diet for 21 days.
Change your exercise for 21 days.
Change your pattern for 21 days and you change your habits.

Permanent Weight Loss Success Rate
You can assess you rate of successful out come with this quick and easy self-assessment quiz. If you answer no to any of these questions it is time to make behavior modifications that will help ensure your successful outcome of permanent weight loss.

Stay Active
"Keep the "Go & Do" mind-set of your youth. Commit to do it and, just do it. Youthful people are busy and active.

Let's go for a walk
Let's go jogging

THE BALANCE DIET & LIFESTYLE

Let's go work out

Let's go to the gym

Let's go play ball

Let's go to the beach

Let's go for a swim

Let's go dancing

Let's go make love

Let's give each other a massage (take turns doing the work)

Let's go help our friends, family or neighbor (move, plant a garden, ect...)

Stay Success Oriented

I am constantly learning all that I can, to prevent and overcome my health issues.

I accept the responsibility and sometimes burden of being a leader.

It is a top priority for me to loose all of my excess weight.

I do not make it a habit of allowing others behavior influence me.

I do not allow others behavior to change my standards of behavior.

I have strong will power.

I really want to loose my excess weight.

I work hard on a daily basis to try to achieve my goals and dreams.

I have a habit of keeping the promises that I make to myself.

The promises I make to myself are not easily broken.

I accept responsibility for my behaviors.

I accept responsibility for my mistakes.

I never put off doing important things, which result in negative consequences.

I never put off getting check-ups regarding my health.

I work my way through a problem quickly and move on to other things.

I have a habit of not allowing others to solve my problems for me.

I realize that I have the power to create my own reality.

If I discover that something is bad for me, I usually, do not have a habit of continuing doing It.

If you answered no to any of these questions the following section can help you to increase your potential of successful weight loss and decrease your risk of failure. Take this quiz after reading and implementing the techniques described in the behavior modification section of this book. I can offer you these words of wisdom on your path to permanent weight loss success. After you have achieved your weight loss goals always remember this:

If you remember these things and the answer to why you don't want to go down that path again, you will be less likely to revert back to your old habits that made you overweight in the first place.

Mind Body Weight Management Daily Tips

☺ Eat a balance of healthy, filling, bulky, fiber rich, natural foods that keep you satisfied and feeling full.

☺ Eat high energy foods that keep your energy levels up.

☺ Cleanse and detoxify your system on a daily basis.

☺ Exercise on a daily basis and increase your exercise levels.

☺ Get adequate rest and sleep to reduce fatigue.

☺ Take food supplements and herbs that increase or enhance mental focus and clarity keeps the mind feeling alert and functioning clearly.

☺ Preventing the mind and body from feeling fatigue, hungry and deprived. This is one of the most important keys to weight management success.

Changing for Good

Make a contract with your higher self. It is hard to break contracts, which we have made with our higher self after a wounding experience. What we subconsciously promise our selves and what we believe becomes our reality. If we can see and feel it, we can know it and believe it, it becomes our reality. Using expanded awareness is important in overcoming any health condition including achieving successful weight loss and permanent healthy weight maintenance. Before making the contract with yourself consider the following and ask yourself if you have any old contracts from childhood, that you must break that may be sabotaging your successful lifelong weight management goals if there are it is time to update your contract. Your self-contracts should support your best interest and your personal goals. The following is a Mind Body Weight Loss Self Contract. Make a copy for your records the day you start your program so that you may keep up with your progress. Keep this in a safe place so that you may monitor your progress and commit to achieving your goal in a timely manner.

THE BALANCE DIET & LIFESTYLE

Personal Weight Loss Vow
I vow to myself to know these truths

If I do not put it in my mouth, it will not put weight on my body.
I will not gain excess weight on my body unless I am consuming something that creates weight.

There is no way that I can gain weigh unless I am overeating or consuming more calories than I am using on a daily basis

Staying Aware Of When and Why People Binge and Over Eat

Food Oriented Social Habits – when hanging out with family and friends, making a habit of socially gathering around food and drink, movie, watching the game, hot dogs popcorn, soda's, beer, candy, birthday cake and ice cream, valentines chocolates, Easter basket candy, Halloween candy, Hanukkah, thanksgiving feast, Christmas cakes and pies, 4th of July barbeque, wedding cakes, funeral feast, reception parties, baby shower, New Years day and other celebrations centered around food.

Food Rewarding – receiving food as a prize, good grade, good behavior treat, doing chores. Usually learned in childhood by being good receiving a reward.

Pleasure Gratification – to satisfy the neo-cortex or pleasure oriented brain.

Poor Self-Control – knowing that overeating and eating the wrong foods is bad for your health and doing it anyway because it taste good to you and you want it.

Dissatisfying relationships – eating when alone and bored or while feeling depressed or lonely.

Bad habits – eating while watching television or movies.

After negative relationship experiences – a break-up in a relationship, using food as emotional comfort.

After negative or suppressed anger experiences – mindlessly eating when stewing over something that happened or something that someone did, eating junk snacks while stressed in traffic, eating when upset, eating to ease tension, eating to feel calm.

After negative work stress – eating while working in a craze at work, eating too much before work for an upcoming hectic day, after a long day "junking-out" Instead of coming home and having a healthy meal, snacking on junk until bedtime while unwinding.

Medical Reasons – There are also medical reasons for overeating, such as, over stimulated amygdala areas in the brain due to Bio-Chemical or Genetic Imbalances

Denial – avoiding thinking about the consequences of food consumption.

Realizing that all of the following behavior examples are forms of self-sabotaging behaviors that require effective modification techniques.

All excessive behavior is bad for your health.

Over weight and obesity is as bad for you, as other addictive or excessive compulsive behaviors.

Health wise, addiction to food is as bad for your health as addiction to alcohol or drugs.

Being overweight indicates imbalance and excessive behaviors.

Excessive behaviors can be an indication of other mental disorders such as, obsessive-compulsive disorder.

Taking a serious and realistic look at the reality of our diet situation in America is important. We should realize that it is important to acknowledge that over indulgent or binge eating habits may be a form of obsessive-compulsive behavior. The following tips may help you break out of this viscous cycle.

Easy Tips to Break Binge Eating Habits
1) Recognize the trigger, why do you do it? Identify the problem, access the cause, and eliminate the behavior source.
2) Get in touch with your emotions and feelings – eating is suppressing the source of your moods and the emotions you are truly feeling.
3) Freeze leftovers so that you do not feel that you have to finish them off before they ruin.
4) Do not feel that you have to take advantage of all free food. Pass up free food unless you are hungry. Do not binge at events where there is free food.

5) Assess if your true needs and desires are being met, water, sleep, love, sex, fresh air, satisfying relationships.

6) The next time you are tempted to binge eat do something you enjoy before eating. If you still feel hungry then eat in moderation.

7) You can create your own aversion therapy by taking ipecac with the food that is sabotaging your weight loss goals to create a distaste for the food until you are able to avoid the food. This is not intended as a permanent solution, the ipecac should not be taken in a quantity that induces vomiting. The preferred method is to use only a few drops to create nausea until behavior modification is achieved. The repeated nausea creates enough pain to kill the desire for the food because the pleasure seeking brain will associate pain with the food item by triggering the discomfort of feeling nauseated.

8) Start a twelve-step support group program similar to AA to stop your food addiction, if you are quitting "cold turkey". If you are addicted to a food, such as sweets. Count the days of sobriety and reward yourself on anniversaries with a smaller clothing item with the money you saved from not purchasing the junk food.

9) Change your instinctive memory that allows the bad eating habit to be continued. Any habit that becomes painful looses its appeal, eventually. When people get salmonella, they will usually avoid the food along time and sometimes for life. Remember these experiences, as most people have been sick on food at some point and can relate to the feeling and recall the memory. Use this negative experience as a positive tool in your weight loss and as a reminder to avoid the sabotaging food item.

10) Eliminate food addictions, under proper supervision, arrange an "ipecac food exorcism" make yourself sick of the taste of the sabotaging food, forever. It is not recommended for bulimics or anorexic people. It is not recommended as a form of habit control in daily eating. It is only recommended under supervision, for food addicts only. If the addicting food is chocolate, for example, you cannot eat or drink anything for twelve hours but, water, ipecac and the addicting food. Addicting foods usually contain caffeine, white sugar or flour, such as; chocolate, cola, donuts, cake, ice cream, caffienated drinks or even coffee or tobacco. These foods must be avoided during weight loss and used only in extreme moderation at any other time.

Ultimately, each individual has full control and power over their own weight. We each decide on a daily basis, what to put in out mouth and swallow.

Make your self-discovery; deal with reality in a healthy manner. Alternatively, find someone who will work through your discovery with you so that you can put it in the past and move on into a healthier future. Self-reflection allows you to discover the source and then it is up to you to forgive and forget. We cannot change the past, but, we do not have to allow it to ruin our future happiness, because, every individual has the power within themselves to allow positive change. Just ahead are the stories of two patients, male and female who overcame their learned negative childhood behaviors. With both of these patients, we used subtle, yogic meditations to make subconscious behavior modifications of the negative learned behaviors and to replace them with healthier new thoughts. The following are examples of mantras or you may write words of your own.

MIND BODY WEIGHT LOSS MANTRAS:

1) "My mind and body, now work together to achieve my weight loss goal".
2) "I release all obstacles so that I will achieve my weight loss goal"
3) "I have renewed powers in my mind & body to control my weight"
4) "I see myself at my ideal weight, I can, I am and I will easily achieve my weight loss goals"
5) "I am achieving the greatest health fitness accomplishment that I can achieve by loosing excess weight".
6) "I am losing all of my excess weight".
7) "I am successful in managing my weight"
8) "I am full of radiant energy that makes me look and feel great"
9) "I am persistent in maintaining my ideal weight"
10) "Victory is mine, I have won the battle of the bulge"
11) "I only eat foods that help me lose my excess weight"
12) "I am achieving my weight loss goals"
13) "Healthy sized portions totally satisfy me"
14) "I enjoy exercise, it helps me lose my excess weight"
15) "I am fully in control of my own weight"
16) "I am creating the me that I have always wanted to be"
17) "I am successfully achieving my weight-loss goals"
18) "Cravings for fattening foods non-longer are a problem"
19) "Fatty bulges are gone, forever"
20) "I am happy and healthy"

THE BALANCE DIET & LIFESTYLE

SELF DISCOVERY FORM

Name: _____ age: _____ Date: _____

Who was the primary caregiver that influenced my eating behaviors most?

_____

What are my learned eating behaviors: _____

Who are my siblings and How many of my siblings are overweight? _____

What foods do I most associate with home:

_____

Snacks/Drinks _____

What foods do I most associate with eating out:

_____

_____

Snacks/Drinks _____

What foods have I consumed on a regular basis that cause fat formation:

_____

I was most happy when I weighed: _____

What foods and drinks should I avoid to lose weight:

_____

_____

_____

What foods should I eat to lose weight and stay healthy:

_____

How much water am I drinking on a daily basis? How much do I need?

_____

My current weight is _____ I want to weigh _____

What Behaviors Do I Most Need To Modify and Change?

_____

_____

_____

314 •

The most important thing to believe in is to believe in yourself! You must have self-confidence and confidence in yourself to be a success in anything. If you have self-confidence, you have all you need to achieve your goals of success. Permanent change requires a life long commitment. It is important, believing that you can successfully make a life long change. It is important to make a commitment to yourself, that you are going to achieve your health goals and that you will be capable of maintaining your ideal weight for life.

"To thine own self, be true"… Shakespeare

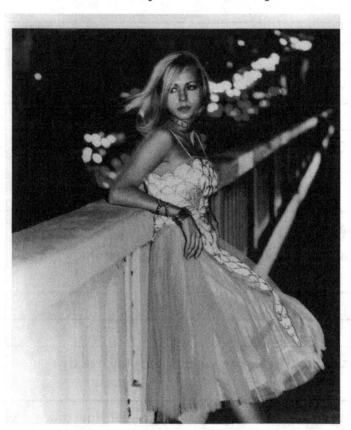

"The outer self is a reflection of the inner-self"

Value the hard work and accomplishment of your weight loss success and realize that all you gave up were excesses that you really did not need in the first place because we only become overweight by excess and imbalance and neither one is healthy for the mind, body or spirit. You are a better person today, than you were ever before. Just by looking back on the path you had to take in overcoming the battle of the bulge, it

THE BALANCE DIET & LIFESTYLE

should serve as a reminder that you do not want to go down that path again. Being able to keep a commitment with yourself. A commitment that you pledge to keep and believe that you will honor, at a deep level of consciousness, for the rest of your life. If you know this one thing in detail, you will know everything you need in order to be successful in your weight loss and management goal. If you adopt this mentality there is nothing that can stop you from achieving your goal.

"Don't forget who you are, where you came from, where you have been, where you are going and why you don't want to go back down that path again."

MIND BODY WEIGHT LOSS SELF CONTRACT

Name: _____ Date: _____

My Current weight is: _____ My Ideal Weight is: _____

Personal Goal: _____

I want to look like: _____

Commitment to Change The Following Habits and Behaviors:

I plan to achieve my goal by this date:

_____

I am committing to myself to do this because, _____ and

because, I realize that I alone control the look and appearance of my body.

I will be rewarded by the look and feel of my new body and because,

I deserve to achieve my health and fitness goals, because:

_____

_____

I plan to manage my weight in these ways to keep my weight loss

permanent: _____

_____

_____

Self-Signature: _____

316 •

DR. JOYCE PETERS

Positive Thinking

Gandhi suggested that there is power in positive thinking and having a positive outlook on your future. The energetic power of positive energetic thought projection is karmic the energy we send out we receive back, therefore, our innate awareness of the true essence of our inner connection with all that is in existence should be a positive interaction. Live out your positive thoughts.

In other words, visualize yourself having lost all of your excess weight. Believe you can lose all of your excess weight, know that you can lose all of your excess weight, think it, say it, act out the steps to make it happen, make these steps your habits, and before you know it your thoughts become your reality, your habits are your values and then what you value becomes your destiny. Meditate on this. Write down your primary health goal and make a mantra out of it so that you can meditate daily on achieving this goal. Set aside a time each day and night to focus on your mantras. Post a list of weight management goals and mantras in a place that you will see as you arise or retire each day and night.

Positive Affirmations

I no longer over eat
I only crave foods that are healthy for me and help me loose weight.
I only eat foods that help me achieve my weight loss goals
My body is becoming slimmer and more physically attractive each day
I have renewed my powers to control my weight
I release all blocks mental emotional physical and spiritual that may prevent me from loosing my excess weight.
Petite size portions satisfy me completely
Exercises is now easier than ever before
The "Mind Body Weight Loss Program" is working for me
I crave and hunger for fresh fruits and veggies
My taste buds have came alive for healthy low calorie foods
My mind body and spirit work together and are achieving my weight loss goals
Food cannot be substituted for any other emotional need
I only eat when I am truly hungry
I stop eating before I feel full and allow my body time to send the signal that I am full.
I am finished craving foods that are not healthy
The old me that ate unhealthy food is gone

THE BALANCE DIET & LIFESTYLE

I have developed a distaste for junk food
Junk food is no longer appealing to me.
The new me, only eats a healthy balanced diet
I am, I can and I will achieve my weight loss goals
I am physically fit, attractive and full of radiant energy
Now nutritional foods excite my taste buds like never before

GIVING UP CHILD'S MINDSET & LEARNING TO PRACTICE MODERATION

As children, we learn positive and negative beliefs and behaviors that are locked into our subconscious mind just as they were originally programmed in. But we are mature adults, now and come to realize that the subconscious mind is without will power, logic or reason. The subconscious mind is literal. We accept information we are given and told as truth because our caregivers were our gods, in the eyes of an infant and young child. We trust and believe that the information taught to us is truthful and correct without question, because our survival is in their hands. To trust wholeheartedly, is the nature of being a child. We all have an inner child that believes things that we would find ridiculous to the adult conscious mind. When we realize that these beliefs can be the hidden reason why we cannot successfully lose weight and keep it off then we also, realize that it is time to change beliefs that no longer work for us.

The interfering blocks can be of the mental, emotional, physical, spiritual or psychological nature. These blocks are usually untruths that we have learned and believe because it is what we have been taught to be correct. They hold a metaphysical energy pattern that can manifest as obstacles in many physical forms to alert us to seek truth and deal with these hidden and unresolved issues and to become truthful with our inner – self. Awareness dissolves the negative energy patterns created by the negative energy of the struggle of our conscious and unconscious mind must eventually become replaced or they continue to create metaphysical obstacles that will perpetually keep repeating in unpleasant occurrences or on our body's physical form until we effectively break the cycle and stop living with the untruth. These obstacles usually stem from learned beliefs and behaviors that we subconsciously know are untruths and our inner and higher-selves can no longer dwell inside with the imbalanced energy that it is creating from within. The energy becomes like magnetic energy. The energy builds up to the surface like a solar flare on the surface of the sun. The longer the truth is denied the greater the potential for the explosion to go super nova. In very spiritually attuned people who thrive in the light of truth and knowledge, it can send them in to a dark phase until the truth is recognized. The two negative magnetic currents will repel greatly against each other. The same inner struggle occurs when we know or believe that we are living a lie. A change must take place for the energies to become balanced. By simply turning a magnet to its positive polarity, the magnetic currents will attract each other and stick together in harmony.

Everything in life has to have balance and our animal magnetism can attract anything we seek. Staying mindful that following a life of falsehoods caused us to be living a lie, which we don't want to repeat just because when we consciously believed falsehoods to be truths it caused imbalance and inner turmoil within ourselves, that we don't wish to repeat again. It is a choice to live a new life. Letting go of the negative untruths that once created self-doubt was the hidden reason that we previously could not control our weight. The behavior that is acceptable to the society that we indulge in may not be acceptable to our inner self. Unconsciously we may be very uncomfortable with our true feelings and emotions and when we continually deny these feelings, our higher self can no longer keep accepting it inside. Our weight and body size can be an indicator of this expanding energy inside. A behavior modification must be made when our subconscious mind recognizes the truth and the conscious mind refuses to recognize the truth. Our intelligent, innate, inner-self will give us warning signs, until we can no longer avoid the expanding problem. It is then that we have to make a conscious choice to adjust our deep belief system and make a truthful change. Our inner self and inner child are always seeking truth. Our corrected belief then emanates an energy, which reflects in our behavior as a positive and growthful change in our lives so that we utilize our energies to achieve goals instead of toward maintaining inner turmoil and imbalanced emotions.

Living out the positive change that has occurred in our life from healthy change, creates happiness and peace and brings us closer to our true purpose in life. Our inner self wants to help us be all that we can be. Our inner self wants us to be content and happy with our life and ourselves. Our inner self wants us to achieve our full potential in truth and light. Our higher self wants us to feel our purpose and the true meaning of life. We will sabotage our self from achieving our goals if we do not remove the blocks that are between our higher self and

THE BALANCE DIET & LIFESTYLE

us. We cannot accomplish our goals and dreams with these obstacles blocking our path to success. Our higher self wants us to achieve our true purpose in life and it will use metaphysical and physical warnings to alert us and bring the true answers to our conscious reality when we believe a lie and when we are living a lie. Beliefs and Behaviors that have a negative influence on our self-esteem or that dis-empower us and make us feel incapable must be eliminated. Beliefs and behaviors that are detrimental to our successful outcome in weight loss and other ventures in life must be eliminated.

Living out a lifestyle filled with the behavior modification we made is the key to making permanent change. The Balance Diet & Lifestyle is designed to give us back our power and restore our energy wherever and whenever we believe that we have lost it along the way or been robbed of it or have had it stolen from us. Powerful positive thinking empowers the individual and gives the power, energy and control back to us where behavior modification is making a healthy change and conscious awareness that we each hold the power in ourselves and in our mind, body and spirit to achieve our goals. It helps us to recognize our abilities to independently utilize and harness the powerful energy within ourselves and direct our power in any area that it is needed in order to successfully achieve our weight loss and other personal goals in life. A positive mental attitude is essential in maintaining your results, permanently. Having the courage to maintain your results is what will set you apart from the rest of the crowd. An effective way to relieve these types of hunger is through journaling, poetry, and spoken word. It is a way of getting the thoughts and feelings onto paper and releasing them. When a person is feeling disconnected from loved ones, society, and even their own emotions and feelings. Greater self-awareness and understanding can be achieved through journaling theses thoughts and feelings on paper and sharing them with others when needed. This is a great self-therapy opposed to stuffing these thoughts and feelings deep down inside with food.

Poetry:

Poetry is this a wonderful way to express anything in rhyme. Most poets write about love and the hunger for love reciprocated. Try writing a poem to fulfill the hidden "hungers" though open and honest communication.

Dr. Joyce Peters

"Fall"

Leaves are falling like tear drops.
Grieving-Summer is leaving
Days are getting shorter
The chill of autumn in the air.
Hear the trees moaning,
Like a lonely soul in despair.

In early fall, traveling down winding country roads
Admiring wild flowers growing everywhere
The radiant color of purple, blue yellow white and gold
Painted on a canvas of green
Round bales of hay dot the fields
Corn hanging from brown stalks, waiting to be pulled

Blonde cat-tails waving in the air
Golden rod swaying in the breeze
Our soul stirs in awe,
By the magnificence of it all.

"Memory Recall"

Oh, tell me sunny golden rods growing everywhere,
Did fairies come from fairylands and weave the dress you wear?
Or did you get from mines of gold your bright and sunny hue?
Or did the baby stars fall down one night and color you?

Lillian Cole
My lifelong friend & mother.

Weight Loss Maintenance Chants & Incantations – Repeating a chant, incantation can help bring mental focus and clarity to your weight loss goals and aspirations. To make your dreams become a reality, it starts with a thought. When we are born, we are fully aware of our desires, it doesn't take an infant very long to realize that all of our desires are not immediately met in human existence. However, what we concentrate on with intent becomes our reality.

THE BALANCE DIET & LIFESTYLE

Relating back to the earlier reference to Mahatma Gandhi's quote, watch your thoughts carefully; your thoughts become your reality. What ever we believe we can achieve at a deep level of consciousness, can be achieved and maintained. Words are powerful.

Express your desires as if you have already achieved them, the intent to achieve your goals and desire is the key. The true intention and intent is the most powerful power in the conscious realm. Whatever you meditate, coming from a loving consciousness and self love can manifest in physical form. The mind over body concept is powerful as well, but your true intention is what will create the reality you choose. If you create a mental image in your head or mind and really think you are fat and ugly every time you look at yourself in the mirror, you will likely become just that thought and visualization. Break the pattern of negative self-thought. Write loving incantations on your mirror to remind yourself of the power of visualization and thought. Chant the following positive weight loss incantations out loud three times each, on a daily basis for a month and once a week there after until you achieve the desired result. Remember your thoughts become your reality. Read these sentences each night before you go to sleep, the last thing you read is the first thing to drop into the sub-conscious mind when you go into sleep state.

Make a mantra drawing box. Make a copy of these mantras and cut each one of the daily affirmations and place them in your daily mantra drawing box. Each day, draw one out as a thought for the day. Repeat your daily mantra to yourself all day and use it as a mantra in your daily meditations. Place the other one on your bed side table, dining room table, and refrigerator or paste them on your mirror. This will serve as a daily motivational reinforcement to keep you on track during your weight management phase.

Mind Body Mantra or Fortune Cookie Draw Box

I love myself and I deserve to have the physical appearance that I desire.

I am dedicated and determined to stay lean and healthy

DR. JOYCE PETERS

I realize my choices create the shape of my body

I give my subconscious mind permission to curb hunger.

Healthy foods satisfy me completely

I no longer cave sugar candy or sweets

I only eat foods that are healthy for me.

I am creating smooth muscle as opposed to fatty bulges on my body

I have broken away from the vicious cycle of yo-yo fad dieting

I am becoming the best that I can be

I love me, I am a beautiful human being, I am a unique work of art.

I released unhealthy behaviors that sabotage my diet

I release all excuses for being over weight.

I release the old me and the excessive behavior.

I welcome the physically fit me to come out.

I welcome a positive transformation into my life

I welcome a stronger healthier me

I welcome a more attractive me

I welcome a slender more physically fit me

THE BALANCE DIET & LIFESTYLE

I deserve to achieve my weight loss goals

I no longer use food to fill the void when other areas of my life appear empty

I am letting the slender me out forever

I feel joy and alive to see the slender me

If I get of track I get back on track and I never look back

My clothing sizes are getting smaller and smaller.

I am powerful and have the energy within me to achieve my goals

I control my own health

I control my thoughts and opinions

I am very powerful

It is all up to me I make the choices, which result in my own destiny

I control my own appearance

I control what I put in my mouth

I control what I swallow

I control what I consume

I control what I can become

DR. JOYCE PETERS

I have the power within me to create the body image that I want.

I have more energy and less baggage without the excess weigh

I look good, I am happy, I feel good, I love the new me.

I am satisfied in a way that no food would ever satisfy me

I create new friends that encourage and create positive energy

I am active and energetic, again

Everyday I will make the metal choice to keep my health and slender body

My success is perpetual and never ending

I am excited about my healthy new life

I really do look good, My excess fat is gone

I really am satisfied with myself

I deserve the best that life has to offer

Balance in my mind and body ensures my continued success.

I am creating the slender me with every breathe I take

I eat smaller portions and I am satisfied.

I love exerting my will power over food

THE BALANCE DIET & LIFESTYLE

I am creating my new image in my mind.

I am manifesting my new image in physical form.

I avoid all foods that cause extra fat to accumulate on my body

I find creative alternatives to fattening foods.

I believe in myself I believe in the power within me

Victory is mine, I am slender forever, I have won the battle of the bulge!

Mind Body Math Equation:

$$
\begin{array}{rl}
1 & \text{Motivated Over Weight Person} \\
+\ 1 & \text{Balanced Diet \& Daily Exercise Plan} \\
\hline
=\ 1 & \text{Slimmer Happier, Healthier More Balanced Person}
\end{array}
$$

On a Weekly Basis, Ask your self these questions:

What will I do to keep myself self thin, now?

_____

How will I keep trying to stay thin, forever?

_____

What will I do when others quit their weight loss plan?

_____

How can I keep my positive mental outlook?

_____

DR. JOYCE PETERS

QUESTION: What do you get when you cross an overweight person with A positive motivated outlook and A healthy balanced diet & lifestyle plan, plus A little dose of daily exercise?

ANSWER: A Happy, Healthy, Slender, Balanced Person.

LIVING WORDS OF WISDOM FROM THE DALAI LAMA

The Dalai Lama said "when you lose, don't lose the lesson".

In weight management, do not forget the lessons of the past. Remember what made you become overweight in the first place and avoid those patterns and behaviors like the plague. Do not allow your self to fall back into your old ways and lifestyle. Dalai Lama also said, "open your arms to change" Thank the universe for the lessons of the past no matter how painful they may be and release the energy of them. Once you release the bonds of obesity from your mind, body and spirit and no longer identify yourself as being overweight or fat, you have made a permanent change. The Dalai Lama also suggested that we follow the three R's and that is not reading, writing and arithmetic. The three R's the Dalai Lama referred to is Respect for self, Respect for others and Responsibility of ones actions. You are responsible for your weight and by doing the things that are necessary to keep your self healthy and physically fit you are respecting yourself and the others around you and you can maintain a healthy weight for life. The Dalai Lama said "Judge your success by what you had to give up to get it".

Getting & Keeping In Touch With Your Inner Hungers Through Journaling

In some cases, people may overeat to stuff down suppressed thoughts and feelings. Keeping a journal is an effective way to get in touch with your inner hungers. These are most often from suppression of our individual thoughts and feelings that may not be acceptable according to the guidelines of acceptable social behaviors and opinions. These that are not related to the hungers for food but hunger for expression. A hunger to be heard and understood. When our needs are not being met, our minds are constantly at work to resolve the issues. Most of our dreams are about resolving these issues. We all have needs and desires. When those needs are not being met, it creates an imbalance. The subconscious mind will not allow us to continue ignoring these needs for very long. Oftentimes, the solution will show up in dreams. Keeping a dream journal can help you realize more quickly, what your conscious mind is discovering. There are books on dream analysis that may help you achieve greater understanding or there are counselors that specialize in dream analysis. Deep psychological needs have to be expressed or we start compensating in other areas of waking consciousness. We all have the need to feel supported and understood by those around us. Writing allows us to identify the areas we are having problems so that we may greater understand ourselves and express ourselves to others to gain the support and understanding we all hunger for.

Solutions:
Choose to concentrate on your slender self-image as a major life long goal. Choose to be positive and maintain your successful weight management Adopt a can do attitude. I can maintain my weight loss, permanently. Take charge of your life and create a lifestyle that accommodates your weight management plan.

It all comes back to choices that we make. Make the decision to make healthier choices by adopting a healthier lifestyle. Make healthier changes for the greater good of your life and health. Low level constant stress is a culprit in weight gain. Fast paced lifestyles are another culprit in the contribution to the development of obesity. Rushing through life is stressful. Slow down and enjoy your life. Adopting a healthy lifestyle is the best permanent solution to weight management. Education is a key component that is necessary to maintain your results on your new Mind Body Health Program as new developments in research occur, as your individual needs change your management plan will change. There are products and dietary supplements available for this program and there are certified healthcare facilities that can assist you in your journey through healthy weight management ask your doctor for more information. If you are a health professional and wish to become involved in the Mind Body referral network, to learn how to help your patients and others visit our website at: www.mindbody-healthprograms.com Good luck and Congratulations on your quest for helping yourself and the people you care about to achieve the best level of natural health possible in Mind, Body & Spirit. Visit the Mind Body Web Site regularly for tips and updates. Keep yourself motivated and remember that the greatest reward that you receive is from the sense of self accomplishment and in the results you will see in your health, appearance and in the way you feel about your new self image.

"The outer self is a reflection of the inner-self, the body is a reflection of the mind. Over weight & almost every other mysterious symptom is caused by Imbalances in the Body or in the Mind". Balance is the Key...

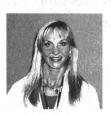

Love & Light, Dr Joyce

ABOUT THE AUTHOR

"Dr. Joyce Peters is a teacher of balanced living practices who has written 17 lifestyle training programs that are available through a vast Medical network of international medical sites. Dr. Joyce holds many certifications in health care and completed a 5 year course of study, receiving her Traditional Naturopathic Doctorate degree from Trinity School in Health Sciences and completed specialty studies in continuing education with the Mind Body Medical Institute at Harvard University Medical School in Clinical Applications of Mind Body Medicine, Positive Psychology and Lifestyle & Weight Management Counseling. Dr. Peters is a Nutritionist, Naturalist, Naturopath, Health Educator and Health Minister who believes inspiration and motivation are the two primary keys That enables anyone to achieve their health goals. Dr. Peters has a certification in Anti- Aging and is an integrative Scientist with interest in DNA and Stem Cell Research. DNA medicine is still in an infant stage. Dr. Joyce offers natural solutions to this growing area of interest and is Involved in international product developments. Dr. Peters is Often quoted as a weight management specialist in Newspapers and magazines and has appeared on many radio and television Shows. She is a health and fitness correspondent for Living Additions, a lifestyle television show that has aired on Oxygen and ION Life networks to millions of households, nationwide. Dr. Peters has studied wellness practices in the U.S., Australia, England, France, Ireland and Germany and is a Member of several health organizations around the world."

A Balanced Lifestyle Accommodates a Healthy Balance in Your Mind, Body & Spirit

---

Equal Time Spent Between Activities

Family, Friends & Loving Relationships
Education, Business & Career
Exercise, Exploration & Play
Beauty, Health & Hygiene
Rest, Relaxation & Sleep

Mental
Physical
Spiritual

INDEX

DR. JOYCE PETERS

THE BALANCE DIET & LIFESTYLE

THE BALANCE DIET & LIFESTYLE

Printed in the United States
By Bookmasters